TENTH EDITION

STUDY GUIDE FOR ESSENTIALS OF NURSING RESEARCH

Appraising Evidence for Nursing Practice

Denise F. Polit, PhD, FAAN

President, Humanalysis, Inc.
Saratoga Springs, New York
Adjunct Professor,
Griffith University School of Nursing
Brisbane, Australia
www.denisepolit.com

Cheryl Tatano Beck, DNSc, CNM, FAAN

Distinguished Professor, School of Nursing
University of Connecticut
Storrs, Connecticut

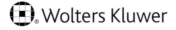 Wolters Kluwer

Philadelphia • Baltimore • New York • London
Buenos Aires • Hong Kong • Sydney • Tokyo

Vice President, Nursing Segment: Julie K. Stegman
Manager, Nursing Education and Practice Content: Jamie Blum
Acquisitions Editor: Michael Kerns
Senior Development Editor: Meredith L. Brittain
Editorial Coordinator: Julie Kostelnik
Marketing Manager: Brittany Clements
Editorial Assistant: Molly Kennedy
Production Project Manager: Barton Dudlick
Design Coordinator: Steve Druding
Art Director: Jennifer Clements
Manufacturing Coordinator: Karin Duffield
Prepress Vendor: Absolute Service, Inc.

Tenth edition

Printed in China

Library of Congress Cataloging-in-Publication Data

ISBN-13: 978-1-9751-4639-9

ISBN-10: 1-9751-4639-5

shop.lww.com

Preface

This *Study Guide* has been prepared to complement the 10th edition of *Essentials of Nursing Research: Appraising Evidence for Nursing Practice*. It contains material designed to further bridge the gap between the passive reading of abstract materials and the active development of skills needed to critically appraise studies and use the findings in practice.

This guide provides you with opportunities to reinforce the acquisition of basic research skills through systematic learning exercises. Please note that some of the articles that are mentioned in the exercises appear on thePoint website and are identified by ☀. Another important feature is that the appendices include eight research reports in their entirety. We deliberately selected some studies that are directly relevant to evidence-based practice (EBP), such as a study on the results of an EBP implementation project, and two systematic reviews. There are activities in each chapter of this *Study Guide* (the Application Exercises) geared around these studies.

The *Study Guide* consists of 18 chapters—1 chapter corresponding to every chapter in the textbook. Each of the 18 chapters (with a few exceptions) consists of four sections:

- **A. Fill in the Blanks.** Terms and concepts presented in the textbook are reinforced by having students complete each sentence. All answers are at the back of the book (Appendix I) for easy reference and cross-checking.
- **B. Matching Exercises.** Further reinforcement for key new terms is offered in matching exercises, which often involve matching the concrete (e.g., an actual research hypothesis) with the abstract (e.g., the term for a specific type of hypothesis). Again, answers are at the back of the book (Appendix I).
- **C. Study Questions.** Each chapter contains two to five short individual exercises relevant to the materials in the textbook. The answers to study questions for which there are objective answers are at the back of the book (Appendix I).
- **D. Application Exercises.** These exercises are geared specifically to help students read, comprehend, and critically appraise nursing studies. In each chapter, the application exercises focus on two or more of the studies in the appendices, and for each study, there are two sets of questions—Questions of Fact and Questions for Discussion.
  - **Questions of Fact** will help students read the report and find specific types of information related to the content covered in the textbook. For these questions, there are "right" answers, which we provide at the back of the book (Appendix I). For example, an application question might ask: How many people participated in this study?
  - **Questions for Discussion**, by contrast, require an assessment of the merits of various features of the study. For example, a question might ask: Did a sufficient number of people participate in this study? The second set of questions can be the basis for classroom discussions.

We hope that you will find these activities rewarding, enjoyable, and useful in your effort to develop skills for evidence-based nursing practice.

Denise F. Polit
Cheryl Tatano Beck

Contents

PART 1

Overview of Nursing Research and Its Role in Evidence-Based Practice

CHAPTER 1

Introducing Nursing Research for Evidence-Based Practice

A. FILL IN THE BLANKS

How many terms have you learned in this chapter? Fill in the blanks in the sentences below to find out.

1. Research that is designed to inform nursing practice is referred to as _____ nursing research.

2. Nurses in practice settings often read and evaluate studies in the context of a journal _____.

3. A(n) _____ is a worldview, a way of looking at natural phenomena.

4. A principle that is believed to be true without proof or verification is a(n) _____.

5. The techniques used by researchers to structure a study are called research _____.

6. _____ is the worldview that assumes that there is an orderly reality that can be studied objectively.

7. The positivist assumption that phenomena are not random, but rather have antecedent causes, is called _____.

8. _____ research involves the collection and analysis of numeric information and is associated with the traditional scientific method.

9. The scientific method involves procedures to reduce bias that could distort the results by enhancing _____ —that is, minimizing subjectivity.

10. _____ evidence is rooted in objective reality and is gathered through the senses.

11. The degree to which research findings can be applied to people who did not participate in a study concerns its _____.

12. The worldview that holds that there are multiple interpretations of reality is _____.

13. The type of research that analyzes narrative, subjective materials is _____ research.

14. Many studies seek to understand determinants of phenomena and are referred to as _____-probing studies.

3

15. In terms of an EBP-related purpose, studies that address _____ questions seek to identify effective treatments for addressing health problems.

16. In terms of an EBP-related purpose, studies that address _____ questions seek to identify the consequences of health problems.

17. In terms of an EBP-related purpose, studies that address _____ questions seek to understand how clients feel about illness and health.

18. The three "legs" or components of EBP are (1) research evidence, (2) clinical expertise, and (3) _____.

19. The most well-respected type of research synthesis used in evidence-based practice is called a(n) _____.

20. Syntheses that involve the statistical integration of findings from quantitative studies are called _____.

21. Evidence _____ rank evidence sources in terms of their risk of bias.

22. In the PICO format for asking well-worded clinical questions, the "O" stands for _____.

23. In the PICO format for asking well-worded clinical questions, the "P" stands for _____.

24. In the PICO format for asking well-worded clinical questions, the "I" stands for _____.

25. In the PICO format for asking well-worded clinical questions, the "C" stands for _____.

B. MATCHING EXERCISES

Match each statement in Set B with one of the paradigms in Set A. Indicate the letter corresponding to the appropriate response next to each entry in Set B.

SET A

a. Positivist/postpositivist paradigm
b. Constructivist paradigm
c. Neither paradigm
d. Both paradigms

SET B   RESPONSES

1. Assumes that reality exists and that it can be objectively studied and known   _____

2. Subjectivity in inquiries is considered inevitable and desirable.   _____

3. Inquiries rely on external (empirical) evidence collected through human senses.   _____

4. Assumes reality is a construction and that many constructions are possible   _____

5. Method of inquiry relies primarily on collecting and analyzing quantitative information.   _____

6. Method of inquiry relies primarily on collecting and analyzing narrative, qualitative information.   _____

7. Provides an overarching framework for inquiries undertaken by nurse researchers   _____

8. Inquiries give rise to emerging interpretations that are grounded in people's experiences.   _____

9. Inquiries are not constrained by ethical issues.   _____

10. Inquiries focus on discrete, specific concepts while attempting to control others.   _____

C. STUDY QUESTIONS

1. Why is it important for nurses who will never conduct their own research to understand research methods?

2. What are some potential consequences to the nursing profession if nurses stopped conducting their own research?

3. Below are descriptions of several research problems. Indicate whether you think the problem is best suited to a qualitative or quantitative approach and explain your rationale.
   a. What is the decision-making process of patients with AIDS seeking treatment?
   b. What effect does room temperature have on the colonization rate of bacteria in urinary catheters?
   c. What are the sources of daily stress among nursing home residents, and what do these stressors mean to the residents?
   d. Does therapeutic touch affect the vital signs of hospitalized patients?
   e. What is the meaning of *hope* among patients with stage IV cancer?
   f. What are the health care needs of the homeless, and what barriers do they face in having those needs met?
   g. What are the effects of a formal exercise program on high blood pressure and cholesterol levels of middle-aged men?

4. What are the PICO elements for question 3.G?

5. What are some of the limitations of quantitative research? What are some of the limitations of qualitative research? Which approach seems best suited to address problems in which you might be interested? Why is that?

D. APPLICATION EXERCISES

Exercise D.1: Study in Appendix A

Read the abstract and introduction to the report by Stephens and colleagues ("Smartphone technology and text messaging for weight loss in young adults") in Appendix A on pages 115–122 and then answer the following questions:

Questions of Fact
   a. Does this report describe an example of a "disciplined research"?
   b. Is this a qualitative or quantitative study?
   c. What is the underlying paradigm of the study?

d. Does the study involve the collection of empirical evidence?
e. Could this study be described as *cause probing?*
f. Which EBP-focused purpose does this study address?
g. Phrase a research question addressed in this study using the PICO format.

Questions for Discussion

a. How relevant is this study to the actual practice of nursing?
b. Could this study have been conducted as *either* a quantitative or qualitative study? Why or why not?

Exercise D.2: Study in Appendix B

Read the abstract and introduction to the report by Ottosen and colleagues ("An ethnography of parents' perceptions of patient safety in the neonatal intensive care unit") in Appendix B on pages 123–133 and then answer the following questions:

Questions of Fact

a. Does this report describe an example of a "disciplined research"?
b. Is this a qualitative or quantitative study?
c. What is the underlying paradigm of the research?
d. Does the study involve the collection of empirical evidence?
e. Could this study be described as *cause probing?*
f. Which EBP-focused purpose does this study address?

Questions for Discussion

a. How relevant is this study to the actual practice of nursing?
b. Could this study have been conducted as *either* a quantitative or qualitative study? Why or why not?
c. Would the PICO format be appropriate for the clinical question posed in this study?
d. Which of the two studies cited in these exercises (the one in Appendix A or Appendix B) is of greater interest and/or relevance to you personally? Why?

Exercise D.3: Study in Appendix C

Skim the report by Saqe-Rockoff and colleagues ("Improving thermoregulation for trauma patients in the emergency department") in Appendix C on pages 135–141 and then answer the following questions:

Questions of Fact

a. Does this report describe an example of a "disciplined research"?
b. Did the team develop a PICO question? If yes, what was it? If no, what might such a question be?
c. Did the team search for relevant systematic reviews to guide their project?
d. Did the report say anything about the level of evidence they found?

Questions for Discussion

a. Discuss the practice change that was implemented. Did the practice change seem appropriate?
b. Discuss how this project and projects like it have importance to the practice of nursing.

CHAPTER 2

Understanding Key Concepts and Steps in Quantitative and Qualitative Research

A. FILL IN THE BLANKS

How many terms have you learned in this chapter? Fill in the blanks in the sentences below to find out.

1. A person who provides information to researchers in a study is often called a(n) _____ in a quantitative study.
2. A(n) _____ is a somewhat more complex abstraction than a concept.
3. A systematic, abstract explanation of phenomena is a(n) _____.
4. In quantitative research, a concept is usually referred to as a(n) _____.
5. Another name for outcome variable is _____ variable.
6. The presumed influence on a dependent variable is the _____ variable.
7. The _____ definition indicates how a variable will be measured.
8. Information gathered in a study is called _____.
9. A(n) _____ is a bond, connection, or pattern of association between variables.
10. A relationship in which one variable directly induces changes in another is a(n) _____ relationship.
11. The type of research that involves the testing of an intervention is called _____ research.
12. Another name for nonexperimental research, often used in the medical literature, is _____ research.
13. In the medical literature, a study that tests the effect of an intervention is called a clinical _____.
14. A qualitative tradition that focuses on social psychological processes within a social setting is called _____ theory.
15. The qualitative research tradition that focuses on lived experiences is _____.
16. The type of qualitative research that focuses on understanding cultures is _____.

17. Some qualitative researchers do not undertake an upfront _____ review to avoid having their conceptualization influenced by the work of others.
18. A research _____ is the basic architecture of a study.
19. The _____ is the entire aggregate of people in which a researcher is interested (the "P" in PICO).
20. A(n) _____ is a subset of a population from which data are gathered.
21. Quantitative researchers perform _____ analyses of their data.
22. To get access to a site and its inhabitants is to gain _____ into the site.
23. Qualitative researchers typically use a(n) _____ design in their studies.
24. _____ is a principle used to decide when to stop sampling in a qualitative study on the basis of redundancy of information.
25. Qualitative analyses usually involve a search for recurrent _____ or _____.

B. MATCHING EXERCISES

1. Match each statement in Set B with one of the paradigms in Set A. Indicate the letter corresponding to the appropriate response next to each entry in Set B.

SET A

a. Term used in quantitative research
b. Term used in qualitative research
c. Term used in both qualitative and quantitative research

SET B   RESPONSES

1. Subject   _____
2. Study participant   _____
3. Informant   _____
4. Variable   _____
5. Phenomenon   _____
6. Saturation   _____
7. Theory   _____
8. Data   _____
9. Emergent design   _____
10. Data analysis   _____

2. Match each term in Set B with one of the terms in Set A. Indicate the letter corresponding to your response next to each item in Set B.

SET A

a. Independent variable
b. Dependent variable
c. Either/both independent/dependent variable
d. Neither independent nor dependent variable

SET B   **RESPONSES**

1. The variable that is the presumed effect   _____
2. The variable involved in a cause-and-effect relationship   _____
3. The variable that is the presumed cause   _____
4. The variable, "length of stay in hospital"   _____
5. The variable that requires an operational definition   _____
6. The variable that is the outcome of interest in the study   _____
7. The variable that is constant   _____
8. The variable in a grounded theory study   _____

3. Match each activity in Set B with one of the options in Set A. Indicate the letter corresponding to your response next to each item in Set B.

SET A

a. An activity in quantitative research
b. An activity in qualitative research
c. An activity in both qualitative and quantitative research
d. An activity in neither quantitative nor qualitative research

SET B   **RESPONSES**

1. Choosing between an experimental or nonexperimental design   _____
2. Ending data collection once saturation has been achieved   _____
3. Developing or selecting measuring instruments   _____
4. Doing a literature review   _____
5. Collecting and analyzing data concurrently   _____
6. Taking steps to ensure protection of human rights   _____
7. Developing strategies to avoid data collection   _____
8. Disseminating research results   _____
9. Analyzing the data for major themes or categories   _____
10. Formulating hypotheses to be tested statistically   _____

C. STUDY QUESTIONS

1. Suggest operational definitions for the following concepts.
    a. Stress:
    b. Prematurity of infants:
    c. Fatigue:
    d. Pain:
    e. Prolonged labor:
    f. Dyspnea:

2. In each of the following research questions, identify the independent variable and the dependent/outcome variable.

    a. Does assertiveness training improve the effectiveness of psychiatric nurses?

        Independent: _____

        Dependent: _____

    b. Does the postural positioning of patients affect their respiratory function?

        Independent: _____

        Dependent: _____

    c. Is the psychological well-being of patients affected by the amount of touch received from nursing staff?

        Independent: _____

        Dependent: _____

    d. Is the incidence of decubitus reduced by more frequent turnings of patients?

        Independent: _____

        Dependent: _____

    e. Are people who were abused as children more likely than others to abuse their own children?

        Independent: _____

        Dependent: _____

    f. Is tolerance for pain related to a patient's age?

        Independent: _____

        Dependent: _____

    g. Is the number of prenatal visits of pregnant women associated with labor and delivery outcomes?

        Independent: _____

        Dependent: _____

    h. Are levels of depression higher among children who experience the death of a sibling than among other children?

        Independent: _____

        Dependent: _____

    i. Is compliance with a medical regimen higher among women than among men?

        Independent: _____

        Dependent: _____

    j. Does participation in a support group enhance coping among family caregivers of patients with AIDS?

        Independent: _____

        Dependent: _____

    k. Is hearing acuity of the elderly affected by the time of day?

        Independent: _____

        Dependent: _____

l. Does home birth affect the parents' satisfaction with the childbirth experience?

Independent: _____

Dependent: _____

m. Does a neutropenic diet in the outpatient setting decrease the positive blood cultures associated with chemotherapy-induced neutropenia?

Independent: _____

Dependent: _____

3. Below is a list of variables. For each, think of a research question for which the variable would be the independent variable, and a second for which it would be the dependent variable. For example, take the variable "birth weight of infants." We might ask, "Does the age of the mother affect the birth weight of her infant?" (dependent variable). Alternatively, our research question might be, "Does the birth weight of infants (independent variable) affect their sensorimotor development at 6 months of age?" HINT: For the dependent variable problem, ask yourself, "What factors might affect, influence, or cause this variable?" For the independent variable, ask yourself, "What factors does *this* variable influence, cause, or affect—what might be the consequences of this variable?"

a. Body temperature

Independent: _____

Dependent: _____

b. Amount of sleep

Independent: _____

Dependent: _____

c. Frequency of practicing breast self-examination

Independent: _____

Dependent: _____

d. Level of hopefulness in cancer patients

Independent: _____

Dependent: _____

e. Stress among victims of domestic violence

Independent: _____

Dependent: _____

4. Look at the table of contents of a recent issue of *Nursing Research* or another nursing research journal. Pick out a study title (without looking at the abstract or the brief description of the study at the beginning) that implies that a relationship between variables was studied. Indicate what you think the independent and dependent variable might be and what the title suggests about the nature of the relationship (i.e., causal or not).

5. Describe what is wrong with the following statements:

a. Koretsky's experimental study was conducted within the ethnographic tradition.

b. Forman's experimental study examined the effect of relaxation therapy (the dependent variable) on pain (the independent variable) in cancer patients.

    c. O'Connor's grounded theory study of the caregiving process for caretakers of patients with dementia was a clinical trial.

    d. In Aldrich's phenomenological study of the meaning of futility among patients with AIDS, subjects received an intervention designed to sustain hope.

    e. In her experimental study, Spence developed her data collection plan after she introduced her intervention to a group of patients.

6. Which qualitative research tradition do you think would be most appropriate for the following research questions? Justify your response.

    a. How do the health beliefs and customs of Chinese immigrants influence their health-seeking behavior?

    b. What is the lived experience of being a recovering alcoholic?

    c. What is the process by which husbands adapt to the sudden loss of their wives?

D. APPLICATION EXERCISES

Exercise D.1: Study in Appendix D

Read the abstract, introduction, and first few subsections of the "Methods" section) of the report by Eckhardt and colleagues ("Fatigue in the presence of coronary heart disease") in Appendix D on pages 143–153 and then answer the following questions:

Questions of Fact

    a. Who were the researchers and what are their credentials and affiliation?

    b. Who were the study participants?

    c. What were the site and setting for this study?

    d. What is the independent variable (or variables) in this study? What is the dependent variable (or variables)? Did the report actually use the terms *independent variable* or *dependent variable*?

    e. How was *fatigue* operationally defined? Was a conceptual definition provided?

    f. Were the data in this study quantitative or qualitative?

    g. Were any relationships under investigation? What type of relationship?

    h. Is this an experimental or nonexperimental study?

    i. Was there any intervention? If so, what was it?

    j. Did the study involve statistical analysis of data?

Questions for Discussion

    a. How relevant is this study to the actual practice of nursing?

    b. How good a job did the researchers do in summarizing their study in the abstract?

    c. How long do you estimate it took for this study to be completed?

Exercise D.2: Study in Appendix E

Read the abstract and introduction to the report by Langegård and colleagues ("The art of living with symptoms") in Appendix E on pages 155–162 and then answer the following questions:

Questions of Fact

    a. Who were the researchers and what are their credentials and affiliation?

    b. Who were the study participants?

c. In what type of setting did the study take place?
d. What was the key concept in this study?
e. Were there any *independent variables* or *dependent variables* in this study?
f. Were the data in this study quantitative or qualitative?
g. Were any relationships under investigation?
h. Could the study be described as an ethnographic, phenomenological, or grounded theory study?
i. Is this an experimental or nonexperimental study?
j. Does the study involve an intervention? If so, what is it?
k. Did the study involve statistical analysis of data? Did the study involve qualitative analysis of data?

Questions for Discussion

a. How relevant is this study to the actual practice of nursing?
b. How good a job did the researchers do in summarizing their study in the abstract?
c. How long do you estimate it took for this study to be completed?
d. Which of the two studies cited in these exercises (the one in Appendix D or Appendix E) is of greater interest and/or relevance to you personally? Why?

Reading and Critically Appraising Research Articles

A. FILL IN THE BLANKS

How many terms have you learned in this chapter? Fill in the blanks in the sentences below to find out.

1. A(n) _____ is an influence that results in a distortion or error.

2. "The lived experience of caring for a dying spouse" is an example of the section of a research report called the _____.

3. The process of reflecting critically on one's self, used by many qualitative researchers, is _____.

4. Qualitative researchers strive to enhance the likelihood that their findings are _____, which includes enhancing credibility, authenticity, and dependability.

5. If the results of a statistical test indicated a probability of .001, the results would be considered statistically _____.

6. _____ is the format used to structure most research reports.

7. To address biases stemming from *awareness*, researchers may use a procedure that is usually called _____.

8. A summary of a study, also known as a(n) _____, appears at the beginning of a report.

9. A(n) _____ variable is a variable that is extraneous to the research question but that needs to be controlled.

10. Research reports are most likely to be accessed as _____ articles.

11. Quantitative researchers strive for findings that are reliable and _____.

12. A(n) _____ is a conclusion drawn from the evidence in a study that takes into account the research methods used.

13. _____ is a criterion for evaluating study evidence (mostly in quantitative study) that concerns the accuracy and consistency of information.

14. Research _____ is used by researchers to hold constant outside influences on the dependent variable so that the relationship under study can be better understood.

14

15. _____ is a broad bias-reducing strategy used by quantitative researchers that involves having aspects of the study established by chance rather than by personal choices.

16. _____ is to qualitative research what generalizability is to quantitative research.

B. MATCHING EXERCISES

Match each statement in Set B with one of the report sections in Set A. Indicate the letter corresponding to the appropriate response next to each entry in Set B.

SET A

a. Abstract
b. Introduction
c. Method
d. Results
e. Discussion

SET B   RESPONSES

1. Describes the research design   _____

2. In quantitative studies, presents findings from statistical analyses   _____

3. Identifies the research questions or hypotheses   _____

4. Presents a brief summary of the major features of the study   _____

5. Provides information on how study participants were selected   _____

6. Offers an interpretation of the study findings   _____

7. In qualitative studies, describes the themes or categories that emerged from the data   _____

8. Presents a rationale for the significance of the study   _____

9. Describes how the research data were collected   _____

10. Identifies the study's main limitations   _____

11. This sentence would appear there: "The purpose of this study was to explore the process by which patients cope with a cancer diagnosis."   _____

12. Includes raw data, in the form of excerpts from participants, in qualitative reports   _____

C. STUDY QUESTIONS

1. Why are qualitative research reports typically easier to read than quantitative research reports?

_____

_____

_____

2. Most journals now instruct contributing authors to prepare "new" style abstracts that organize material within specific headings (usually, Background, Objective, Methods, Results, Conclusions/Discussion). The two abstracts presented at the end of Chapter 3 of the textbook were in this "new" style. Read the following "traditional" (one paragraph) abstract for a qualitative study by Tarabeih and Bokek-Cohen (2020) and rewrite it as a "new style" abstract with specific headings:

While extensive scholarship has been dedicated to the emotional experiences of transplant patients, little is known about the emotional experiences of transplant co-ordinators. Semi-structured face-to-face interviews were conducted with ten transplant co-ordinators who have worked for more than 20 years in this job. The transplant co-ordinators spoke of negative feelings and moral distress with regard to futile care of deceased donor family members as well as of living donors. Transplant co-ordinators experience intense negative feelings, emotional pain, and moral distress on a daily basis. Transplant co-ordinators play a pivotal role in the process of obtaining consent for live or dead donation of organ; however, their well-being and job satisfaction are impaired by contradictions between their moral values and the tasks they are instructed to perform. The study exposes the silent emotional suffering of transplant co-ordinators; main findings show that the transplant co-ordinators are torn between contradictory expectations and a gap between values and praxis. It is recommended to offer them training and support for the sake of their retention.

Reprinted with permission from Tarabeih, M., & Bokek-Cohen, Y. (2020). Between health and death: The intense emotional pain experienced by transplant nurses. *Nursing Inquiry, 27*, e12335.

3. Read the titles of the journal articles appearing in the most recent issue of the journal *Nursing Research* (or another nursing research journal). Evaluate the titles of the articles in terms of length and adequacy in communicating essential information about the studies.

4. Below is a brief abstract of a fictitious study, followed by a brief critical appraisal. Do you agree with the appraisal? Can you add other comments relevant to issues discussed in Chapter 3 of the textbook?

FICTITIOUS STUDY
Solomons (2021) prepared the following abstract for her study.

Abstract. Family members often experience considerable anxiety while their loved ones are in surgery. This study examined the effectiveness of a nursing intervention that involved providing oral intraoperative progress reports to family members. Surgical patients undergoing elective procedures were selected either to have family members receive the intervention or to have them not receive it. The findings indicated that the family members in the intervention group were less anxious than family members who received usual care.

Critical Appraisal. This brief abstract provides a general overview of the nature of Solomons' study. It indicates a rationale for the study (the high anxiety level of surgical patients' family members) and summarizes what the researcher did. However, the abstract could have provided more information while still staying within a 100 or 125-word guideline (the abstract only contains 75 words). For example, the abstract could have better described the nature of the intervention (e.g., At what point during the operation was information given to family members? How much detail was provided in the progress reports?). For a reader to have a preliminary assessment of the worth of the study—and therefore to make a decision about whether to read the entire report—more information about the methods would have been helpful. For example, the abstract should have indicated how many families were in the sample, how anxiety was measured, and whether group differences were statistically significant. Also missing is information about how families were allocated to receive the intervention—that is, was *randomness* used? Some mention of the study's implications might also have enhanced the usefulness of the abstract.

D. APPLICATION EXERCISES

Exercise D.1: Study in Appendix A

Read the abstract and introduction to the report by Stephens and colleagues ("Smartphone technology and text messaging for weight loss in young adults") in Appendix A on pages 115–122 and then answer the following questions:

Questions of Fact
a. Does the structure of this article follow the IMRAD format?
b. Does the abstract summarize information about the study purpose, how the study was done, what the key findings were, and what the findings mean?
c. Skim the Method section. Is the presentation in the active or passive voice?
d. Is this study experimental or nonexperimental?
e. Was the principle of *randomness* used in this study?

Questions for Discussion
a. What parts of the abstract were most difficult to understand? Identify words that you consider to be research "jargon."
b. Comment on the organization *within* the method section of this report.

Exercise D.2: Study in Appendix E

Read the abstract and introduction to the report by Langegård and colleagues ("The art of living with symptoms") in Appendix E on pages 155–162 and then answer the following questions:

Questions of Fact
a. Does the structure of this article follow the IMRAD format?
b. Does the abstract include information about the study purpose, how the study was done, what the findings were, and what the findings mean?

c. Skim the Method section. Is the presentation in the active or passive voice?

d. Is the study in one of the three main qualitative traditions described in Chapter 2? If so, which tradition?

Questions for Discussion

a. What parts of the abstract were most difficult to understand?

b. Comment on the organization *within* the Results section of this report.

c. Compare the level of difficulty of the abstracts for the two studies used in these exercises—that is, the studies in Appendix A and E. Why do you think the level of difficulty differs?

CHAPTER 4

Attending to Ethics in Research

A. FILL IN THE BLANKS

How many terms have you learned in this chapter? Fill in the blanks in the sentences below to find out.

1. Most disciplines have developed formal _____ of ethics.

2. _____ is the best method of protecting participants' confidentiality but is not always possible.

3. Researchers should conduct a _____/benefit assessment to evaluate the ethical aspects of their research plan.

4. _____ is a major ethical principle concerning maximizing benefits of research.

5. _____ _____ refers to the type of consent procedure that may be required in qualitative research involving multiple points of data collection.

6. A(n) _____ is a payment sometimes offered to participants as an incentive to take part in a study.

7. The _____ *Report* is the basis for ethical regulations for studies funded by the U.S. government.

8. The return of a questionnaire is often assumed to demonstrate _____ consent.

9. Informal agreement to participate in a study (e.g., by minors) is called _____.

10. Participants' privacy is often protected by _____ procedures, even though the researchers know participants' identities.

11. People can make informed decisions about research participation when there is full _____ of relevant information.

12. A(n) _____ is a formal institutional committee (in the United States) that reviews the ethical aspects of a study.

13. A conflict between the rights of participants and the demands for rigorous research creates an ethical _____.

14. Prisoners and children involved in research are examples of _____ _____.

19

15. _____ _____ procedures offer prospective participants information needed to make a reasonable decision about study participation.

16. _____ sessions at the conclusion of a study offer participants an opportunity to learn more about a study, ask questions, and air complaints.

17. A risk no greater than those ordinarily experienced in everyday life is called a(n) _____ risk in research parlance.

B. MATCHING EXERCISES

Match each description in Set B with one of the procedures used to protect human subjects listed in Set A. Indicate the letter corresponding to the appropriate response next to each entry in Set B.

SET A

a. Freedom from harm or exploitation
b. Informed consent
c. Anonymity
d. Confidentiality

SET B   RESPONSE

1. A questionnaire distributed by mail bears an identification number in one corner. Respondents are assured their responses will not be individually divulged.   _____

2. Hospitalized children included in a study, and their parents, are told the study's aims and procedures. Parents are asked to sign an authorization.   _____

3. Participants in a study in which the same people will participate twice by completing questionnaires are asked to place their own four-digit identification number on the questionnaire and to memorize the number for use in the next round. Participants are assured their answers will remain private.   _____

4. Study participants in an in-depth study of family members' coping with a natural disaster renegotiate the terms of their participation at successive interviews.   _____

5. The psychological consequences of a recent mastectomy are being studied. In the interviews, sensitive questions are carefully worded. After the interview, debriefing with the respondent is used to assess the need for psychological support.   _____

6. Women interviewed in the above study (question 5) are told that the information they provide will not be individually divulged.   _____

7. Subjects who volunteered for an experimental treatment for AIDS are warned of potential side effects and are asked to sign an agreement.   _____

8. After determining that a new intervention resulted in participant discomfort, the researcher discontinued the study. _____

9. Unmarked questionnaires are distributed to a class of nursing students. The instructions indicate that responses will not be individually divulged. _____

10. The researcher assures participants that they will be interviewed at a single point in time and adheres to this promise. _____

11. A questionnaire distributed to a sample of nursing students includes a statement indicating that completion and submission of the questionnaire will be construed as voluntary participation in a study. _____

12. The names, ages, and occupations of study participants whose interviews are excerpted in the research report are not divulged. _____

C. STUDY QUESTIONS

1. Below are brief descriptions of several studies. Suggest some ethical dilemmas that could emerge for each.
   a. A study of coping behaviors among rape victims
   b. An unobtrusive observational study of fathers' behavior in the delivery room
   c. An interview study of the factors contributing to heroin addiction
   d. A study of dependence among children with developmental delays
   e. An investigation of verbal interactions among schizophrenic patients
   f. A study of the effects of a new drug on humans
   g. A study of the relationship between sleeping patterns and acting-out behaviors in hospitalized psychiatric patients

2. Evaluate the ethical aspects of one or more of the following studies using the critical appraisal guidelines in Box 4.2 in the textbook and available in the Student Resources on thePoint. Pay special attention (if relevant) to the manner in which the participants' heightened vulnerability was handled.

   - Gaffney, K., Kermer, D., Kitsantas, P., Brito, A., Ramos, K., Pereddo, G., & Villatoro, L. (2019). Early life factors for overweight risk among infants of Hispanic immigrant mothers. *Journal of Pediatric Health Care, 33*, 35–41.

   - *Ploeg, J., Canesi, M., Fraser, K., McAiney, C., Kaasalainen, S., Markle-Reid, M., . . . Chambers, T. (2019). Experiences of community-dwelling older adults living with multiple chronic conditions: A qualitative study. *BMJ Open, 9*, e023345.

   - *Santa Maria, D., Breeden, K., Drake, S., Narendorf, S., Barman-Adhikari, A., Petering, R., . . . Bender, K. (2020). Gaps in sexual assault health care among homeless young adults. *American Journal of Preventive Care, 58*, 191–198.

   - *Stajduhar, K., Mollison, A., Giesbrecht, M., McNeil, R., Pauly, B., Reimer-Kirkham, S., . . . Rounds, K. (2019). "Just too busy living in the moment and surviving": Barriers to accessing health care for structurally vulnerable populations at end-of-life. *BMC Palliative Care, 18*, 11.

---

*A link to this open-access article is provided in the Internet Resources for this chapter on thePoint website.

3. In the textbook, an actual study with ethical problems was described—that is, the Tuskegee study of syphilis among black men. Identify which ethical principles were transgressed in this study. (Do an Internet search for more information about the Tuskegee experiment, if desired.)

4. Below is a brief description of the ethical aspects of a fictitious study, followed by a critique. Do you agree with the critique? Can you add other comments relevant to the ethical dimensions of the study?

FICTITIOUS STUDY

Walsh conducted an in-depth study of nursing home residents to explore whether their perceptions about personal control over decision making differed from the perceptions of the nursing staff. The investigator studied 25 nurse–patient dyads to assess whether there were conflicting perceptions and experiences regarding control over activities of daily living, such as arising, eating, and dressing. All the nurses in the study were employed by the nursing home in which the patients resided. Because the nursing home had no Institutional Review Board (IRB), and because Walsh's study was not funded by an organization that required IRB approval, the project was not formally reviewed. Walsh sought permission to conduct the study from the nursing home administrator. She also obtained the consent of the legal guardian or responsible family member of each patient. All study participants were fully informed about the nature of the study. The researcher assured the nurses and the legal guardians and family members of the patients of the confidentiality of the information and obtained their written consent. Data were gathered primarily through in-depth interviews with the patients and the nurses separately. The researcher also observed interactions between the patients and nurses. The findings from the study suggested that patients perceived that they had more control over all aspects of the activities of daily living (except eating) than the nurses perceived that they had. Excerpts from the interviews were used verbatim in the research report, but Walsh did not divulge the location of the nursing home, and she used fictitious names for all participants.

CRITICAL COMMENTS

Walsh did a reasonably good job of adhering to ethical principles in undertaking her research. She obtained written permission to conduct the study from the nursing home administrator, and she obtained informed consent from the nurse participants and the legal guardians or family members of the patients. The study participants were not put at risk in any way, and the patients who participated may have enjoyed the opportunity to converse with the researcher. Walsh also took appropriate steps to maintain the confidentiality of participants. It is still unclear, however, whether the patients knowingly and willingly participated in the research. Nursing home residents are a vulnerable group. They may not have been aware of their right to refuse to be interviewed without fear of repercussion. Walsh could have enhanced the ethical aspects of the study by taking more vigorous steps to obtain the informed, voluntary consent of the nursing home residents themselves or to exclude patients who could not reasonably be expected to understand the researcher's request. Given the vulnerability of the group, Walsh should have pursued opportunities for a formal review with an institution with which she was affiliated—or she should have established her own review panel composed of peers and interested lay people to review the ethical dimensions of her project. Debriefing sessions with study participants might also have been appropriate.

D. APPLICATION EXERCISES

Exercise D.1: Study in Appendix D

Read the Method section of the report by Eckhardt and colleagues ("Fatigue in the presence of coronary heart disease") in Appendix D on pages 143–153 and then answer the following questions:

Questions of Fact

a. Does the report indicate that the study procedures were reviewed by an IRB or other similar institutional human subjects review group?
b. Would the participants in this study be considered "vulnerable"?
c. Were participants subjected to any physical harm or discomfort or psychological distress as part of the study? What efforts did the researchers make to minimize harm and maximize good?
d. Were participants deceived in any way?
e. Were participants coerced into participating in the study?
f. Were appropriate informed consent procedures used? Was there full disclosure?
g. Does the report discuss steps that were taken to protect the privacy and confidentiality of study participants? Were data collected anonymously?

Questions for Discussion

a. Do you think the benefits of this research outweighed the costs to participants—what is the overall risk/benefit ratio?
b. Do you consider that the researchers took adequate steps to protect study participants? If not, what else could they have done?
c. The report did not indicate that the participants were paid a stipend. Do you think they should have been?
d. Is there any evidence of discrimination in this study, with regard to people recruited to participate?
e. How comfortable would you feel about having a parent or grandparent participate in this study?

Exercise D.2: Study in Appendix B

Read the Method section of the report by Ottosen and colleagues ("An ethnography of parents' perceptions of patient safety in the neonatal intensive care unit") in Appendix B on pages 123–133 and then answer the following questions:

Questions of Fact

a. Does the report indicate that the study procedures were reviewed by an IRB or other similar ethical review committee?
b. Would the study participants in this study be considered "vulnerable"?
c. Were participants subjected to any physical harm or discomfort or psychological distress as part of this study? Did the researcher make efforts to minimize harm and maximize good?
d. Were participants deceived in any way?
e. Were participants coerced into participating in the study?

f. Were appropriate informed consent procedures used? Was there full disclosure? Was participation voluntary?

g. Does the report discuss steps that were taken to protect the privacy and confidentiality of study participants?

h. Did the researchers offer participating parents a stipend?

Questions for Discussion

a. Do you think the benefits of this research outweighed the costs to participants—what is the overall risk/benefit ratio? Would you characterize the study as having *minimal risk*?

b. Do you consider that the researchers took adequate steps to protect the study participants? If not, what else could they have done?

PART 2

Preliminary Steps in Quantitative and Qualitative Research

CHAPTER 5

Identifying Research Problems, Research Questions, and Hypotheses

A. FILL IN THE BLANKS

How many terms have you learned in this chapter? Fill in the blanks in the sentences below to find out.

1. A research _____ is an enigmatic or troubling condition.

2. A(n) _____ _____ _____ in a quantitative study states an aim and indicates the key study variables and the population of interest.

3. A research _____ is what researchers wish to answer through a systematic study.

4. A(n) _____ is a statement of the researcher's prediction about variables in the study.

5. Hypotheses predict a(n) _____ between the independent and dependent variables.

6. Hypotheses are typically put to a statistical _____ .

7. A hypothesis stipulates the expected relationship between a(n) _____ variable and a dependent variable.

8. A research hypothesis in which the specific nature of the predicted relationship is not stipulated is a(n) _____ hypothesis.

9. The results of hypothesis testing never constitute _____ that a hypothesis is or is not correct.

10. Hypotheses typically involve at least _____ variables.

11. The *actual* hypothesis of an investigator is the _____ hypothesis.

12. The hypothesis that posits the absence of a relationship between variables is called a(n) _____ hypothesis.

B. MATCHING EXERCISES

1. Match each sentence in Set B with one of the phrases listed in Set A. Indicate the letter corresponding to the appropriate response next to each entry in Set B.

SET A

 a. Statement of purpose—qualitative study
 b. Statement of purpose—quantitative study
 c. Not a statement of purpose for a research study

SET B   RESPONSE

1. The purpose of this study is to test whether the removal of physical restraints results in behavioral changes in elderly patients.   _____

2. The purpose of this project is to facilitate the transition from hospital to home among women who have just given birth.   _____

3. The goal of this project is to explore the process by which an elderly person adjusts to placement in a nursing home.   _____

4. The investigation was designed to describe the prevalence of smoking, alcohol use, and drug use among urban preadolescents aged 10 to 12 years.   _____

5. The study's purpose was to describe the nature of touch used by parents in touching their preterm infants.   _____

6. The goal is to develop guidelines for spiritually related nursing interventions.   _____

7. The purpose of this project is to examine the relationship between social support and the use of over-the-counter medications among community-dwelling elders.   _____

8. The purpose is to develop an in-depth understanding of patients' feelings of powerlessness in hospital settings.   _____

2. Match each sentence in Set B with one of the phrases listed in Set A. Indicate the letter corresponding to the appropriate response next to each entry in Set B.

SET A

 a. Research hypothesis—directional
 b. Research hypothesis—nondirectional
 c. Null hypothesis
 d. Not a testable hypothesis as stated

SET B   RESPONSE

1. First-born infants have higher concentrations of estrogens and progesterone in umbilical cord blood than do later-born infants.   _____

2. There is no relationship between women's participation in prenatal classes and the health outcomes of their infants.   _____

3. Many nursing students are interested in obtaining advanced degrees. _____

4. Functional disability after a cardiac event is higher among patients with comorbidities than among those without comorbidities. _____

5. A person's income is related to his or her difficulty in accessing health care. _____

6. Glaucoma can be effectively screened by means of tonometry. _____

7. Higher noise levels result in increased anxiety among hospitalized patients. _____

8. Media exposure regarding the health hazards of smoking is unrelated to the public's smoking habits. _____

9. Patients' compliance with their medication regimens is related to their perceptions of the consequences of noncompliance. _____

10. Many patients delay seeking health care for symptoms of myocardial infarction because they are afraid. _____

11. Patients from hospitals in urban and rural areas differ with respect to their level of satisfaction with their nursing care. _____

12. A cancer patient's degree of hopefulness regarding the future is unrelated to his or her religiosity. _____

13. The degree of attachment between infants and their mothers is associated with the infant's status as low birth weight or normal birth weight. _____

14. The presence of homonymous hemianopia in stroke patients negatively affects their length of stay in hospital. _____

15. Adjustment to hemodialysis does not vary by the patient's gender. _____

C. STUDY QUESTIONS

1. Below is a list of general topics that could be investigated. Develop at least one research question for each, making sure that some are questions that could be addressed through qualitative research and others are ones that could be addressed through quantitative research. (HINT: For quantitative research questions, think of these concepts as potential independent or dependent variables, then ask, "What might cause or affect this variable (outcome)?" and "What might be the consequences or effects of this variable on other outcomes?" This should lead to some ideas for research questions.)
    a. Patient comfort _____.
    b. Psychiatric patients' readmission rates _____.
    c. Anxiety in hospitalized children _____.
    d. Elevated blood pressure _____.
    e. Incidence of sexually transmitted diseases _____.

   f. Patient cooperativeness in the recovery room _____.
   g. Caregiver stress _____.
   h. Mother–infant bonding _____.
   i. Menstrual irregularities _____.

2. Below are five nondirectional hypotheses. Restate each one as a directional hypothesis. Your hypotheses do not need to be "right"—this exercise is designed to encourage familiarity with wording hypotheses.

NONDIRECTIONAL   **DIRECTIONAL**

   a. Tactile stimulation is associated with   a.
      comparable physiological arousal as verbal
      stimulation among infants with congenital
      heart disease.
   b. The risk of hypoglycemia in term newborns is   b.
      related to the infant's birth weight.
   c. The use of isotonic sodium chloride solution   c.
      before endotracheal suctioning is related to
      oxygen saturation.
   d. Fluid balance is related to degree of success in   d.
      weaning older adults from mechanical
      ventilation.
   e. Nurses administer the same amount of   e.
      narcotic analgesics to male and female patients.

3. Below are five research hypotheses. Reword them as null hypotheses.

RESEARCH HYPOTHESIS   **NULL HYPOTHESIS**

   a. First-time blood donors experience greater   a.
      anxiety during the donation than donors
      who have given blood previously.
   b. Nurses who initiate more conversation with   b.
      patients are rated as more effective in their
      nursing care by patients than those who initiate
      less conversation.
   c. Surgical patients who give high ratings to the   c.
      informativeness of nursing communications
      experience less preoperative stress than do
      patients who give low ratings.
   d. Appendectomy patients who are pregnant are   d.
      more likely to experience peritoneal infection
      than female patients who are not pregnant.
   e. Women who give birth by cesarean delivery are   e.
      more likely to experience postpartum depression
      than women who give birth vaginally.

4. In study questions 2 and 3, 10 research hypotheses were provided. Identify the independent and dependent (outcome) variables in each.

INDEPENDENT VARIABLE(S)	DEPENDENT (OUTCOME) VARIABLE(S)
2a	
2b	
2c	
2d	
2e	
3a	
3b	
3c	
3d	
3e	

5. Below are five statements that are *not* testable research hypotheses as currently stated. Suggest modifications to these statements that would make them testable hypotheses.

ORIGINAL STATEMENT	HYPOTHESIS
a. Relaxation therapy is effective in reducing hypertension.	a.
b. The use of bilingual health care staff produces high utilization rates of health care facilities by ethnic minorities.	b.
c. Nursing students are affected in their choice of clinical specialization by interactions with nursing faculty.	c.
d. Sexually active teenagers have a high rate of using male methods of contraception.	d.
e. In-use intravenous solutions become contaminated within 48 hours.	e.

D. APPLICATION EXERCISES

Exercise D.1: Study in Appendix D

Read the abstract and introduction to the report by Eckhardt and colleagues ("Fatigue in the presence of coronary heart disease") in Appendix D on pages 143–153 and then answer the following questions:

Questions of Fact

a. In which paragraph(s) of this report is the research problem stated? Summarize the problem in a few sentences.

b. Did the researchers present a statement of purpose? If so, what *verb* did they use in the purpose statement, and is that verb consistent with the type of research that was undertaken?

c. Did the researchers specify a research question? If so, was it properly stated? If not, how would you state what the question was?

d. Did the researchers specify hypotheses? If there are hypotheses, were they appropriately worded? Are they directional or nondirectional? Simple or complex? Research or null? If no hypotheses were stated, what would one be?

e. Were any hypotheses *tested* in this study by means of statistical tests?

Questions for Discussion

a. Did the researchers do an adequate job of describing the research problem? Suggest ways in which the problem statement could be improved.

b. Comment on the significance of the study's research problem for nursing.

c. Did the researchers adequately explain the study purpose, research questions, and/or hypotheses? Were they well-worded?

Exercise D.2: Study in Appendix B

Read the abstract and introduction to the report by Ottosen and colleagues ("An ethnography of parents' perceptions of patient safety in the neonatal intensive care unit") in Appendix B on pages 123–133 and then answer the following questions:

Questions of Fact

a. In which paragraph(s) of this report is the research problem stated? Summarize the problem in a few sentences.

b. Did the researchers present a statement of purpose? If so, what *verb* did they use in the purpose statement, and is that verb consistent with the type of research that was undertaken?

c. Did the researchers specify a research question? If so, was it properly stated? If not, how would you state what the question was?

d. Did Ottosen and colleagues specify hypotheses? If there are hypotheses, were they appropriately worded? Are they directional or nondirectional? Simple or complex? Research or null?

e. Were any hypotheses *tested*?

Questions for Discussion

a. Did the researchers do an adequate job of describing the research problem? Suggest ways in which the problem statement could be improved.

b. Comment on the significance of the study's research problem for nursing.

c. Did the researchers adequately explain the study purpose, research questions, and/or hypotheses? Were they well-worded?

Finding and Reviewing Research Evidence in the Literature

A. FILL IN THE BLANKS

How many terms have you learned in this chapter? Fill in the blanks in the sentences below to find out.

1. A research journal article written by the researchers who conducted a study is a(n) _____ source for a research review.

2. Descriptions of studies prepared by someone other than the investigators are considered _____ sources.

3. A search strategy sometimes called "footnote chasing" is the _____ approach.

4. When a reviewer identifies a pivotal study and then searches forward for studies that cited that pivotal study, the strategy is called the _____ approach.

5. A major resource for finding research reports are _____ databases.

6. A feature called _____ allows people to search for topics using their own words, rather than needing to know subject codes in the database.

7. When doing a database search, one begins with one or more _____.

8. _____ is an especially important bibliographic database for nurses and the allied health professions.

9. Examples of _____ operators include "AND" and "OR."

10. The controlled vocabulary used to code entries in MEDLINE is called _____.

11. The MEDLINE database can be accessed for free through _____.

12. If a researcher has been prominent in an area, it is useful to do a(n) _____ search in bibliographic databases.

B. MATCHING EXERCISES

Match each statement in Set B with one of the types of databases listed in Set A. Indicate the letter corresponding to the appropriate response next to each entry in Set B.

SET A

a. CINAHL
b. MEDLINE
c. Neither CINAHL nor MEDLINE
d. Both CINAHL and MEDLINE

SET B   RESPONSES

1. An important bibliographic database for nurses   _____
2. Can be accessed on the Internet through PubMed   _____
3. Does not allow the use of Boolean operators   _____
4. Uses MeSH to index entries   _____
5. Focuses on nursing and allied health   _____
6. Does not provide abstracts, only citations   _____
7. Has more than 26 million records   _____
8. The articles in the appendices to this *Study Guide* could
   be retrieved in this database   _____

C. STUDY QUESTIONS

1. Below are several research questions. Indicate one or more keywords that you would use to begin a literature search on this topic.

   ## RESEARCH QUESTIONS   KEY WORDS

   a. What is the lived experience of being a survivor of a
      suicide attempt?   _____
   b. Do weekly text messages improve patient compliance
      with a treatment regimen?   _____
   c. What is the decision-making process for a woman
      considering having an abortion?   _____
   d. Is the use of silk-like synthetic fabrics for the linens
      of postsurgical patients effective in reducing the risk
      of pressure ulcers?   _____
   e. Do children raised on vegetarian diets have different
      growth patterns than other children?   _____
   f. What is the course of appetite loss among cancer
      patients undergoing chemotherapy?   _____
   g. What is the effect of alcohol skin preparation
      before insulin injection on the incidence of local
      and systemic infection?   _____
   h. Are bottle-fed babies introduced to solid foods
      sooner than breastfed babies?   _____

2. Below are fictitious excerpts from research literature reviews. Each excerpt has a stylistic problem. Change each sentence to make it acceptable stylistically, inventing citations if necessary.

ORIGINAL	REVISED
a. Most elderly people do not eat a balanced diet.	_____
b. Patient characteristics have a significant impact on nursing workload.	_____
c. A child's view of appropriate sick role behavior changes as the child grows older.	_____
d. Home birth poses many potential dangers.	_____
e. Traumatic brain injury results in considerable anxiety to the family of the patients.	_____
f. Studies have proved that most nurses prefer not to work the night shift.	_____
g. Life changes are the major cause of stress in adults.	_____
h. Stroke rehabilitation programs are most effective when they involve the patients' families.	_____
i. The traditional pelvic examination is sufficiently unpleasant to many women that they avoid having the examination.	_____

3. Read the literature review section from a research article appearing in a nursing journal about 10 to 15 years ago. Then, search the literature for more recent research on the topic of the article and update the original researchers' review section. If possible, use the descendancy approach as one of your search strategies. (Don't forget to incorporate in your review the findings from the cited research article itself.) Here are a few possible articles—all of them are open-access articles and links to them are provided in the Internet Resources section on thePoint.

- Chen, W., & Bakken, S. (2004). Breast cancer knowledge assessment in female Chinese immigrants in New York. *Cancer Nursing, 27,* 407–412.

- Estrada, C., Danielson, K., Drum, M., & Lipton, R. (2012). Insufficient sleep in young patients with diabetes and their families. *Biological Research for Nursing, 14,* 48–54.

- Given, B., Wyatt, G., Given, C., Gift, A., Sherwood, P., DeVoss, D., & Rahbar, M. (2004). Burden and depression among caregivers of patients with cancer at the end-of-life. *Oncology Nursing Forum, 31,* 1105–1117.

- McDougall, G. (2004). Memory self-efficacy and memory performance among black and white elders. *Nursing Research, 53,* 323–331.

- Sawin, E. M. (2012). "The body gives way, things happen": Older women describe breast cancer with a non-supportive intimate partner. *European Journal of Oncology Nursing, 16,* 64–70.

- Thoyre, S. M., & Carlson, J. (2003). Preterm infants' behavioural indicators of oxygen decline during bottle feeding. *Journal of Advanced Nursing, 43,* 631–641.

D. APPLICATION EXERCISES

Exercise D.1: Study in Appendix G

Read the abstract, introduction, and the first subsection under "Methods" of the report by Chase and colleagues ("The effectiveness of medication adherence interventions among patients with coronary artery disease") in Appendix G on pages 175–184 and then answer the following questions:

Questions of Fact

a. What type of research review did the investigators undertake?
b. Did the researchers begin with a problem statement? Summarize the problem in two or three sentences.
c. Did the researchers provide a statement of purpose? If so, what was it? Did they state research questions? If yes, what were they?
d. Which bibliographic databases did the researchers search?
e. What keywords were used in the search?
f. Did the reviewers use the ancestry approach in their search for studies?
g. Did the researchers restrict their search to English-language reports?
h. How many studies ultimately were included in the review?
i. Were the studies included in the review qualitative, quantitative, or both?

Questions for Discussion

a. Did the researchers do an adequate job of explaining the problem and their purpose in undertaking the review?
b. Did the researchers appear to do a thorough job in their search for relevant studies?
c. Certain studies that were initially retrieved were eliminated. Do you think the researchers provided a sound rationale for their decisions?

Exercise D.2: Study in Appendix H

Read the following abstract, introduction, and study design and methods sections of the report by Carr and colleagues ("Patient information needs and breast reconstruction after mastectomy") in Appendix H on pages 185–197 and then answer the following questions:

Questions of Fact

a. What type of research review did Carr and colleagues undertake?
b. What was the purpose of this metasynthesis?
c. Did this review involve a systematic search for evidence in bibliographic databases?
d. How many studies were included in the metasynthesis?
e. Which qualitative research traditions were represented in the review?

Questions for Discussion

a. Did Carr and colleagues do an adequate job of explaining the problem and the study purpose?
b. Can you think of other databases the reviewers could have used in their search for qualitative studies?

CHAPTER 7

Understanding Theoretical and Conceptual Frameworks

A. FILL IN THE BLANKS

How many terms have you learned in this chapter? Fill in the blanks in the sentences below to find out.

1. The conceptual underpinnings of a study is known as its _____.

2. Abstract concepts assembled because of their relevance to a core theme form a(n) _____ model.

3. A(n) _____ theory thoroughly accounts for or describes a phenomenon, without formal propositions stipulating a logical system of interrelationships.

4. A theory that focuses on a specific aspect of human experience is sometimes called _____ range.

5. A schematic _____ is a mechanism for representing concepts with a minimal use of words; another term for this is a conceptual _____.

6. The four elements in conceptual models of nursing are _____, _____, _____, and _____.

7. The originator of the Health Promotion Model is Nola _____.

8. _____ is the originator of the Humanbecoming Paradigm.

9. Roy conceptualized the _____ Model of nursing.

10. A construct that was fully conceptualized by Bandura and that is a key mediator in many models of health behavior is _____ - _____.

11. The Transtheoretical Model involves a construct called _____ of _____, which concerns a person's motivational readiness to modify behavior.

12. In the Theory of _____ _____, a person's intention to act in a certain way determines his or her actual behavior.

B. MATCHING EXERCISES

1. Match each statement from Set B with one of the phrases in Set A. Indicate the letter corresponding to your response next to each of the statements in Set B.

SET A

a. Classic theory
b. Conceptual model
c. Schematic model
d. Neither a, b, nor c
e. a, b, *and* c

SET B   **RESPONSE**

1. Makes minimal use of language   _____
2. Uses concepts as building blocks   _____
3. Is often created in grounded theory studies   _____
4. Can be used as a basis for generating hypotheses   _____
5. Can be proved through empirical testing   _____
6. Incorporates a system of propositions that assert
   relationships among variables   _____
7. Consists of interrelated concepts organized in a rational
   scheme but does not specify formal relationships among
   the concepts   _____
8. Exists in nature and is awaiting scientific discovery   _____

2. Match each model from Set B with one of the theorists in Set A. Indicate the letter corresponding to your response next to each of the statements in Set B.

SET A

a. Bandura
b. Pender
c. Roy
d. Prochaska
e. Mishel
f. Ajzen

SET B   **RESPONSE**

1. Adaptation Model   _____
2. Transtheoretical Model   _____
3. Uncertainty in Illness Theory   _____
4. Social Cognitive Theory   _____
5. Health Promotion Model   _____
6. Theory of Planned Behavior   _____

C. STUDY QUESTIONS

1. Read some recent issues of a nursing research journal. Identify at least two different theories cited by nurse researchers in these research reports.

2. Select one of the research questions/problems listed below. Could the selected problem be developed within one of the models or theories discussed in this chapter? Defend your answer.
   a. What are the factors contributing to perceptions of fatigue among patients with congestive heart failure?
   b. What effect does the presence of the father in the delivery room have on the mother's satisfaction with the childbirth experience?
   c. The purpose of the study is to explore why some women fail to perform breast self-examination regularly.
   d. What are the factors that lead to poorer health among low-income children compared to higher-income children?

3. Suggest an important health outcome that could be studied using the Health Promotion Model. Identify another theory described in this chapter that could be used to explain or predict the same outcome. Which theory or model do you think would do a better job? Why?

4. Read the following open-access article (a link is provided in the Internet Resources section on thePoint website) and then assess the following: (a) What evidence do the researchers offer to substantiate that their grounded theory is a good fit with their data? and (b) To what extent is it clear or unclear in the article that symbolic interaction was a theoretical underpinning of the study?

   • Hatcher, D., Chang, E., Schmied, V., & Garrido, S. (2019). Holding momentum: A grounded theory study of strategies for sustaining living at home in older persons. *International Journal of Qualitative Studies on Health and Well-being, 14*, 1658333.

D. APPLICATION EXERCISES

Exercise D.1: Study in Appendix D

Read the abstract and introduction (all of the material before "Methods") of the article by Eckhardt and colleagues ("Fatigue in the presence of coronary heart disease") in Appendix D on pages 143–153 and then answer the following questions:

Questions of Fact
   a. Did the study by Eckhardt and colleagues involve a conceptual or theoretical framework? What is it called?
   b. Is this framework one of the models of nursing cited in the textbook? Is it related to one of those models?
   c. Was the theory thoroughly described?
   d. Did the researchers adapt the theory? In what way was it adapted?
   e. Did the report include a schematic model?

f. What are the key concepts in the model?
g. Did this model indicate relationships among the concepts?
h. Did the report present conceptual definitions of key concepts?
i. Did the report explicitly present hypotheses deduced from the framework?

Questions for Discussion

a. Did the link between the problem and the framework seem contrived? Did the hypotheses (if any) naturally flow from the framework?
b. Do you think any aspects of the research would have been different without the framework?
c. Would you describe this study as a model-testing inquiry or do you think the model was used more as an organizing framework?

Exercise D.2: Study in Appendix E

Read the report by Langegård and colleagues ("The art of living with symptoms") in Appendix E on pages 155–162 and then answer the following questions:

Questions of Fact

a. Did this article describe a conceptual or theoretical framework for the study? What is it called?
b. Did the study result in the generation of a theory? What was it called?
c. Did the report include a schematic model? If so, what are the key concepts in the model?
d. Did the report explicitly present hypotheses deduced from the framework? Did they undertake hypothesis-testing statistical analyses?

Questions for Discussion

a. Comment on the ability of the schematic model to capture important processes gleaned from the research. Would a more dynamic model (showing the evolution of symptom management strategies) have been more useful?
b. Could this study have been undertaken within a different qualitative tradition? Defend your answer.

PART 3

Designs and Methods for Quantitative and Qualitative Nursing Research

3

Designs and
Methods for
Quantitative and
Qualitative Nursing
Research

Appraising Quantitative Research Design

A. FILL IN THE BLANKS

How many terms have you learned in this chapter? Fill in the blanks in the sentences below to find out.

1. Good research design in quantitative studies involves achieving four types of _____.

2. A(n) _____ design refers to a study design in which the same people are exposed to two or more conditions in random order.

3. The loss of participants from a study over time is called _____.

4. A key threat to internal validity stemming from preexisting group differences on the outcome is the _____ threat.

5. The allocation of study participants to groups by chance is called _____ assignment.

6. Researchers use the strategy of _____ (or masking) to guard against expectation biases.

7. Techniques of research _____ include randomization, homogeneity, and matching.

8. _____ is the threat to internal validity stemming from differential loss of participants from groups.

9. In a(n) _____ design, data about a cause are collected before data about effects.

10. Demonstrating the existence of a relationship between an independent variable and an outcome contributes to _____ conclusion validity.

11. The degree to which it can be inferred that the independent variable caused or affected the outcome variable is _____ validity.

12. The type of validity referring to the generalizability of results is _____ validity.

13. Data are collected at a single point in time in a(n) _____-_____ study.

14. A(n) _____ is what would have happened to the same people simultaneously exposed and not exposed to a hypothesized causal factor.

15. A(n) _____-_____ study uses a retrospective nonexperimental design involving the comparison of a *case* and a matched counterpart.

16. A(n) _____ design involves the collection of data over an extended period of time.

17. _____ involves the deliberate pairing of participants in different groups as a method of controlling confounding variables.

18. Statistical _____ refers to the capacity to detect true relationships among variables.

19. A(n) _____ threat is an internal validity problem that concerns the effect of other possible causes co-occurring with the independent variable.

20. In a delayed treatment design, control group members are _____-listed for the intervention.

21. In an intervention study, the outcome data collected before implementing the intervention are often called _____ data.

22. Intervention studies in which there is no randomization to treatment conditions are called _____-_____.

23. Correlational studies examine _____ between variables but involve no intervention.

24. In _____ studies, researchers search for antecedent causes of an effect occurring in the present.

B. MATCHING EXERCISES

Match each research question from Set B with one (or more) of the phrases from Set A that indicates a potential reason for using a nonexperimental design. Indicate the letter(s) corresponding to your response next to each statement in Set B.

SET A

a. Independent variable cannot be manipulated
b. Possible ethical constraints on manipulation
c. No constraints on manipulation

SET B   RESPONSE

1. Does the use of certain tampons cause toxic shock syndrome?   _____

2. Does heroin addiction among mothers affect Apgar scores of infants?   _____

3. Is the age of a patient who is on dialysis related to the incidence of the disequilibrium syndrome?   _____

4. What body positions aid respiratory function?   _____

5. Does the ingestion of saccharin cause cancer in humans?   _____

6. Does a nurse's attitude toward the elderly affect his or her choice of a clinical specialty?   _____

7. Does the use of touch by nursing staff affect patient satisfaction? _____

8. Does a nurse's gender affect his or her salary and rate of promotion? _____

9. Does extreme athletic exertion in young women cause amenorrhea? _____

10. Does assertiveness training affect a psychiatric nurse's job performance? _____

C. STUDY QUESTIONS

1. Suppose you wanted to study self-efficacy among successful dieters who lost 20 or more pounds and maintained their weight loss for at least 6 months. Specify at least two different types of comparison strategies that might provide a useful comparative context for this study. Do your strategies lend themselves to experimental manipulation? If not, why not?

2. Refer to the 10 hypotheses in Chapter 5 Exercises C.2 on page 30 and C.3 on page 30. Indicate below whether these hypotheses could be tested using an experimental/quasi-experimental approach, a nonexperimental approach, or both/either.

Question Number	Experimental/ Quasi-Experimental	Nonexperimental	Both/Either
2a			
2b			
2c			
2d			
2e			
3a			
3b			
3c			
3d			
3e			

3. A nurse researcher found a relationship between teenagers' level of knowledge about birth control and their level of sexual activity. That is, teenagers with higher levels of sexual activity knew more about birth control than teenagers with less sexual activity. Suggest at least three interpretations for this finding. Is this a research problem that is *inherently* nonexperimental? Why or why not?

4. Suppose that you were studying the effects of range-of-motion exercises on radical mastectomy patients. You start your randomized controlled trial (RCT)

with 50 experimental patients and 50 control patients. Your intervention requires the experimental group members to come for daily sessions over a 2-week period, whereas control participants come only once at the end of 2 weeks. Your final group sizes are 40 for the experimental group and 49 for the control group. The results of your study indicate that women in the experimental group did better in raising the arm of the affected side above head level than those in the control group. What effects, if any, do you think the attrition might have on the internal validity of your study?

5. Suppose that you were interested in testing the hypothesis that regular ingestion of aspirin reduced the risk of colon cancer. Describe how such a hypothesis could be tested using a retrospective case-control design. Now describe a prospective cohort design for the same study. Compare the strengths and weaknesses of the two approaches.

D. APPLICATION EXERCISES

Exercise D.1: Study in Appendix A

Read the Methods section of the report by Stephens and colleagues ("Smartphone technology and text messaging for weight loss in young adults") in Appendix A on pages 115–122 and then answer the following questions:

Questions of Fact
a. Was there an intervention in this study?
b. What were the independent and dependent variables?
c. Is the design for this study experimental, quasi-experimental, or nonexperimental?
d. Was randomization used? If yes, what method was used to assign participants to groups?
e. In terms of the control group strategies described in the textbook, what approach did the researchers use?
f. What is the specific name of the research design used in this study?
g. Was any masking/blinding used in this study?
h. Would this study be described as longitudinal?
i. Which of the methods of research control described in this chapter were used to control confounding variables?
j. What confounding variables were controlled?
k. Was there any attrition in this study?
l. Was selection a threat to the internal validity of this study?
m. Was mortality a threat to the internal validity of this study?

Questions for Discussion
a. What was the intervention? Comment on how well the intervention was described, including a description of how it was developed and refined.
b. Comment on the researchers' control group strategy. Could a more powerful or effective strategy have been used?
c. Discuss ways in which this study achieved or failed to achieve the criteria for making causal inferences.

d. Comment on the researchers' use or nonuse of blinding.
e. Comment on the timing of postintervention data collection.
f. Comment on the external validity of this study.

Exercise D.2: Study in Appendix D

Read the Methods section of the report by Eckhardt and colleagues ("Fatigue in the presence of coronary heart disease") in Appendix D on pages 143–153 and then answer the following questions:

Questions of Fact

a. Was there an intervention in this study?
b. Is the design for this study experimental, quasi-experimental, or nonexperimental?
c. Was this a cause-probing study?
d. What were the independent and dependent variables in this study?
e. Was the independent variable amenable to manipulation?
f. Was randomization used? If yes, what method was used to assign subjects to groups?
g. What is the specific name of the research design used in this study?
h. Was any blinding (masking) used in this study?
i. Would this study be described as longitudinal? Would it be described as prospective?

Questions for Discussion

a. Discuss ways in which this study achieved or failed to achieve the criteria for making causal inferences.
b. Comment on the timing of data collection. Would a different time perspective be useful?

9 CHAPTER

Appraising Sampling and Data Collection in Quantitative Studies

A. FILL IN THE BLANKS

How many terms have you learned in this chapter? Fill in the blanks in the sentences below to find out.

1. The aggregate set of people/objects with specified characteristics is a(n) _____.

2. Subdivisions of a population are called _____.

3. Specifications for population characteristics are identified in the _____ criteria.

4. The total number of participants in a study is known as the study's sample _____.

5. _____ sampling involves recruiting *every* eligible person over a specified period of time.

6. _____ sampling involves sampling by convenience, but within specified subgroups of the population, to enhance representativeness.

7. The broad class of sampling in which every element of a population has an equal chance of being selected is _____ sampling.

8. In quantitative studies, the key criterion for evaluating a sample is its _____ of the population.

9. _____ sampling is the most widely used type of sampling in quantitative health care research.

10. Probability sampling involves the selection of sample members at _____.

11. Sampling _____ is the systematic overrepresentation or underrepresentation of some segment of the population.

12. In _____ sampling, the researcher samples every *k*th case (e.g., every 10th case).

13. In quantitative studies, researchers use _____ _____ to estimate how large a sample they need.

14. The most widely used method of data collection by nurse researchers is by _____-report.

48

15. The type of questions in mailed questionnaires are primarily _____-ended questions.

16. The question, "What is it like to be a cancer survivor?" is a(n) _____-ended question.

17. A composite _____ with multiple items yields a score that places people on a continuum with regard to an attribute.

18. A(n) _____ scale is a type of summated rating scale used to measure agreement or disagreement with statements.

19. The tendency to distort self-report information in characteristic ways is called a response _____ bias.

20. The bias that occurs when a person consistently agrees with statements regardless of their content is known as _____ bias.

21. Methods of collecting data by watching behaviors and events are referred to as _____ methods.

22. In a structured observation, a(n) _____ is used with a category system to record frequencies of observed events or behaviors.

23. _____ sampling in observational studies is used to select periods when observations are made, either systematically or randomly.

24. _____ involves assigning numbers to attributes according to established rules.

25. _____ is the extent to which scores for people *who have not changed* are the same for repeated measurements.

26. An assessment of a composite scale's _____ _____ involves evaluating whether there is consistency across items designed to measure the same trait.

27. The method used to assess an instrument's stability is _____–_____ reliability.

28. _____ is a measurement property that concerns the extent to which an instrument is actually measuring what it purports to measure.

29. _____ validity concerns the extent to which the scores on a measure are a good reflection of a "gold standard."

30. One means of assessing construct validity is through the known-_____ technique.

B. MATCHING EXERCISES

1. Match each statement relating to sampling for quantitative studies from Set B with one of the phrases from Set A. Indicate the letter corresponding to your response next to each of the statements in Set B.

SET A

a. Probability sampling
b. Nonprobability sampling
c. Both probability and nonprobability sampling
d. Neither probability nor nonprobability sampling

SET B   **RESPONSE**

1. Includes purposive sampling   _____
2. Allows an estimation of the magnitude of sampling error   _____
3. Guarantees a representative sample   _____
4. Includes quota sampling   _____
5. Requires a sample size of at least 100 subjects   _____
6. Elements are selected by nonrandom methods.   _____
7. Can be used with entire populations or with selected
   strata from the populations   _____
8. Used to select populations   _____
9. Elements have an equal chance of being selected.   _____
10. Is most widely used by nurse researchers   _____

2. Match each descriptive statement regarding data collection methods from
   Set B with one (or more) of the statements from Set A. Indicate the letter(s)
   corresponding to your response next to each item in Set B.

SET A

a. Self-reports
b. Observations
c. Biomarkers/biophysiological measures
d. None of the above

SET B   **RESPONSE**

1. Cannot easily be gathered unobtrusively   _____
2. Can be biased by the participants' desire to "look good"   _____
3. Can be used to gather data from infants   _____
4. Is a good way to obtain information about human behavior   _____
5. Can be biased by the researcher's values and beliefs   _____
6. Can be combined with other data collection methods in
   a single study   _____
7. Can yield quantitative information   _____
8. Is the most widely used method of collecting data by
   nurse researchers   _____

3. Match each descriptive statement regarding self-report methods from Set B
   with one of the statements from Set A. Indicate the letter corresponding to
   your response next to each item in Set B.

SET A

a. Interviews
b. Questionnaires
c. Both interviews and questionnaires
d. Neither interviews nor questionnaires

SET B	RESPONSE
1. Can provide participants the protection of anonymity	_____
2. Can be used with illiterate participants	_____
3. Can include both open- and closed-ended questions	_____
4. Is the best way to measure human behavior	_____
5. Is generally an inexpensive method of data collection	_____
6. Can be distributed by mail	_____

C. STUDY QUESTIONS

1. Identify the type of quantitative sampling design used in the following examples:
   a. A sample of 250 members randomly selected from a roster of American Nurses Association members
   b. All the oncology nurses participating in a continuing education seminar
   c. Every 20th patient admitted to the emergency room
   d. Twenty male and 20 female patients admitted to the hospital with hypothermia
   e. Twenty-five internationally renowned experts in critical care nursing
   f. All patients receiving hospice services from Capital District Hospice in 2021

2. Suppose you were interested in studying the attitude of nurse practitioners toward autonomy in work situations. Suggest a possible target and accessible population. What strata might be useful if quota sampling were used?

3. Below are several research problems. Indicate which quantitative methods of data collection (self-report, observation, biomarkers, records) you might recommend using for each. Defend your response.
   a. What are the predictors of intravenous site symptoms?
   b. What are the health and mental health consequences of a sedentary lifestyle among community-dwelling elders?
   c. To what extent and in what manner do nurses interact differently with older and younger patients?
   d. What are the effects of an HIV-prevention intervention on the risk-taking behavior of urban adolescents?

4. Which of the following measures could be assessed with respect to internal consistency?
   a. Infants' Apgar scores
   b. Blood pressure measurements
   c. A 10-item scale to measure resilience
   d. A visual analog scale measuring dyspnea

5. What types of groups might be useful for a known-groups approach to assessing construct validity for measures of the following:
   a. Emotional maturity
   b. Children's aggressiveness
   c. Quality of life
   d. Compliance with a medication regimen
   e. Subjective pain

D. APPLICATION EXERCISES

Exercise D.1: Quantitative Appendix Studies

Which of the studies in Appendix A (by Stephens et al.) on pages 115–122, Appendix C (by Saqe-Rockoff et al.) on pages 135–141, and Appendix D (by Eckhardt et al.) on pages 143–153 used the following sampling methods?
a. Probability sampling
b. Convenience sampling
c. Consecutive sampling

Exercise D.2: Quantitative Appendix Studies

Which of the studies in Appendix A (by Stephens et al.) on pages 115–122, Appendix C (by Saqe-Rockoff et al.) on pages 135–141, and Appendix D (by Eckhardt et al.) on pages 143–153 used the following data collection methods?
a. Self-reports
b. Observational methods
c. Biomarkers
d. Records

Exercise D.3: Study in Appendix D

Read the Methods and first part of the Results sections of the report by Eckhardt and colleagues ("Fatigue in the presence of coronary heart disease") in Appendix D on pages 143–153 and then answer the following questions:

Questions of Fact

a. What was the target population of this study? How would you describe the accessible population?
b. What were the eligibility criteria for the study?
c. Was the sampling method probability or nonprobability? What specific sampling method was used?
d. How were study participants recruited?
e. What efforts did the researchers make to ensure a diverse (and hence more representative) sample?
f. What was the sample size that the research team achieved?
g. Was a power analysis used to determine sample size needs? If yes, what number of participants did the power analysis estimate as the minimum needed number?
h. Were sample characteristics described? If yes, what were the main characteristics of study participants?
i. Did the researchers develop their own measures, or did they use instruments or scales that had been developed by others?
j. What did the article say about the reliability and validity of key measures?

Questions for Discussion

a. Comment on the adequacy of the researchers' sampling plan and recruitment strategy. How representativeness was the sample of the target population? What types of sampling biases might be of special concern?
b. Do you think the sample size was adequate? Why or why not?

c. Comment on the adequacy of the data collection approaches used in this study. Did Eckhardt and her colleagues operationalize their outcome measures in the best possible manner?

d. Did the researchers' description of their measures inspire confidence in data quality in this study?

10 CHAPTER

Appraising Qualitative Designs and Approaches

A. FILL IN THE BLANKS

How many terms have you learned in this chapter? Fill in the blanks in the sentences below to find out.

1. Qualitative designs are usually _____ designs that require an ongoing analysis of data to suggest profitable new strategies.

2. _____ was Leininger's phrase for research at the interface between culture and nursing.

3. Ethnographers typically undertake _____ observation as a data collection strategy during their fieldwork.

4. Ethnographers rely on one or more key _____ to help them understand and interpret a culture.

5. An ethnography that studies the culture of small units, groups, or institutions is called a(n) _____ ethnography.

6. Phenomenologists study _____ experiences.

7. A descriptive phenomenological question is: What is the _____ of this phenomenon?

8. _____ phenomenology focuses on the *meaning* of experiences; another term used for this type of phenomenology is _____.

9. Descriptive phenomenologists use the strategy called _____ to hold in abeyance their presuppositions about a phenomenon.

10. Grounded theory researchers often identify a _____ social process (BSP) that explains how people resolve a problem.

11. The two originators of grounded theory were _____ and _____.

12. Grounded theorists use an analytic strategy called _____ comparison.

13. In a(n) _____ study, a single person or group (or a small number) is at center stage.

14. In _____ analysis, the focus is on a *story*.

15. Research that seeks to be transformative is based on _____ theory.

16. Participatory _____ research is designed to be empowering for the group under study.

54

B. MATCHING EXERCISES

Match each descriptive statement from Set B with one of the research traditions from Set A. Indicate the letter corresponding to your response next to each item in Set B.

SET A

a. Ethnography
b. Phenomenology
c. Grounded theory
d. Ethnography, phenomenology, and grounded theory

SET B   RESPONSES

1. Is rooted in a philosophical tradition developed by
   Husserl and Heidegger   _____

2. Involves the study of both broadly defined cultures and
   more narrowly defined ones   _____

3. Uses qualitative data to address questions of interest   _____

4. Is an approach to the study of social processes and
   social structures   _____

5. Is concerned with the lived experiences of humans   _____

6. Strives to achieve an emic perspective on the members
   of a group   _____

7. Is closely related to a research tradition called
   hermeneutics   _____

8. Requires the use of a procedure called *constant
   comparison*   _____

9. Stems from a discipline other than nursing   _____

10. Developed by the sociologists Glaser and Strauss   _____

11. Is a tradition that is particularly well suited to a critical
    theory perspective   _____

12. Typically involves in-depth interviews with study
    participants.   _____

C. STUDY QUESTIONS

1. For each of the research questions below, indicate the qualitative research tradition that would likely guide the inquiry and why you think that would be the case.
   a. What is the social psychological process through which couples deal with the sudden loss of an infant through SIDS?
   b. How does the culture of a suicide survivors' self-help group adapt to a successful suicide attempt by a former member?

    c. What is the lived experience of spousal caretakers of patients with Alzheimer's disease?

    d. What is the meaning of loneliness to childless widows with chronic health problems?

2. Skim the following two qualitative studies, both of which are available as open-access articles (links to these articles are included in the Internet Resources section on thePoint® website). Both studies are examples of qualitative studies (grounded theory and qualitative description) that focused on cancer survivors. What were the central phenomena under investigation? Compare and contrast the methods used in these two studies (e.g., How were data collected? How many study participants were there? To what extent did the design unfold while the researchers were in the field?).

   • *Grounded Theory Study:* Brauer, E., Pieters, H., Ganz, P., Landier, W., Pavlish, C., & Heilemann, M. (2018). Coming of age with cancer: Physical, social, and financial barriers to independence among emerging adult survivors. *Oncology Nursing Forum, 45,* 148–158.

   • *Qualitative Descriptive Study:* Howard, A., Kazanjian, A., Pritchard, S., Olson, R., Hasan, H., Newton, K., & Goddard, K. (2018). Healthcare system barriers to long-term follow-up for adult survivors of childhood cancer in British Columbia, Canada: A qualitative study. *Journal of Cancer Survivorship, 12,* 277–290.

3. Skim the following open-access article about a participatory action research (PAR) study and comment on the roles of participants and researchers. (A link to this article is included in the Internet Resources section on thePoint® website.) How might the study have been different if a participatory approach had not been used?

   • Smith-MacDonald, L., Venturato, L., Hunter, P., Kaasalainen, S., Sussman, T., McCleary, L., . . . Sinclair, S. (2019). Perspectives and experiences of compassion in long-term care facilities within Canada: A qualitative study of patients, family members and health care providers. *BMC Geriatrics, 19,* 128.

4. Read the following open-access journal article about a grounded theory study and evaluate the extent to which the problem was amenable to the grounded theory tradition. (A link to this article is included in the Internet Resources section on thePoint® website.) Which school of grounded theory thought was followed in this study? Did the report explicitly discuss how the constant comparative method was used?

   • McCullough, K., Whitehead, L., Bayes, S., Williams, A., & Cope, V. (2020). The delivery of primary health care in remote communities: A grounded theory study of the perspective of nurses. *International Journal of Nursing Studies, 102,* 103474.

D. APPLICATION EXERCISES

Exercise 1: Study in Appendix B

Read the Methods section of the report by Ottosen and colleagues ("An ethnography of parents' perceptions of patient safety in the neonatal intensive care unit") in Appendix B on pages 123–133 and then answer the following questions:

Questions of Fact

a. Within which tradition was this study based?
b. What was the central phenomenon under study?
c. Was the study longitudinal?
d. What was the setting for this research?
e. Did the researchers make explicit comparisons?
f. Did the researchers use methods that were congruent with the chosen qualitative research tradition?
g. Did this study have an ideological perspective?

Questions for Discussion

a. How well did Ottosen and colleagues describe their research design? Were design decisions explained and justified?
b. Does it appear that the researchers made all design decisions up front, or did the design emerge during data collection, allowing them to capitalize on early information?
c. Could this study have been undertaken within an ideological perspective? Why or why not?
d. Could the researchers have used narrative analysis in this study?

Exercise 2: Study in Appendix E

Read the report by Langegård and colleagues ("The art of living with symptoms") in Appendix E on pages 155–162 and then answer the following questions:

Questions of Fact

a. Within which tradition was this study based?
b. Which specific approach was used—that of Glaser and Strauss, Strauss and Corbin, or Charmaz?
c. What was the central phenomenon under study?
d. Was the study longitudinal?
e. What was the setting for this research?
f. Did the report indicate or suggest that constant comparison was used?
g. Was a core variable or basic social process identified? If yes, what was it?
h. Did the researchers use methods that were congruent with the chosen qualitative research tradition?
i. Did this study have an ideological perspective? If so, which one?

Questions for Discussion

a. How well is the research design described in the report? Were design decisions explained and justified?

b. Does it appear that the researchers made all design decisions up front, or did the design emerge during data collection, allowing them to capitalize on early information?

c. Were there any elements of the design or methods that appear to be more appropriate for a qualitative tradition other than the one the researchers identified as the underlying tradition?

CHAPTER 11

Appraising Sampling and Data Collection in Qualitative Studies

A. FILL IN THE BLANKS

How many terms have you learned in this chapter? Fill in the blanks in the sentences below to find out.

1. _____ sampling is a type of sampling based on referrals from early participants.

2. _____ sampling is preferred by grounded theory researchers.

3. A sampling approach in which participants are intentionally selected by the researchers to fulfill the needs of the study is known as _____ sampling.

4. A type of purposive sampling that involves deliberate attempts to draw from diverse groups is _____ _____ sampling.

5. The principle used by qualitative researchers to determine when to stop sampling is called _____ _____.

6. A(n) _____ guide is used in some qualitative studies to ensure that important question areas are covered in an interview.

7. An interview that is guided by an established list of topics or broad questions is _____-structured.

8. A completely unstructured interview typically begins with a(n) _____ _____ question to initiate an undirected conversation.

9. _____ is a technique that involves participants taking pictures of their own environments and then explaining and interpreting the pictures to the researcher.

10. A technique for gathering in-depth information from 5 to 10 informants simultaneously is called a(n) _____ _____ interview.

11. In ethnographic studies, researchers rely on _____ _____ to provide insights about the culture and to offer guidance about activities and events to observe.

12. Participant observers record their observations, thoughts, and interpretations in _____ notes; they also maintain a daily _____ to record activities and events.

59

B. MATCHING EXERCISES

1. Match each type of sampling approach from Set B with one of the phrases from Set A. Indicate the letter corresponding to your response next to each of the statements in Set B.

SET A

a. Sampling approach for quantitative studies
b. Sampling approach for qualitative studies
c. Sampling approach for either quantitative or qualitative studies
d. Sampling approach for neither quantitative nor qualitative studies

SET B   RESPONSE

   1. Typical case sampling   _____
   2. Purposive sampling   _____
   3. Weighted sampling   _____
   4. Consecutive sampling   _____
   5. Extreme case sampling   _____
   6. Stratified random sampling   _____
   7. Maximum variation sampling   _____
   8. Quota sampling   _____
   9. Theoretical sampling   _____
  10. Power sampling   _____

2. Match each descriptive statement regarding data collection methods from Set B with one of the statements from Set A. Indicate the letter corresponding to your response next to each item in Set B.

SET A

a. Self-reports
b. Observations
c. Both self-reports and observations
d. Neither self-reports nor observations

SET B   RESPONSE

   1. Is the primary source of data in phenomenological research   _____
   2. Data are recorded in logs and field notes.   _____
   3. Ethnographies rely on this as a data source.   _____
   4. Photovoice is one approach.   _____
   5. Mobile positioning is a strategy for collecting such data.   _____
   6. Can be either structured for quantitative inquiries or
       unstructured for qualitative inquiries   _____

7. Usually relies on transcriptions in qualitative studies   _____
8. Can involve active participation of researchers   _____
9. Can be collected in focus groups   _____
10. Can rely on a topic guide   _____

C. STUDY QUESTIONS

1. Below are several research questions. Indicate which method of sampling you might recommend using for each and what you think the sample size might be. Defend your response.
   a. How does an elderly person manage the transition from a nursing home to a hospital and then back again?
   b. What is it like to be an in vitro fertilization patient and not get pregnant after many months of treatment?
   c. What is the process by which patients adjust to postdischarge life following a spinal cord injury?
   d. What are the health beliefs and risk-taking behaviors of adolescent members of a vampire cult?
2. Suppose a qualitative researcher wanted to study the quality of life of cancer survivors. Suggest what the researcher might do to obtain a maximum variation sample and an extreme case sample.
3. Read the following open-access article (a link is provided in the Internet Resources section of thePoint®). Identify specific examples of what could be called *thick description*:

   • McCaughan, D., Sheard, L., Cullum, N., Dunville, J., & Chetter, I. (2018). Patients' perceptions and experiences of living with a surgical wound healing by secondary intention: A qualitative study. *International Journal of Nursing Studies*, *77*, 29–38.

4. The following open-access study relied primarily on a sample of convenience and snowball sampling (a link to the article is provided in the Internet Resources section on thePoint®). Suggest ways in which the researchers might have improved the study by using a different sampling approach:

   • Kool, L., Schellevis, F., Jaarsma, D., & Feijen-De Jong, E. (2020). The initiation of Dutch newly qualified hospital-based midwives in practice, a qualitative study. *Midwifery*, *83*, 102648.

5. Below are several research questions. Indicate which type of unstructured self-report approach you might recommend using for each. Defend your response.
   a. How do parents of children with autism manage their frustration and fears?
   b. What are the barriers to preventive health care practices among the urban poor?
   c. What stresses does the spouse of a patient who is terminally ill experience?
   d. What are the coping mechanisms and perceived barriers to coping among patients with severely disfigured burn?

6. Suppose you were interested in studying patients' impatience and anxiety waiting for treatment in the waiting area of an emergency department. Develop a topic guide for a semi-structured interview on this topic.

7. Suggest how you might collect data to address the following research question: *To what extent and in what manner do male and female nurses interact differently with male and female patients?* Would *participant* observation be appropriate? What are the possible advantages and drawbacks of such an approach?

D. APPLICATION EXERCISES

Exercise 1: Study in Appendix B

Read the Methods sections of the report by Ottosen and colleagues ("An ethnography of parents' perceptions of patient safety in the neonatal intensive care unit") in Appendix B on pages 123–133 and then answer the following questions:

Questions of Fact

a. What were the eligibility criteria for this study?
b. How were study participants recruited?
c. What type of sampling approach was used?
d. How many participants comprised the sample?
e. Was data saturation achieved?
f. Were sample characteristics described? If yes, what were those characteristics?
g. Did the researcher collect any self-report data? If no, could self-reports have been used? If yes, what concepts were captured by self-report?
h. What specific types of qualitative self-report methods were used?
i. Were examples of interview questions included in the report?
j. Did the report provide information about how long interviews took on average?
k. How were the self-report data recorded?
l. Did this study collect any data through observation? If no, could observation have been used? If yes, what concepts were captured through observation?
m. If there were observations, how were observational data recorded?
n. Who collected the data in this study?

Questions for Discussion

a. Comment on the adequacy of the researchers' sampling plan and recruitment strategy for achieving the goals of this study.
b. Do you think the sample size in this study was adequate? Why or why not?
c. Ottosen and colleagues selected parents who matched the characteristics of parents in the NICU. Comment on this strategy.
d. Comment on the adequacy of the researchers' description of their data collection methods.
e. Comment on the data collection approaches the research team used. Did they fully capture the concepts of interest in the best possible manner? Were adequate steps taken to ensure the highest possible quality data?

Exercise 2: Study in Appendix E

Read the report by Langegård and colleagues ("The art of living with symptoms") in Appendix E on pages 155–162 and then answer the following questions:

Questions of Fact

a. What were the eligibility criteria for this study?
b. How were study participants recruited?
c. What type of sampling approach was used?
d. How many study participants comprised the sample?
e. Was data saturation achieved?
f. Did the sampling strategy include confirming and disconfirming cases?
g. Were sample characteristics described? If yes, what were those characteristics?
h. Did the researcher collect any self-report data? If no, could self-reports have been used? If yes, what concepts were captured by self-report?
i. What specific types of qualitative self-report methods were used?
j. Were examples of interview questions included in the report?
k. Did the report provide information about how long interviews took on average?
l. How were the self-report data recorded?
m. Did this study collect any data through observation? If no, could observation have been used? If yes, what concepts were captured through observation?

Questions for Discussion

a. Comment on the adequacy of the researchers' sampling plan and recruitment strategy for achieving the goals of a grounded theory study.
b. Do you think the sample size in this study was adequate? Why or why not?
c. Consider what the researchers might have done if they had also collected observational data. How might observational data have enriched the study?

12

Understanding Mixed Methods Research, Quality Improvement, and Other Special Types of Research

A. FILL IN THE BLANKS

How many terms have you learned in this chapter? Fill in the blanks in the sentences below to find out.

1. The type of research that integrates qualitative and quantitative data is called _____ _____ research.

2. Mixed methods designs can be characterized by decisions with regard to _____ and _____.

3. In the notation QUAL + quan, the dominant strand is the _____ component.

4. The notation QUAL → quan signifies a design in which _____ data are collected first.

5. In mixed methods research, the design notation of an arrow (→) designates a design that is _____.

6. In mixed methods research, the design notation of a plus sign (+) designates a design that is _____.

7. The paradigm most often associated with mixed methods research is called _____.

8. _____ _____ involves the assessment of a patient care problem in a health care organization, with the aim of introducing changes to improve patient outcomes.

9. An important planning tool in QI projects is to undertake a(n) _____ _____ _____ to identify factors contributing to a patient care problem.

10. The most frequently used model used to guide QI projects is called _____-_____-_____-_____.

11. A(n) _____ _____ is a multiphase effort to refine and test the effectiveness of a clinical treatment.

12. Phase IV clinical trials are sometimes called _____ studies.

13. Phase III of a clinical trial is typically a(n) _____ controlled trial.

14. In nursing intervention research, the construct validity of a new intervention is enhanced by using a(n) _____ _____ as the basis for intervention features.

15. An evaluation of how a new intervention gets implemented is called a(n) _____ analysis.

16. In a(n) _____ analysis, the focus of the evaluation is on whether a program's benefits outweigh its monetary costs.

17. In _____ _____ research, researchers make direct comparisons of two or more interventions.

18. _____ research involves efforts to understand the end results of health care practices.

19. In the Donabedian framework, the three key factors are process, outcomes, and _____.

20. A(n) _____, which involves collecting self-report data about people's opinions, characteristics, and intentions, can be administered by telephone, mail, Internet, or in person.

21. A(n) _____ analysis involves undertaking a study using an existing dataset to answer new questions.

22. The type of research that focuses on improving research strategies is called _____ research.

B. MATCHING EXERCISES

1. Match each feature from Set B with one (or more) of the phrases from Set A that indicates a type of quantitative research. Indicate the letter(s) corresponding to your response next to each statement in Set B.

SET A

a. Clinical trial
b. Evaluation research
c. Survey research
d. Outcomes research

SET B   **RESPONSE**

1. Can involve an experimental design   _____
2. Examines the global effectiveness of nursing services   _____
3. Data are always from self-reports.   _____
4. Often designed in a series of phases (often four)   _____
5. Includes process analyses   _____
6. Donabedian's framework is often used in this research.   _____
7. May include an economic analysis   _____
8. Data from this can be used in a secondary analysis.   _____

C. STUDY QUESTIONS

1. Read one of the following open-access articles (a link is provided in the Internet Resources section on thePoint® website) describing a study in which quantitative data were gathered and analyzed to address a research question. Suggest ways in which the collection of qualitative data might have enriched the study, strengthened its validity, or enhanced its interpretability:

   • Lopes, A., & Nihei, O. (2020). Burnout among nursing students: Predictors and association with empathy and self-efficacy. *Revista Brasileira de Enfermagen, 73*, e20180280.

   • Wang, X., Liu, M., Li, Y., Guo, C., & Yeh, C. (2020). Community canteen services for the rural elderly: Determining impacts on general mental health, nutritional status, satisfaction with life, and social capital. *BMC Public Health, 20*, 230.

2. Read one of the following open-access articles (a link is provided in the Internet Resources section on thePoint® website) describing a study in which qualitative data were gathered and analyzed to address a research question. Suggest ways that the findings could be validated or the emergent hypotheses could be tested in a quantitative component:

   • Amponsah, A., Kyei, E., Agyemang, J., Boakye, H., Kyei-Dompim, J., Ahoto, C., & Oduro, E. (2020). Nursing-related barriers to children's pain management at selected hospitals in Ghana: A descriptive qualitative study. *Pain Research and Management, 2020*, 7125060.

   • Ghafoori, F., Dehghan-Nayeri, N., Khakbazan, Z., Hedayatnejad, M., & Nabavi, S. (2020). Pregnancy and motherhood concerns surrounding women with multiple sclerosis: A qualitative content analysis. *International Journal of Community Based Nursing and Midwifery, 8*, 2–11.

3. Identify a nursing-sensitive outcome. Propose a research question that would use the outcome as the dependent variable. Would you consider the research to address this question to be outcomes research?

4. Below is a brief description of a mixed methods study, followed by some critical comments. Do you agree with the comments? Can you add other critical appraisal comments regarding the study design?

FICTITIOUS STUDY

Aldrich conducted a study to examine the emotional well-being of women who had a mastectomy. Aldrich wanted to develop an in-depth understanding of the emotional experiences of women as they recovered from their surgery, including the process by which they handled their fears, their concerns about their sexuality, their levels of anxiety and depression, their methods of coping, and their social supports.

Aldrich's basic study design was a descriptive qualitative study. She gathered information from a sample of 26 women, primarily by means of in-depth interviews with the women on two occasions. The first interviews were scheduled within 1 month after the surgery. Follow-up interviews were conducted about 12 months later.

Several women in the sample participated in a support group, and Aldrich attended and made observations at several meetings. Additionally, Aldrich decided to interview the "significant other" (usually the husbands) of most of the women, when it became clear that the women's emotional well-being was linked to the manner in which the significant other reacted to the surgery.

In addition to the rich, in-depth information she gathered, Aldrich wanted to be able to better interpret the emotional status of the women. Therefore, at both the original and follow-up interview with the women, she administered a psychological scale known as the Center for Epidemiological Studies Depression Scale (CES-D), a quantitative measure with scores that can range from 0 to 60. This scale has been widely used in community populations and has cut-off scores designating when a person is at risk of clinical depression (i.e., a score of 16 and above).

Aldrich's qualitative analysis showed that the basic process underlying psychological recovery from the mastectomy was something she labeled "gaining by losing," a process that involved heightened self-awareness and self-respect after an initial period of despair and self-pity. The process also involved, for some, a strengthening of personal relationships with significant others, whereas for others, it resulted in the birth of awareness of fundamental deficiencies in their relationships. The quantitative findings confirmed that a very high percentage of women were at risk of being depressed at 1 month after the mastectomy, but at 12 months, the average level of depression was modestly lower than in the general population of women.

CRITICAL APPRAISAL COMMENTS
In her study, Aldrich embedded a quantitative measure into her fieldwork in an interesting manner. The bulk of data were qualitative—in-depth interviews and in-depth observations. However, she also opted to include a well-known measure of depressive symptoms, which provided her with an important context for interpreting her data. A major advantage of using the CES-D is that this scale has known characteristics in the general population and therefore provided a built-in "comparison group."

Aldrich used a flexible design that allowed her to use her initial data to guide her inquiry. For example, she decided to conduct in-depth interviews with significant others when she learned their importance to the women's process of emotional recovery. Aldrich did do some advance planning, however, that provided general guidance. For example, although her questioning likely evolved while in the field, she had the foresight to realize that to capture a process as it evolved, she would need to collect data longitudinally. She also made the up-front decision to use the CES-D to supplement the in-depth interviews.

In this study, the findings from the qualitative and quantitative portions of the study were complementary. Both portions of the study confirmed that the women initially had emotional "losses," but eventually, they recovered and "gained" in terms of their emotional well-being and their self-awareness. This example illustrates how the validity of study findings can be enhanced by the blending of qualitative and quantitative data. If the qualitative data alone had been gathered, Aldrich might not have gotten a good handle on the degree to which the women had actually "recovered" (*vis à vis* women who had never had a mastectomy). Conversely, if she had collected only the CES-D data, she would have had no insights into the process by which the recovery occurred.

D. APPLICATION EXERCISES

Exercise D.1: All Studies in Appendices

Which of the studies in the appendices of this *Study Guide* (if any) could be considered:
  a. A quality improvement project?
  b. A clinical trial?
  c. An economic analysis?
  d. Outcomes research?
  e. Survey research?
  f. A secondary analysis?
  g. Methodological research?

Exercise D.2: Study in Appendix D

Read the article by Eckhardt and colleagues ("Fatigue in the presence of coronary heart disease") in Appendix D on pages 143–153 and then answer the following questions:

Questions of Fact

  a. Was this a mixed methods study? If yes, what was the purpose of the quantitative strand, and what was the purpose of the qualitative strand?
  b. Which strand had priority in the study design?
  c. Was the design sequential or concurrent?
  d. Using the design names used in the textbook, what would the design be called?
  e. How would the design be portrayed using the notation system described in the textbook? Did the researchers themselves use this notation?
  f. What sampling design was used in this study?
  g. What did the report say about integrating the two strands?

Questions for Discussion

  a. Evaluate the use of a mixed methods approach in this study. Did the approach yield richer or more useful information than would have been achieved with a single-strand study?
  b. Discuss the researchers' choice of a specific research design and the sampling design. Would an alternative mixed methods design have been preferable? If so, why?

Exercise D.3: Study in Appendix F

Read the article by Hountz and colleagues ("Increasing colorectal cancer screening. . .") in Appendix F on pages 163–174 and then answer the following questions:

Questions of Fact

  a. What was the setting for this quality improvement (QI) project?
  b. What health care problem did the QI team decide to address?
  c. What were the goals of the project?

d. Was the QI project approved by an ethics review committee?
e. Did the team use a QI model described in the book? Did the project involve multiple cycles?
f. In planning the interventions to be tested, did the team perform a root cause analysis?
g. What type(s) of QI interventions did Hountz and colleagues implement?
h. Were the interventions evidence-based?
i. What is the basic research design for this study?
j. What were the outcome measures for this project?
k. Were any qualitative data collected?
l. Did the team conclude the interventions were successful?

Questions for Discussion

a. Comment on the team's use of staff input in this project.
b. Comment on the interventions that were implemented. Can you think of others that the team might have tested?
c. Did the team use the strongest possible study design? If not, what other designs might have strengthened the study's internal validity?
d. How would you rate the overall rigor of this project?
e. In what other types of setting might it be possible to use the findings from this study?

PART 4

Analysis, Interpretation, and Application of Nursing Research

CHAPTER 13

Understanding Statistical Analysis of Quantitative Data

A. FILL IN THE BLANKS

How many terms have you learned in this chapter? Fill in the blanks in the sentences below to find out.

1. The _____ level of measurement rank orders attributes but provides no information about distance between values.

2. A(n) _____-level measurement has a rational zero point.

3. The lowest level of measurement is _____ measurement, which places objects into mutually exclusive categories.

4. Psychological scales yield _____-level measures.

5. Variables measured on an interval or ratio scale are often referred to as _____ variables.

6. Distributions with a tail pointing to the left have a(n) _____ skew; those with a tail pointing to the right have a(n) _____ skew.

7. Distributions with a single high point are _____; those with two high points are _____.

8. A bell-shaped curve is a popular name for a(n) _____ distribution.

9. The most stable, and most frequently used, index of central tendency is known as the _____.

10. An index of central tendency that indicates the most "popular" value in a distribution is called the _____.

11. The most widely used index of variability is the _____ deviation.

12. The distributions for two nominal-level variables can be displayed in a(n) _____ table.

13. The _____ _____ is a widely used risk index that summarizes the ratio of two probabilities—the likelihood of occurrence versus nonoccurrence.

14. _____ statistics is the broad class of statistics used to draw conclusions about a population.

15. The criterion used to establish the risk of a Type I error is called _____.

16. A(n) _____ _____ error occurs when a true null hypothesis is incorrectly rejected.

73

Copyright © 2022. Wolters Kluwer.
Study Guide for Essentials of Nursing Research: Appraising Evidence of Nursing Practice, 10e

17. A(n) _____ _____ error is the error committed when a false null hypothesis is accepted.

18. A Type II error can occur when the analysis has insufficient _____, usually reflecting too small a sample.

19. The _____ of significance establishes the researcher's risk of making a Type I error.

20. The statistical test used to compare two group means is the _____-_____.

21. Researchers establish a(n) _____ interval around a statistic to indicate the range within which a population parameter probably lies.

22. The statistical test used to compare means of three or more group means is _____ _____ _____.

23. An effect size index called the _____ _____ captures the magnitude of difference between two group means.

24. The index most often used as a correlation coefficient is called _____ _____.

25. The statistic $r = .85$ indicates a strong, _____ relationship between two variables.

26. The _____ _____ test is used to test hypotheses about differences in proportions.

27. Multiple _____ analysis could be used to predict body weight, based on data about people's height, gender, and daily caloric intake.

28. In regression analysis, the independent variables are often called _____ variables.

29. The _____ of the multiple correlation coefficient (R) is an estimate of the proportion of variance in the outcome variable accounted for by the independent variables.

30. In ANCOVA, the confounding variable being statistically controlled is called a(n) _____.

31. _____ regression is a type of regression used to predict a nominal-level dependent variable from multiple predictors.

32. The index used to estimate internal consistency reliability is _____ _____.

33. The preferred index for assessing test–retest reliability is the _____ _____ coefficient.

34. Interrater reliability is evaluated using _____ _____ when the ratings are dichotomous (e.g., presence vs. absence of a disease).

35. A measure's ability to identify a case correctly is its _____.

B. MATCHING EXERCISES

1. Match each variable in Set B with the level of measurement from Set A that captures the highest possible level for that variable. Indicate the letter corresponding to your response next to each variable in Set B.

SET A

a. Nominal scale
b. Ordinal scale
c. Interval scale
d. Ratio scale

SET B   RESPONSES

   1. Hours spent in labor before childbirth   _____
   2. Religious affiliation   _____
   3. Time to first postoperative voiding   _____
   4. Responses to a single Likert scale item   _____
   5. Temperature on the centigrade scale   _____
   6. Nursing specialty area   _____
   7. Health status on the following scale: poor, fair, good, excellent   _____
   8. Pulse rate   _____
   9. Score on a 25-item Likert scale   _____
10. Highest college degree attained (bachelor's, master's, doctorate)   _____
11. Apgar scores   _____
12. Marital status   _____

2. Match each statement or phrase from Set B with one of the phrases from Set A. Indicate the letter corresponding to your response next to each of the statements in Set B.

SET A

a. Index(es) of central tendency
b. Index(es) of variability
c. Index(es) of neither central tendency nor variability
d. Index(es) of both central tendency and variability

SET B   RESPONSES

   1. The range   _____
   2. In lay terms, an average   _____
   3. A percentage   _____
   4. Descriptor(s) of a distribution of scores   _____
   5. Descriptor(s) of how heterogeneous a set of values is   _____
   6. The standard deviation   _____

7. The mode   _____
8. The median   _____
9. A normal distribution   _____
10. The mean   _____

C. STUDY QUESTIONS

1. Prepare a frequency distribution and frequency polygon for the set of scores below, which represent the ages of 30 women receiving a mammogram:

   47 50 51 50 48 51 50 51 49 51

   54 49 49 53 51 52 51 52 50 53

   49 51 52 51 50 55 48 54 53 52

   Describe the resulting distribution in terms of its symmetry and modality (i.e., whether it is unimodal or multimodal). What is the mode?

2. Calculate the mean, median, and mode for the following pulse rates:

   78 84 69 98 102 72 87 75 79 84 88 84 83 71 73

   Mean:_____ Median:_____ Mode:_____

3. Suppose a researcher has conducted a study concerning lactose intolerance in children. The data reveal that 12 boys and 16 girls have lactose intolerance, out of a sample of 120 children (60 of each gender). Construct a crosstabs table and calculate the column percentages for each cell in the table, with gender listed in the columns (similar to Table 13.8 in the textbook). Discuss the meaning of these statistics. What test would we need to use to test the significance of group differences?

4. Below is a correlation matrix based on real data from a study of 997 low-income mothers. Answer the following questions with respect to this matrix:
   a. What is the correlation between body mass index (BMI) and scores on the physical functioning subscale?
   b. Is the correlation between physical functioning and mental health scores significant at conventional levels?
   c. With which variable(s) is BMI related at the .01 level of significance?
   d. Explain what the correlation between the physical functioning scores and number of doctor visits means.

VARIABLE	1	2	3	4
1 Number of doctor visits	1.00			
2 Body mass index (BMI)	.13**	1.00		
3 Physical functioning	−.32**	−.13**	1.00	
4 Mental health score	−.13**	−.08*	.17**	1.00

$*p < .05.$ $**p < .01$

5. Indicate which statistical tests you would use to analyze data for the following variables:
   a. Variable 1 is psychiatric patients' gender; variable 2 is whether or not the patient has attempted suicide in the past 6 months.
   b. Variable 1 is the participation versus nonparticipation of patients with a pulmonary embolus in a special intervention group; variable 2 is the pH of the patients' arterial blood gases.
   c. Variable 1 is serum creatinine concentration levels; variable 2 is daily urine output.
   d. Variable 1 is patients' marital status (married vs. divorced/separated/ widowed vs. never married); variable 2 is the patients' degree of self-reported depression (measured on a 20-item depression scale).

6. In the following examples, which multivariate procedure is most appropriate for analyzing the data?
   a. A researcher is testing the relationship between self-esteem, age, and the availability of family supports among a group of recently discharged psychiatric patients on the one hand and recidivism (i.e., whether or not they will be readmitted within 12 months after discharge) on the other.
   b. A researcher is comparing daily hours of sleep of recently widowed versus divorced individuals, controlling for their age and years of marriage.
   c. A researcher wants to predict hospital staff absentee rates (number of days absent per year) based on salary, shift, number of years with the hospital, and number of children.

7. Below is a list of variables. Assume that you have data from 500 nurses on these variables. Develop two or three hypotheses regarding the relationships among these variables and indicate which statistical tests you would use to test your hypotheses.

   • Number of years of nursing experience

   • Type of employment setting (hospital, nursing home, public school system, other)

   • Annual salary

   • Job satisfaction (as measured on a 10-item Likert-type scale)

   • Number of children under 18 years of age

   • Gender

   • Type of nursing preparation (associate's, bachelor's)

D. APPLICATION EXERCISES

Exercise D.1: Studies in Appendices A, C, D, and F

Which of the studies in Appendix A (Stephens et al.), Appendix C (Saqe-Rockoff et al.), Appendix D (Eckhardt et al.), and Appendix F (Hountz et al.) reported the following descriptive statistics:
  a. Percentages?
  b. Means and standard deviations?
  c. Medians?
  d. Mode?

Exercise D.2: Studies in Appendices A, C, and D

Which of the studies in Appendix A (Stephens et al.), Appendix C (Saqe-Rockoff et al.), and Appendix D (Eckhardt et al.) reported the following bivariate inferential statistics?
  a. *t*-Test
  b. Chi-squared test
  c. Pearson's *r*

Exercise D.3: Study in Appendix D

Read the Results section of the article by Eckhardt and colleagues ("Fatigue in the presence of coronary heart disease") in Appendix D. Then, answer the following questions:

Questions of Fact

  a. Referring to Table 1, answer the following questions:

  - Which variables described in the tables, if any, was measured as a nominal-level variable?

  - Which variables described in the tables, if any, was measured as an ordinal-level variable?

  - Which variables described in the tables, if any, was measured as an interval-level variable?

  - Which variables described in the tables, if any, was measured as a ratio-level variable?

  - State in one sentence what the "typical" participant was like demographically.

  - What percentage of the *total* sample had a graduate degree?

  b. Referring to Table 2, answer the following questions:

  - With which variables were fatigue intensity scores correlated at statistically significant levels?

  - Were better educated people *more likely* or *less likely* to have high fatigue intensity?

  - Were men or women more likely to have high scores on fatigue interference?

  c. Which multivariate statistical analysis did the researchers use in this study?
  d. Did the researchers report any values for R^2?

Questions for Discussion

a. Evaluate the statistical tests used in this research. Were the tests appropriate, given the level of measurement of the research variables? Should other statistics have been used as an alternative or as a supplement?

b. Some of the researchers' statistical results were nonsignificant. Is it possible that the study was underpowered (i.e., that a Type II error was committed)? Did the researchers undertake a power analysis?

c. Comment on the adequacy of the statistical tables. Were they easy to understand? Did they communicate important information effectively?

14 CHAPTER

Interpreting Quantitative Findings and Evaluating Clinical Significance

A. FILL IN THE BLANKS

How many terms have you learned in this chapter? Fill in the blanks in the sentences below to find out.

1. Both researchers and consumers of quantitative research must develop a(n) _____ of the accuracy, meaning, and importance of the study results.

2. A famous research precept is that _____ does not prove that one variable caused another.

3. _____ size estimates such as *d* help to better understand the importance of the results.

4. The _____ guidelines for preparing research reports include a flow chart documenting participant flow in a study.

5. Researchers should take both the strengths and the _____ of their study into account when interpreting their findings.

6. A research _____ that is actually null is difficult to evaluate through standard statistical methods.

7. An important aspect of interpretation for clinical decision making is the degree of _____ of results, usually communicated through confidence intervals (CIs).

8. Researchers' interpretations are presented in the _____ section of a report.

9. Results that are non_____ are especially difficult to interpret because of the possibility of a Type II error.

10. The _____ significance of research results is their importance to patients' daily lives or to health care decision making.

11. A widely used benchmark for clinical significance at the individual level is the _____ _____ _____.

12. Individuals' change scores in different groups can be classified as exceeding or not exceeding the MIC threshold and then compared in a(n) _____ analysis.

80

B. MATCHING EXERCISES

Match each statement or phrase from Set B with one or more of the phrases from Set A. Indicate the letter(s) corresponding to your response next to each of the statements in Set B.

SET A

a. Credibility of results
b. Precision of results
c. Magnitude of effects and importance
d. Generalizability of results
e. Implications of results

SET B   RESPONSE

1. Confidence intervals provide information about this.   _____

2. An analysis of threats to study validity is a way to
   explore this.   _____

3. A consideration of how study limitations could be
   corrected in subsequent research is part of this.   _____

4. In assessing this, consideration is given to the
   characteristics of the study sample and the research
   setting and to any sampling biases.   _____

5. Effect size information can be especially useful for
   considering this.   _____

6. An analysis of the success of the researcher's "proxies"
   is an approach to this.   _____

7. Biases can reduce this.   _____

8. Statements about the utility of findings for clinical
   practice are part of this.   _____

C. STUDY QUESTIONS

1. Read one of the following open-access articles (a link is provided in the Internet Resources on thePoint˚) and evaluate the extent to which the researchers assessed and considered possible biases and commented on them in their discussions.

   • Alharbi, M. (2019). Influence of individual and family factors on physical activity among Saudi girls: A cross-sectional study. *Annals of Saudi Medicine, 39*, 13–21.

   • Bennetts, S., Hokke, S., Crawford, S., Hackworth, N., Leach, L. Nguyen, C., . . . Cooklin, A. (2019). Using paid and free Facebook methods to recruit Australian parents to an online survey: An evaluation. *Journal of Medical Internet Research, 21*, e11206.

- Öhlin, J., Ahlgren, A., Folkesson, R., Gustafson, Y., Littbrand, H., Olofsson, B. & Toots, A. (2020). The association between cognition and gait in a representative sample of very old people—The influence of dementia and walking aid use. *BMC Geriatrics, 20*, 34.

2. In the following open-access research article (a link is provided on thePoint®), a team of researchers reported that they obtained some nonsignificant results that were not consistent with expectations. Review and appraise the researchers' interpretation of the findings and suggest some possible alternatives:

   - Szanton, S., Xue, Q., Leff, B., Guralnik, J., Wolff, J., Tanner, E., . . . Gitlin, L. (2019). Effect of a biobehavioral environmental approach on disability among low-income older adults: A randomized clinical trial. *JAMA Internal Medicine, 179*, 204–211.

3. Skim one of the following articles, the titles for which imply a causal connection between phenomena. Do you think a causal inference is warranted? Why or why not?

   - Albdour, M., Hong, J., Lewin, L., & Yarandi, H. (2019). The impact of cyberbullying on physical and psychological health of Arab American adolescents. *Journal of Immigrant and Minority Health, 21*, 706–715.

   - Gasior, S., Forchuk, C., & Regan, S. (2018). Youth homelessness: The impact of supportive relationships on recovery. *The Canadian Journal of Nursing Research, 50*, 28–36.

   - *Jeon, G., Choi, K., & Cho, S. (2017). Impact of living alone on depressive symptoms in older Korean widows. *International Journal of Environmental Research & Public Health, 14*(10), E1191.

   - *Lambert, S., Bowe, S., Livingston, P., Heckel, L., Cook, S., Kowal, P., & Orellana, L. (2017). Impact of informal caregiving on older adults' physical and mental health in low-income and middle-income countries: A cross-sectional, secondary analysis based on the WHO's Study on global AGEing and adult health (SAGE). *BMJ Open, 7*(11), e017236.

4. Following is a fictitious research report and a critical appraisal of various aspects of it. This example is designed to highlight features about the form and content of both a written report and a written evaluation of the study's worth. To economize on space, the report is brief, but it incorporates essential elements for a meaningful appraisal. Read the report and appraisal and then determine whether you agree with the critique. Can you add other comments relevant to a critical appraisal of the study?

THE REPORT
The Role of Health Care Providers in Teenage Pregnancy by Dana Clinton (2021)

Background. Of the 20 million teenagers living in the United States, about one in four is sexually active by age 14 years; more than half have had sexual intercourse

---

by age 17 years (Kelman & Saner, 2011).* Despite increased availability of contraceptives, the number of teenage pregnancies has remained fairly stable over the past two decades. About 1 million girls under age 20 years become pregnant each year and, of these, about 500,000 become teenage mothers (U.S. Bureau of the Census, 2014).

Public concern regarding teenage pregnancy stems not only from the high rates but also from the extensive research that has documented the adverse consequences of early parenthood in the health arena. Pregnant teenagers have been found to receive less prenatal care (Tremain, 2010), to be more likely to develop toxemia (Schendley, 2012; Waters, 2014), to be more likely to experience prolonged labor (Curran, 1999), to be more likely to have low-birth-weight babies (Beach, 2014; Tremain, 2009), and to be more likely to have babies with low Apgar scores (Beach, 2014) than older women. The long-term consequences to the teenage mothers themselves are also bleak: Teenage mothers get less schooling, are more likely to be on public assistance, are likely to earn lower wages, and are more likely to get divorced if they marry than women who postpone parenthood (Jamail, 2009; North, 2012; Smithfield, 2008).

The 1 million teenagers who become pregnant each year have a difficult emotional decision—to carry the pregnancy to term and keep the baby, to have an abortion, or to deliver the baby and surrender it for adoption. Despite the widely reported adverse consequences of young parenthood cited above, most young women today are opting for delivery and child-rearing, often out of wedlock (Henderson, 2011; Jaffrey, 2009). Relatively few young mothers in recent years have been relinquishing their babies for adoption, forcing many couples with fertility problems to seek adoption options overseas (Smith, 2016).

The purpose of this study was to test the effect of a special intervention based in an outpatient clinic of a Chicago hospital on improving the health outcomes of a group of pregnant teenagers. Specifically, it was hypothesized that pregnant teenagers who were in the special program would receive more prenatal care, be less likely to develop toxemia, be less likely to have a low-birth-weight baby, spend fewer hours in labor, have babies with higher Apgar scores, and be more likely to use a contraceptive at 6 months postpartum than pregnant teenagers not enrolled in the program.

The theoretical model on which this research was based is an ecological model of personal behavior (Brandenburg, 1984). A schematic diagram of the ecological model is presented in Figure A. In this framework, the actions of the person are the focus of attention, but those actions are believed to be a function not only of the person's own characteristics, attitudes, and abilities but also of other influences in their environment. Environmental influences can be differentiated according to their proximal relationship with the target person. Health care workers and institutions are, according to the model, more distant influences than family, peers, and boyfriends. Yet, it is assumed that these less immediate forces are real and can intervene to change the behaviors of the target person. Thus, it is hypothesized that pregnant teenagers can be influenced by increased exposure to a health care team providing a structured program of services designed to promote improved health outcomes.

Method. A special program of services for pregnant teenagers was implemented in the outpatient clinic of an inner-city public hospital in Chicago. The intervention involved 8 weeks of nutrition education and counseling, parenting education, instruction on prenatal health care, preparation for childbirth, and contraceptive counseling.

---

*All references in this example are fictitious.

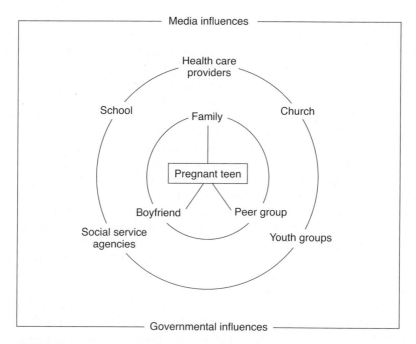

FIGURE A Model of ecological contexts.

All teenagers with a confirmed pregnancy attending the clinic were asked if they wanted to participate in the special program. The goal was to enroll 150 pregnant teenagers during the program's first year of operation. A total of 276 teenagers attending the clinic were invited to participate; of these, 59 had an abortion or miscarriage, and 108 declined to participate, yielding an experimental group sample of 109 girls.

To test the effectiveness of the special program, a comparison group of pregnant teenagers was needed. Another inner-city hospital agreed to cooperate in the study. Staff obtained information on the labor and delivery outcomes of the 120 teenagers who delivered at the comparison hospital, where no special teen-parent program was available. For both experimental group and comparison group subjects, a follow-up telephone interview was conducted 6 months postpartum to determine if the teenagers were using birth control.

The outcome variables in this study were the teenagers' labor and delivery and postpartum outcomes and their contraceptive behavior. Operational definitions of these variables are as follows:

Prenatal care: Number of visits made to a physician or nurse-midwife during the pregnancy, exclusive of the visit for the pregnancy test

Toxemia: Presence versus absence of preeclamptic toxemia as diagnosed by a physician or nurse-midwife

Labor time: Number of hours elapsed from the first contractions until birth of the baby, to the nearest half hour

Low infant birth weight: Infant birth weights of less than 2,500 g versus those of 2,500 g or greater

Apgar score: The summary rating (from 0 to 10) of the health of the infant, taken at 1 minute after birth

Contraceptive use postpartum: Self-reported use of any form of birth control 6 months postpartum versus self-reported nonuse

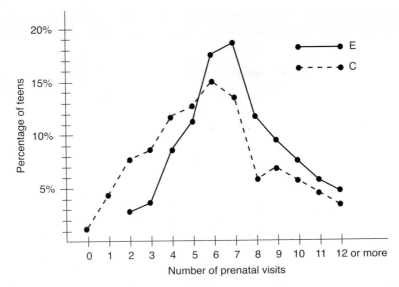

FIGURE B   Frequency distribution of prenatal visits, by experimental versus comparison group. E, experimental group; C, comparison group.

The two groups were compared on these six outcome measures using *t*-tests and chi-squared tests.

Results. The teenagers in the sample were, on average, 17.6 years old at the time of delivery. The mean age was 17.0 in the experimental group and 18.1 in the comparison group (*p* < .05).

By definition, all the teenagers in the experimental group had received prenatal care. Two of the teenagers in the comparison group had no health care treatment before delivery. The distribution of visits for the two groups is presented in Figure B. The experimental group had a higher mean number of prenatal visits than the comparison group, as shown in Table A, but the difference was not statistically significant at the .05 level, using a *t*-test for independent groups.

In the sample as a whole, about 1 girl in 10 was diagnosed as having preeclamptic toxemia. The difference between the two groups was in the hypothesized direction, with 1.6% more of the comparison group teenagers developing this complication, but the difference was not significant.

The hours spent in labor ranged from 3.5 to 29.0 in the experimental group and from 4.5 to 33.5 in the comparison group. On average, teenagers in the experimental group spent 14.3 hours in labor, compared with 15.2 for the comparison group teenagers. The difference was not statistically significant.

With regard to low-birth-weight babies, a total of 43 girls out of 229 in the sample gave birth to babies who weighed less than 2,500 g (5.5 pounds).[†] More of the comparison group teenagers (20.9%) than experimental group teenagers (16.5%) had low-birth-weight babies, but, once again, the group difference was not significant.

The 1-minute Apgar score in the two groups was similar—7.3 for the experimental group and 6.7 for the comparison group. This difference was nonsignificant.

[†]All mothers gave birth to live infants; however, there were two neonatal deaths within 24 hours of birth in the comparison group.

TABLE A   Summary of Experimental and Comparison Group Differences

| | Group | | | |
| | Experimental | Comparison | | |
Outcome Variable	(n = 109)	(n = 120)	Difference	Test Statistic
Mean number of prenatal visits	7.1	5.9	1.2	t = 1.83, df = 227, NS
Percentage with toxemia	10.1	11.7	−1.6	χ^2 = 0.15, df = 1, NS
Mean hours spent in labor	14.3	15.2	−.09	t = 1.01, df = 227, NS
Percentage with low-birth-weight baby	16.5	20.9	−4.4	χ^2 = 0.71, df = 1, NS
Mean Apgar score	7.3	6.7	.6	t = 0.98, df = 227, NS
Percentage adopting contraception postpartum	81.7	62.5	19.2	χ^2 = 10.22, df = 1, p < .01

Finally, the teenagers were compared with respect to their use of birth control 6 months after giving birth to their babies. For this variable, teenagers were coded as users of contraception if they were either using some method of birth control at the time of the follow-up interview or if they were nonusers but were sexually inactive (i.e., were using abstinence to prevent a repeat pregnancy). The results of the chi-squared test revealed that a significantly higher percentage of experimental group teenagers (81.7%) than comparison group teenagers (62.5%) reported using birth control after delivery. This difference was significant beyond the .01 level.

Discussion. The results of this evaluation were disappointing but not discouraging. There was only one outcome for which a significant difference was observed. The experimental program significantly increased the percentage of teenagers who used birth control after giving birth. Thus, one highly important result of participating in the program is that an early repeat pregnancy will be postponed. There is abundant research that has shown that repeat pregnancy among teenagers is especially damaging to their educational and occupational attainment and leads to particularly adverse labor and delivery outcomes in the higher order births (Jackson, 2007; Klugman, 2002).

The experimental group had more prenatal care but not significantly more. Perhaps part of the difficulty is that the program can only begin to deliver services once pregnancy has been diagnosed. If a teenager does not come in for a pregnancy test until her fourth or fifth month, this puts an upper limit on the number of visits she will have; it also gives less time for her to eat properly, avoid smoking and drinking, and take other steps to enhance her health during pregnancy. Thus, one implication of this finding is that the program needs to do more to encourage early pregnancy screening. Perhaps a joint effort between the clinic personnel and school nurses in neighboring middle schools and high schools could be launched to publicize the need for a timely pregnancy test and to inform teenagers where such a test could be obtained. The two groups performed similarly with respect to the various labor and delivery outcomes chosen to evaluate the effectiveness of the new program. The issue of timeliness is again relevant here. The program may have been delivering services too late in the pregnancy for the instruction to have made much of an impact on the health of the mother and her child. This interpretation is supported, in part, by the fact that the one variable for which timeliness was *not* an issue (postpartum contraception) was positively affected by program participation. Another possible implication is that the program itself should be made more powerful, for example, by lengthening or adding to instructional sessions.

Given that the experimental and comparison group differences were all in the hypothesized direction, it is also tempting to criticize the study's sample size. A larger sample (which was originally planned) might have yielded some significant differences.

In summary, the experimental intervention is not without promise. A particularly exciting finding is that participation in the program resulted in better contraceptive use, which will presumably lower the incidence of repeat pregnancy. It would be interesting to follow these teenagers 2 years after delivery to see if the groups differ in the rates of repeat pregnancy. It appears that more needs to be done to get these teenagers into the program early in their pregnancies. Perhaps then the true effectiveness of the program would be demonstrated.

CRITICAL APPRAISAL OF THE RESEARCH REPORT

In the following critique, we present some comments on various aspects of this research report. You are urged to read the report and form your own opinion about its strengths and weaknesses before reading our appraisal. An evaluation of a study is necessarily partly subjective. Therefore, you might disagree with some of the points made below, and you might have additional criticisms and comments. We believe, however, that most of the serious methodological flaws of the study are highlighted in our critical appraisal.

Title. The title for the study is misleading. The research does *not* investigate the role of health care professionals in serving the needs of pregnant teenagers. A more appropriate title would be "Effects of an Educational Intervention for Pregnant Teenagers on Health-Related Outcomes."

Background. The background section of this report consists of three distinct elements that can be analyzed separately: a literature review, statement of the problem, and a theoretical framework.

The literature review is relatively clearly written and well organized. It serves the function of establishing a need for an intervention by documenting the prevalence of teenage pregnancy and some of its adverse consequences. However, the literature review could be improved. First, an inspection of the citations suggests that the author is likely not up-to-date on research relating to teenage pregnancy. Most of the references date before 2015, and so the review might be different if more recent studies were cited. Second, there is material in the literature review section that is not relevant and should be removed. For example, the paragraph on the options with which a pregnant teenager is faced (paragraph 3) is not germane to the research problem. A third and more critical flaw is what the review did *not* cover. Given the research problem, there are probably four main points that should be addressed in the review:

1. How widespread is teenage pregnancy and parenthood?
2. What are the social and health consequences of early childbearing?
3. What has been done by health care researchers to address the problems associated with teenage parenthood?
4. How successful have other interventions been?

The review adequately handles the first question: The need for concern is established. The second question is covered in the review, but perhaps more depth and more recent research is needed here. The new study is based on an assumption of negative health outcomes in teenage mothers. The author has strung together a series of references without giving the reader any clues about the reliability of the information. The author would have been more convincing by adding a sentence such as "For example, in a carefully executed prospective study involving nearly 4,000 pregnant women, Beach (2014) found that young maternal age was significantly associated with higher rates of prematurity and other negative neonatal outcomes." The third and fourth points that should have been covered are totally absent from the review. Surely, the author's intervention does not represent the first attempt to address the needs of pregnant teenagers. How is Clinton's intervention different from or better than other interventions? What reason is there to believe that such an intervention might be successful? Clinton has provided a rationale for addressing the problem but no justification for the manner in which it was addressed. If, in fact, there is little information about other interventions and their effectiveness in improving health outcomes, then the review should say so.

The problem statement and hypothesis were stated succinctly and clearly. The hypothesis is complex (there are multiple dependent variables) and directional (it predicts better outcomes among teenagers participating in the special program).

The third component of the background section of the report is the theoretical framework. In our opinion, the theoretical framework chosen does little to enhance the research. The hypothesis is not generated on the basis of the model, or does the intervention itself grow out of the model. One gets the feeling that the model might have been slapped on as an afterthought to try to make the study seem more theoretical. Actually, if more thought had been given to this conceptual framework, it might have proved useful. According to this model, the most immediate and direct influences on a pregnant teenager are her family, friends, and sexual partner. One programmatic implication of this is that the intervention should involve one or more of these influences. For example, a workshop for the teenagers' parents could have been developed to reinforce the teenagers' need for adequate nutrition and prenatal care. A research hypothesis that could have been tested in the context of the model is that teenagers who are missing one of the direct influences would be especially susceptible to the influence of less proximal health care providers (i.e., the program). For example, it might be hypothesized that pregnant teenagers who do not live with both parents have to depend on alternative sources of social support (such as health care personnel) during the pregnancy. Thus, it is not that the theoretical context selected is far-fetched but rather that it was not convincingly linked to the actual research problem.

Method. The design used to test the research hypothesis was a quasi-experimental design. Two groups, whose equivalence is assumed but not established, were compared on several outcome measures. The design is one that has serious problems because the preintervention comparability of the groups is unknown.

The most serious threat to the internal validity of the study is selection bias. Selection bias can work both ways—either to mask true treatment effects or to create the illusion of a program effect when none exists. This is because selection bias can be either positive (i.e., the experimental group can be initially advantaged in relation to the comparison group) or negative (i.e., the experimental group can have pretreatment disadvantages). In the present study, it is possible that the two hospitals served clients of different economic circumstances, for example. If the average income of the families of the experimental group teenagers was higher, then these teenagers would probably have a better opportunity for adequate prenatal nutrition than the comparison group teenagers. Or the comparison hospital might serve older teens, or a higher percentage of married teens, or a higher percentage of teens attending a special school-based program for pregnant students. None of these confounding variables, which could affect the mother's health outcomes, has been controlled.

Another way in which the design was vulnerable to selection bias is the high refusal rate in the experimental group. Of the 217 eligible teenagers, half declined to participate in the special program. We cannot assume that the 109 girls who participated were a random sample of the eligible girls. Again, biases could be either positive or negative. A positive selection bias would be created if, for example, the teenagers who were the most motivated to have a healthy pregnancy selected themselves into the intervention group. A negative selection bias would result if the teenagers from the most disadvantaged households or from families offering little support elected to participate in the program.

The researcher could have taken a number of steps to either control selection biases or, at the least, estimate their direction and magnitude. The following are among the most critical confounding variables: social class and family income, age, race and ethnicity, parity, participation in another pregnant teenager program, marital status, and prepregnancy experience with contraception (for the postpartum contraception outcome). The researcher should have attempted to gather information on these variables from experimental group and comparison group teenagers and from eligible teenagers in the experimental hospital who declined to participate in the program. To the extent that these groups were similar on these variables, the internal validity of the study, and thus the credibility of the results, would be enhanced. If sizable differences were observed, the researcher would at least know or suspect the direction of the biases and could factor that information into the interpretation and conclusions.

Had the researcher gathered information on the confounding variables, another possibility would have been to match experimental and comparison group subjects on one or two variables, such as family income and age. Matching is not an ideal method of controlling confounding variables; for one thing, matching on two variables would not equate the two groups in terms of the other confounding variables. However, matching is preferable to doing nothing to control extraneous variation.

So far we have focused our attention on the research design, but other aspects of the study are also problematic. Let us consider the decision the researcher made about the population. The target population is not explicitly defined by the researcher, but we can infer that the target population is pregnant young women younger than 20 years who carry their infants to delivery. The accessible population is pregnant teenagers from one area in Chicago. It cannot reasonably be assumed that the accessible population is representative of the target population. It is likely that the accessible population is quite different with regard to health care, family intactness, and many other characteristics. The researcher should have more clearly discussed who the target population of this research was.

Clinton would have done well, in fact, to delimit the target population; had this been done, it might have been possible to control some of the confounding variables discussed previously. For example, Clinton could have established eligibility criteria that excluded multigravidas, very young teenagers (e.g., younger than 15 years), or married teenagers. Such a specification would have limited the generalizability of the findings, but it would have enhanced the internal validity of the study because it probably would have increased the comparability of the experimental and comparison groups.

The sample was a sample of convenience, the least effective sampling design for a quantitative study. There is no way of knowing whether the sample represents the accessible and target populations. Although probability sampling likely was not feasible,

5

the researcher might have improved the sampling design by using a quota sampling plan. For example, if the researcher knew that in the accessible population, half of the families received public assistance, then it might have been possible to enhance the representativeness of the samples by using a quota system to ensure that half of the research subjects came from welfare-dependent families.

Sample size is a difficult issue. Many of the reported results were in the hypothesized direction but were nonsignificant. When this is the case, the adequacy of the sample size is always suspect, as Clinton pointed out. Each group had about 100 participants. In many cases, this sample size would be considered adequate, but in the present case, it is not. One of the difficulties in testing the effectiveness of new interventions is that, generally, the experimental group is not being compared with a no-treatment group. Although the comparison group in this example was not getting the special program services, it cannot be assumed that this group was getting no services at all. Some comparison group members may have had ample prenatal care during which the health care staff may have provided much of the same information as was taught in the special program. The point is not that the new program was not needed but rather that unless an intervention is extremely powerful and innovative, the incremental improvement will typically be small. When relatively small effects are anticipated, the sample must be large for differences to be statistically significant. Indeed, power analysis can be performed using the study findings. For example, a power analysis indicates that to detect a significant difference between the two groups with respect one outcome—the incidence of toxemia—a sample of over 5,000 pregnant teenagers would have been needed. A power analysis performed before conducting the study might have alerted the researcher to the insufficiency of the sample for some of the outcomes.

The third major methodological decision concerns the measurement of the research variables. For the most part, the researcher did a good job in selecting objective, reliable, and valid outcome measures. Also, the operational definitions were clearly worded and unambiguous. Two comments are in order, however. First, it might have been better to operationalize two of the variables differently. Infant birth weight might have been more sensitively measured as actual weight (a ratio-level measurement) instead of as a dichotomous variable. The contraceptive variable could also have been operationalized to yield a more sensitive (i.e., more discriminating) measure. For example, rather than measuring contraceptive use as a dichotomy, Clinton could have measured frequency of using contraception (e.g., never, sometimes, usually, or always), effectiveness of the *type* of birth control used, or a combination of these two.

A second consideration is whether the outcome variables adequately captured the effects of program activities. It would have been more directly relevant to the intervention to capture group differences in, say, dietary practices during pregnancy than in infant birth weight. None of the outcome variables measured the effects of parenting education. In other words, Clinton could have added more direct measures of the effectiveness of the intervention.

One other point about the methods should be made and that relates to ethical considerations. The article does not specifically say that participants were asked for their informed consent, but that does not necessarily mean that no written consent was obtained. It is quite likely that the experimental group subjects, when asked to volunteer for the special program, were asked to sign a consent form. But what about the control group subjects? The article implies that comparison group members were given no opportunity to decline participation and were not aware of having their birth outcomes used as data in the research. In some cases, this procedure is acceptable. For example, a hospital or clinic might agree to release patient information without the patients' consent if the release of such information is done anonymously—that is, if it can be provided in such a way that even the researcher does not know the identity of the patients. In the present study, however, it is clear that the names of the comparison subjects were provided since the researcher had to contact the comparison group at 6 months postpartum to determine their contraceptive practices. Thus, this study does not appear to have adequately safeguarded the rights of the comparison group subjects.

In summary, the researcher appears not to have given the new program a particularly fair test. Clinton should have taken a number of steps to control confounding variables and should have measured more proximal outcomes. Attempts should have been made to enlist a larger sample, even if this meant waiting for additional subjects to enroll in the program.

Results. Clinton did an adequate job of presenting the results of the study. The presentation was straightforward and succinct and was enhanced by the inclusion of a good table and figures. The style of this section was also appropriate: It was written objectively and was well organized.

The statistical analyses were also adequate. The descriptive statistics (means and percentages) were appropriate for the level of measurement of the variables. The two types of inferential statistics used (the *t*-test and chi-squared test) were also appropriate, given the levels of measurement of the outcome variables. The results of these tests were efficiently presented in a single table. Of course, more powerful statistics could have been used to control confounding variables (e.g., analysis of covariance). It appears, however, that the only confounding variable that could have been controlled statistically was the participants' age; no data were apparently collected on other confounding variables (social class, ethnicity, parity, and so on).

Discussion. Clinton's discussion section fails almost entirely to take the study's limitations into account in interpreting the data. The one exception is the acknowledgment that the sample size was too small. There seems to be little concern about the many threats to the internal or external validity of the research.

Clinton lays almost all the blame for the nonsignificant findings on the program rather than on the research methods. The researcher suggests that two aspects of the program should be changed: (1) recruitment of teenagers into the program earlier in their pregnancies and (2) strengthening program services. Both recommendations might be worth pursuing, but there is little in the data to suggest these modifications. With nonsignificant results such as those that predominated in this study, there are two possibilities to consider: (1) The results are accurate—that is, the program is not effective for those outcomes examined (although it might be effective for other outcomes), and (2) the results are false—that is, the existing program is effective for the outcomes examined, but the tests failed to demonstrate it. Clinton concluded that the first possibility was correct and therefore recommended that the program be changed. Equally plausible is the possibility that the study methods were too weak to demonstrate the program's true effects.

We do not have enough information about the characteristics of the sample to conclude with certainty that there were substantial selection biases. We do, however, have a clue that selection biases were operative in a direction that would make the program look less effective than it actually is. Clinton noted in the beginning of the results section that the average age of the teenagers in the experimental group was 17.0, compared with 18.1 in the comparison group—a difference that was significant. Age is inversely related to positive labor and delivery outcomes, indeed, that is the basis for having a special program for teenage mothers. Therefore, the experimental group's performance on the outcome measures was possibly depressed by the younger age of that group. Had the two groups been equivalent in terms of age, group differences on the outcomes might have been larger and could have reached levels of statistical significance. Other uncontrolled pretreatment differences could also have masked true treatment effects.

For the one significant outcome, we cannot rule out the possibility that a Type I error was made—that is, that the null hypothesis was in fact true. Selection biases also could have been operative for this outcome. The experimental group might have contained many more girls who had preprogram experience with contraception; it might have contained more highly motivated teenagers, or more teenagers who already had multiple pregnancies than the comparison group. There simply is no way of knowing whether the significant outcome reflects true program effects or merely group differences on confounders that influence the outcome.

Aside from disregard for the problems of internal validity, Clinton overstepped the bounds of scholarly speculation. It was assumed that the program *caused* contraceptive improvements: "The experimental program significantly increased the percentage of teenagers who used birth control. . . ." Worse yet, Clinton went on to conclude that repeat pregnancies will be postponed in the experimental group, although there is no information on whether the teenagers used an effective contraception, whether they used it all the time, or whether they used it correctly.

As another example of going beyond the data, Clinton became overly invested in the notion that teenagers need greater and earlier exposure to the program. It is not that the hypothesis has no merit—the problem is that the researcher built an elaborate rationale for program changes with no apparent empirical support. Clinton probably had information on when in the pregnancy the teenagers entered the program, but that information was not shared with readers. The argument about the need for more publicity on early screening would have had more clout if the researcher had reported that most teenagers entered the program during the fourth month of their pregnancies or later. Additionally, more evidence in support of the proposal could have been marshalled by demonstrating that earlier entry into the program was associated with better health outcomes. For example, Clinton could have compared the outcomes of teenagers entering the program in the first, second, and third trimesters of their pregnancies.

In conclusion, the study has several positive features. As the researcher noted, there is some reason to be cautiously optimistic that the program *could* have some beneficial effects. However, the existing study is too flawed to reach any conclusions, even tentatively. A replication with improved research methods is needed.

D. APPLICATION EXERCISES

Exercise D.1: Study in Appendix A

Read the Results, and Discussion sections of the report by Stephens and colleagues ("Smartphone technology and text messaging for weight loss in young adults") in Appendix A on pages 115–122 and then answer the following questions:

Questions of Fact

a. Was a CONSORT-type flow chart included in this report? If yes, what did it show?
b. Did the researchers provide evidence about the success of randomization—i.e., whether those in the intervention and control groups were equivalent at the outset and, thus, selection biases were absent?

c. Did the researchers report an analysis of attrition biases? Was attrition taken into account in the analysis of group differences on the outcomes?

d. With regard to the primary aim of the study, to compare intervention and control group outcomes on weight-related outcomes following the smartphone intervention, were hypotheses supported, not supported, or mixed?

e. Did the report provide information about the precision of results via confidence intervals?

f. Did the report provide information about magnitude of effects via calculation of effect sizes?

g. In the Discussion section, was there any explicit discussion about the study's internal validity?

h. In the Discussion section, was there any explicit discussion about the study's external validity (generalizability)?

i. In the Discussion section, was there any explicit discussion about the study's statistical conclusion validity?

j. Did the Discussion section link study findings to findings from prior research—i.e., did the authors place their findings into a broader context?

k. Were any study limitations identified in the Discussion section?

l. Did the researchers explicitly comment on the clinical significance of the findings?

Questions for Discussion

a. Do you agree with the researchers' interpretations of their results? Why or why not?

b. What is your assessment of the internal and external validity of the study?

c. To what extent do you think the researchers adequately described the study's limitations and strengths?

Exercise D.2: Study in Appendix D

Read the Results and Discussion sections of the report by Eckhardt and colleagues ("Fatigue in the presence of coronary heart disease") in Appendix D on pages 143–153 and then answer the following questions:

Questions of Fact

a. Were any biases discussed in this study? If yes, what did the researchers say?

b. Did the researchers state or imply any hypotheses? Were hypotheses supported or nonsupported?

c. Did the researchers make any unwarranted causal inferences about the relationship between variables in their study?

d. Did the report provide information about the precision of results via confidence intervals?

e. Did the report provide information about magnitude of effects via calculation of effect sizes?

f. In the Discussion section, was there any explicit discussion about the study's external validity (generalizability)?

g. Were any study limitations identified in the Discussion section?

h. Did the researchers explicitly comment on the clinical significance of any of the findings?

Questions for Discussion

a. Do you agree with the researchers' interpretations of their results? Why or why not?

b. To what extent do you think the researchers adequately described the study's limitations and strengths?

c. How did the inclusion of qualitative data help in interpreting results?

Understanding the Analysis of Qualitative Data

A. FILL IN THE BLANKS

How many terms have you learned in this chapter? Fill in the blanks in the sentences below to find out.

1. A widely used method of data management in a qualitative data set involves _____ the data.

2. Qualitative descriptive studies typically rely on _____ analysis or _____ analysis to discover key themes and patterns.

3. In ethnographies, a broad unit of cultural knowledge is called a(n) _____.

4. The second level of analysis in Spradley's ethnographic method, yielding an organizational structure for the data, is called _____ analysis.

5. Colaizzi's approach is one method used in _____ phenomenological studies.

6. Van Manen's _____-_____-_____ approach involves analyzing every sentence.

7. A(n) _____ is a literary device sometimes used as part of an analytic strategy, especially by interpretive phenomenologists.

8. A hermeneutic _____ involves movement between parts and whole of a text being analyzed.

9. In Benner's hermeneutic approach, the presentation of _____ in reports allows readers to draw conclusions about the validity of the results.

10. _____ cases, in one approach to hermeneutic analysis, are strong examples of ways of being in the world.

11. The first stage of Glaserian grounded theory analysis involves _____ coding.

12. In Glaserian grounded theory, the type of coding focused on the core variable is _____ coding.

13. Grounded theorists document an idea in an analytic _____.

14. The concept of _____ fit in grounded theory involves comparing identified concepts with similar concepts from previous studies.

15. A recent approach to grounded theory analysis, developed by Charmaz, is called _____ grounded theory.

95

B. MATCHING EXERCISE

Match each descriptive statement from Set B with one or more types of qualitative analyses from Set A. Indicate the letter(s) corresponding to your response next to each item in Set B.

SET A

a. Grounded theory analysis
b. Phenomenological/hermeneutic analysis
c. Ethnographic analysis
d. None of the above

SET B   RESPONSES

1. Involves the development of codes   _____
2. Begins with "open coding"   _____
3. One method of analysis was developed by Colaizzi.   _____
4. Data can be organized using computer software.   _____
5. One method of analysis was developed by
   Glaser and Strauss.   _____
6. May involve the development of a taxonomy   _____
7. One analytic approach is called "holistic."   _____
8. Requires computer software   _____

C. STUDY QUESTIONS

1. What is wrong with the following statements?
   a. Perez conducted a grounded theory study about coping with a miscarriage; she identified four major themes.
   b. Marcolin's ethnographic analysis of Haitian clinics involved gleaning related thematic material from French poetry.
   c. Titterton's phenomenological study of the lived experience of Parkinson's disease focused on the domain of fatigue.
   d. Levine's grounded theory study of widowhood yielded a taxonomy of coping strategies.
   e. In her ethnographic study of the culture of a nursing home, Stimpfle used a rural nursing home as a paradigm case.

2. Beck and Watson (2010) conducted a phenomenological study about a subsequent birth following a previous traumatic birth. The coding scheme for that study is presented in Box 1. Use this coding scheme to code the following two segments from actual interviews:

Excerpt 1	Codes
"My pregnancy was planned and initially on discovering I was pregnant again I was happy and excited to be having a baby and I was able to shut out thoughts of the fact I would have to give birth again. However, when I was about 9 weeks pregnant I could no longer contain this anxiety and I spiraled into panic attacks thinking that I could not live like that for another 7 months. I went to see my doctor and he prescribed some medication for my panic attacks. On the whole from 20 weeks on my emotions settled down and I was focused on the birth and the delivery of my baby. I still had periods of anxiety normally around when I went for my OB appointments. When I finally gave birth to my baby I pushed him into the world and I was shocked. All the scenarios for having another baby that I had run through in my mind since the traumatic birth of my first child never ended like this. I had never dreamed for such a perfect delivery. I was there holding my baby and all that anxiety about his birth had been for nothing. I breastfed my baby and had a cuddle before giving him to my husband while my episiotomy was stitched. It was then that it hit me like a brick wall of emotions as my husband held our baby. He looked just like my daughter had the day she was born but I had missed some of her precious first hours being in surgery to have my 4th degree tear repaired and at this moment I just sobbed. It was a mixture of joy that my son was ok and I had achieve what I had dreamt of for his birth and grief for the birth of my first child that had been so very different and so difficult for me to get over. After the birth I felt confident and proud of my body and of what I had come through since my first traumatic birth. My second birth was very positive and did heal me in some ways. But experiencing what childbirth should be like made me realize how hideous my first birth was and my second birth can never erase the past memories of my first traumatic birth."	

Excerpt 2	Codes
"My first birth was horrendous. As soon as I became pregnant with my second child I read absolutely everything I could possibly get my hands on about childbirth from midwifery textbooks to independent research papers. I was determined that this next time was going to be very different. I would be very aware of the facts and I would have a better understanding of my own needs for privacy, control, and emotional support. I then went about choosing an independent midwife. I interviewed 2 lovely women and asked them identical questions. I told them both that I had not dilated beyond 3 cm in my first birth and asked what they would do if I got to 3 cm then progress slowed. Midwife #1 said she would probably transfer me to the hospital. Midwife #2 said she would just wait until things changed. She talked about how much faith she had in the female body. I went with midwife #2. During my pregnancy I bought a copy of *Birthing from Within* and spent a lot of time painting my previous birth experience and how I envisioned birth #2. I truly nurtured myself. I swam, did yoga, walked, and spent lots of time outdoors and enjoyed being with my 2 year old. Over my pregnancy I felt very supported by my midwife and I became able to trust her. My husband and I also hired a doula to make sure both he and I would be supported during this labor and delivery."	

From the author's records for the study reported in the following paper: Beck, C. T., & Watson, S. (2010). Subsequent childbirth after a previous traumatic birth. *Nursing Research, 59*, 241–249.

3. Suppose a researcher was studying people with hypertension who were struggling unsuccessfully for months to manage their weight. The researcher plans to interview 15 to 25 people for this study. Answer the following questions:
   a. What might be the research question that a phenomenologist would ask relating to this situation? And what might the research question be for a grounded theory researcher?
   b. Which do you think would take longer to do—the analysis of data for the phenomenological or the grounded theory? Why?
   c. What would the final "product" of the analyses be for the two different studies?
   d. Which study would have more appeal to you? Why?
4. Read the following open-access article (a link for which is available in the Internet Resources section on **thePoint** website) and critically appraise how well the researchers described the analytic process for this phenomenological study:

   • Hemberg, J., & Wiklund Gustin, L. (2020). Caring from the heart as belonging: The basis for mediating compassion. *Nursing Open, 7*, 660–668.

BOX 1 Beck and Watson's (2010) Coding Scheme for Study on a Subsequent Childbirth After a Previous Traumatic Birth

Theme 1: Riding the Turbulent Wave of Panic During Pregnancy

A. Reactions to learning of pregnancy
B. Denial during the first trimester
C. Heightened state of anxiety
D. Panic attacks as delivery date gets closer
E. Feeling numb toward the baby

Theme 2: Strategizing: Attempts to Reclaim Their Body and Complete the Journey to Motherhood

A. Spending time nurturing self by exercising, going to yoga classes, and swimming
B. Keeping a journal throughout pregnancy
C. Turning to doulas for support during labor
D. Reading avidly to understand the birth process
E. Engaging in birth art exercises
F. Opening up to health care providers about their previous birth trauma
G. Sharing with partners about their fears
H. Learned relaxation techniques

Theme 3: Bringing Reverence to the Birthing Process and Empowering Women

A. Treated with respect
B. Pain relief taken seriously
C. Communicated with labor and delivery staff
D. Reclaimed their body
E. Strong sense of control
F. Birth plan was honored by labor and delivery staff.
G. Mourned what they missed out with prior birth
H. Healing subsequent birth but it can never change the past

Theme 4: Still Elusive: The Longed-For Healing Birth Experience

A. Failed again as a woman
B. Better than first traumatic birth but not healing
C. Hopes of a healing home birth dashed

From the author's records for the study reported in the following paper: Beck, C. T., & Watson, S. (2010). Subsequent childbirth after a previous traumatic birth. *Nursing Research, 59*, 241–249.

D. APPLICATION EXERCISES

Exercise D.1: Studies in Appendices B and D

Did either of the studies in Appendix B (Ottosen et al.) or Appendix D (Eckhardt et al.) report the following?
- a. One or more themes?
- b. A taxonomy?
- c. A grounded theory?
- d. A schematic model/conceptual map?

Exercise D.2: Study in Appendix E

Read the Design and Methods and Findings sections of the report by Langegård and colleagues ("The art of living with symptoms") in Appendix E on pages 155–162 and then answer the following questions:

Questions of Fact

- a. Did the researchers audiorecord and transcribe the interviews? If yes, who did the transcription? Did the report state how many pages of data comprised the data set?
- b. Did data collection and data analysis occur concurrently?
- c. Was a computer used to analyze the data? If yes, what software was used?
- d. Were there any metaphors used to highlight key findings?
- e. Did the researchers prepare any analytic memos?
- f. Did the authors describe the coding process? If so, what did they say?
- g. Whose grounded theory analysis approach was used?
- h. Did the researchers present a schematic model that summarized major findings?
- i. Did the researchers provide supporting evidence for their findings, in the form of excerpts from the data?

Questions for Discussion

- a. Were data presented in a manner that allows you to be confident about the researchers' conclusions? Comment on the inclusion or noninclusion of figures that graphically represent the grounded theory.
- b. Comment on the amount of verbatim quotes from study participants that were included in this report.
- c. Discuss the effectiveness of the researchers' presentation of results. Does the analysis seem sensible, thoughtful, and thorough? Was sufficient evidence provided to support the findings? Were data presented in a manner that allows you to be confident about the conclusions?

Appraising Trustworthiness and Integrity in Qualitative Research

A. FILL IN THE BLANKS

How many terms have you learned in this chapter? Fill in the blanks in the sentences below to find out.

1. _____ is a key criterion for assessing quality in qualitative studies concerning confidence in the truth value of the findings.

2. The stability of data over time and conditions, analogous to reliability, is called _____.

3. The quality criterion concerning the extent to which qualitative findings can be applied to other settings is called _____.

4. The criterion of _____ refers to the potential for congruence between independent coders, analysts, or interpreters of qualitative data; its analog in quantitative studies is objectivity.

5. _____ is a quality criterion indicating the extent to which the researchers fairly and faithfully portray different realities.

6. Use of multiple means of converging on the truth is called _____.

7. The dependability of an inquiry can be enhanced by a(n) _____ trail that documents judgments and choices.

8. Transferability is enhanced through the researcher's use of _____ _____ in a research report.

9. Credibility in qualitative inquiry has been described as analogous to _____ validity in quantitative inquiry.

10. Persistent _____ refers to a focus on the aspects of a situation that are relevant to the phenomena being studied.

11. A process by which researchers revise their interpretations by including cases that appear to disconfirm earlier hypotheses is a(n) _____ case analysis.

12. One method of addressing credibility is to do _____ checks, which involve going back to participants to have them review preliminary findings.

13. _____ triangulation is achieved by having two or more researchers make key decisions and interpretations.

14. The strategy of _____ debriefing involves seeking the input from other researchers regarding the analysis of interpretation of qualitative data.

15. The strategy of _____ engagement involves a researcher's investment of sufficient time collecting and analyzing qualitative data.

B. MATCHING EXERCISES

Match each statement from Set B with one of the phrases from Set A. Indicate the letter corresponding to your response next to each of the statements in Set B.

SET A

a. Data source triangulation
b. Investigator triangulation
c. Method triangulation

SET B   RESPONSE

1. A researcher studying health beliefs of the rural elderly interviews old people and health care providers in the area.   _____

2. Two researchers independently interview 10 informants in a study of adjustment to a cancer diagnosis and debrief with each other to review what they have learned.   _____

3. A researcher studying embarrassment in school-based clinics observes interactions in the clinics and also conducts in-depth interviews with students.   _____

4. A researcher studying the process of resolving an infertility problem interviews husbands and wives separately.   _____

5. Categories emerging in the field notes of an observer on a psychiatric ward are coded and labeled independently by two members of the research team.   _____

C. STUDY QUESTIONS

1. Suppose you were conducting a grounded theory study of couples' struggling to come to terms with a child's diagnosis of cancer. What might you do to incorporate various types of triangulation into your study?

2. What is your opinion about the value of member checking as a strategy to enhance credibility? Defend your position.

3. Read a research report in a recent issue of the journal *Qualitative Health Research*. Identify several examples of "thick description." Also, identify areas of the report in which you feel additional thick description would have enhanced the transferability of the evidence.

4. Read the abstract, and then the method section, of one of the following studies, published as open-access articles (links to these articles are provided in the Internet Resources section on thePoint° website). Comment on the amount of information the researchers provided regarding the integrity and trustworthiness of the study.

   - Dos Santos, E., Eslabão, A., Kantoski, L., & de Pinho, L. (2020). Nursing practices in a psychological care center. *Revista Brasileira de Enfermagem*, *73*, e20180175.

   - Hoog, S., Dautzenberg, M., Eskes, A., Vermeulen, H., & Vloet, L. (2020). The experiences and needs of relatives of intensive care unit patients during the transition from the intensive care unit to a general ward: A qualitative study. *Australian Critical Care*. Advance online publication. doi:10.1016 /j.aucc.2020.01.004.

   - Hussain, L., Kanji, Z., Lalani, S., Moledina, S., & Sattar, A. (2019). Exploring lived experiences of married Pakistani women post-mastectomy. *Asia-Pacific Journal of Oncology Nursing*, *6*, 78–85.

D. APPLICATION EXERCISES

Exercise D.1: Study in Appendix B

Read the report by Ottosen and colleagues ("An ethnography of parents' perceptions of patient safety in the neonatal intensive care unit") in Appendix B on pages 123–133 and then answer the following questions:

Questions of Fact

a. Did the researchers devote a section of the report to describing their quality-enhancement strategies? If so, what was it labeled? If not, where was information about such strategies located?
b. What types of triangulation, if any, were used in this study?
c. Were any of the following methods used to enhance the credibility of the study?

   - Prolonged engagement and/or persistent observation

   - Peer review and debriefing

   - Member checks

   - Search for disconfirming evidence

   - Reflexivity

Questions for Discussion

a. Discuss the thoroughness with which Ottosen et al. described their efforts to enhance and evaluate the quality and integrity of their study.
b. How would you characterize the integrity and trustworthiness of this study based on the researchers' documentation? How would you describe the credibility, dependability, confirmability, authenticity, and transferability of this study?
c. What recommendations would you offer, if any, regarding enhanced member checking in this study?

Exercise D.2: Study in Appendix E

Read the report by Langegård and colleagues ("The art of living with symptoms") in Appendix E on pages 155–162 and then answer the following questions:

Questions of Fact

a. Did the researchers devote a section of their report to describing their quality-enhancement strategies? If so, what was it labeled? If not, where was information about such strategies located?
b. What types of triangulation, if any, were used in this study?
c. What can be said about transferability of the study findings?
d. Were any of the following methods used to enhance the credibility of the study?

- Prolonged engagement
- Member checks
- Disconfirming
- Reflexivity
- Audit trail
- Researcher credibility

Questions for Discussion

a. Discuss the thoroughness with which Langegård and colleagues described their efforts to enhance and evaluate the quality and integrity of their study.
b. How would you characterize the integrity and trustworthiness of this study based on the researchers' documentation? How would you describe the credibility, dependability, confirmability, authenticity, and transferability of this study?

CHAPTER 17

Learning From Systematic Reviews

A. FILL IN THE BLANKS

How many terms have you learned in this chapter? Fill in the blanks in the sentences below to find out.

1. The statistical integration of primary study findings in a systematic review is called a(n) _____.

2. A(n) _____ review is a preliminary exploration of the literature to clarify the evidence base.

3. The body of unpublished studies is sometimes referred to as _____ literature.

4. A concern in a systematic review is the _____ bias that stems from including only studies that are published in journals.

5. An appraisal of primary study's methodological _____ is undertaken in most systematic reviews, although approaches to using appraisal information vary.

6. In a meta-analysis, findings are in the form of a(n) _____ _____ index, such as *d*.

7. In a meta-analysis, statistical _____ concerns the degree of dissimilarity among the estimates of effects in the primary studies.

8. Another name for the effect index *d* for comparing two group means is *standardized mean* _____.

9. In a meta-analysis, a(n) _____ analysis involves examining the extent to which effects differ for different types of studies, people, or intervention elements.

10. A(n) _____ plot is a graphic display of the effect size (including confidence intervals around them) of each primary study in a meta-analysis.

11. An assessment of the degree of confidence that a review team has in its findings typically uses the _____ system.

12. Systematic reviews of qualitative evidence can be characterized as either _____ or _____.

13. The Cochrane Collaboration uses the umbrella term _____ _____ _____ to refer to systematic reviews of qualitative evidence.

14. Systematic reviews that integrate, interpret, and transform qualitative study findings are often called _____.

15. Noblit and Hare developed an approach to synthesizing qualitative findings called _____.

16. A(n) _____, which involves calculating manifest effect sizes, can lay the foundation for a metasynthesis.

17. In a meta-summary, a(n) _____ effect size is the percentage of reports that contain a given thematic finding.

18. The method of integrating qualitative findings used by the Joanna Briggs Institute is called _____.

B. MATCHING EXERCISE

1. Match each of the statements in Set B with the appropriate phrase in Set A. Indicate the letter(s) corresponding to your response next to each of the statements in Set B.

SET A

a. Quantitative review with meta-analysis
b. Qualitative review—metasynthesis
c. Neither meta-analysis nor metasynthesis
d. Both meta-analysis and metasynthesis

SET B   RESPONSES

1. Involves gathering data from human participants   _____
2. Focuses on synthesizing information from prior studies   _____
3. Can use findings from ethnographies and grounded theory studies   _____
4. Can use findings from the grey literature   _____
5. Sandelowski developed an approach for this.   _____
6. Often involves calculating d or OR statistics   _____
7. CINAHL likely would be used for this in searching for primary studies.   _____
8. Relies on a process that is interpretive and transformative   _____

C. STUDY QUESTIONS

1. Read one of the following systematic reviews (with meta-analysis) published several years ago as open-access articles (links to each paper are provided in the Internet Resources section on **thePoint**)

   - Atlantis, E., Fahey, P., & Foster, J. (2014). Collaborative care for comorbid depression and diabetes: A systematic review and meta-analysis. *BMJ Open*, *4*, e004706.

   - Lee, E. N., & Lee, J. H. (2016). The effects of low-dose ketamine on acute pain in an emergency setting: A systematic review and meta-analysis. *PLoS One, 11*(10), e0165461.

   - Li, Z. Z., Li, Y., Lei, X., Zhang, D., Liu, L., Tang, S., & Chen, L. (2014). Prevalence of suicidal ideation in Chinese college students: A meta-analysis. *PLoS One, 9*, e104368.

   - Patil, S., Ruppar, T., Koopman, R., Lindbloom, E., Elliott, S., Mehr, D., & Conn, V. (2016). Peer support interventions for adults with diabetes: A meta-analysis of hemoglobin A1c outcomes. *Annals of Family Medicine, 14*, 540–551.

   Then, search the literature for relevant quantitative primary studies published *after* this systematic review. Are new study results consistent with the conclusions drawn in the meta-analytic report? Are there enough new studies to warrant a new meta-analysis—or has a new systematic review already been completed?

2. Read one of the following metasynthesis reports published several years ago as open-access articles (links to each paper are provided in the Internet Resources section on **thePoint**):

   - Bridges, J., Nicholson, C., Maben, J., Pope, C., Flatley, M., Wilkinson, C., . . . Tziggili, M. (2013). Capacity for care: Meta-ethnography of acute care nurses' experiences of the nurse-patient relationship. *Journal of Advanced Nursing, 69*, 760–772.

   - Flores, D., Leblanc, N., & Barroso, J. (2016). Enrolling and retaining patients with human immunodeficiency virus (HIV) in their care: A metasynthesis of qualitative studies. *International Journal of Nursing Studies, 62*, 126–136.

   - Kemp, K., Griffiths, J., & Lovell, K. (2012). Understanding the health and social care needs of people living with IBD: A meta-synthesis of the evidence. *World Journal of Gastroenterology, 18*, 6240–6249.

   Then, search the literature for related qualitative primary studies published *after* this metasynthesis. Are new study results consistent with the conclusions drawn in the metasynthesis report? Are there enough new studies to warrant a new metasynthesis—or has a new review already been published?

3. Read the following open-access report, which involved a quantitative systematic review without a meta-analysis. Did the authors adequately justify their decision not to conduct a meta-analysis? (A link to this paper is provided in the Internet Resources section on **thePoint**.):

    *   Zhao, Y., Brettle, A., & Qiu, L. (2018). The effectiveness of shared care in cancer survivors—A systematic review. *International Journal of Integrated Care, 18*, 1–17.

D. APPLICATION EXERCISES

Exercise D.1: Study in Appendix G

Read the report on the meta-analysis by Chase and colleagues ("The effectiveness of medication adherence interventions among patients with coronary artery disease") in Appendix G on pages 175–184 and then answer the following questions:

Questions of Fact

a. What was the stated purpose of this review? What were the independent and dependent variables in this review?
b. What inclusion criteria were stipulated? How many studies met all inclusion criteria?
c. What methods did the reviewers use to search for primary studies?
d. Did the authors present a flow chart showing the progression of potential studies through an identification and screening process? If no, was this information presented effectively in the text or in a table?
e. How many participants were there in total, in all included studies combined?
f. What were the key demographic characteristics of study participants in the primary studies?
g. How many of the studies included in this systematic review used an experimental (randomized) design? How many were quasi-experimental?
h. Did the researchers rate each study in the data set for its quality? If yes, what aspects of the study were appraised? How many people evaluated the studies for quality? Was interrater agreement assessed?
i. Did the researchers set a threshold for study quality as part of their inclusion criteria? If yes, what was it?
j. What effect size index was used in the meta-analysis?
k. Did the researchers perform any tests for statistical heterogeneity? Was a fixed effects or random effects model used?
l. Were study-by-study effects presented in a forest plot?
m. Overall, what was the value of the effect size index for the interventions? What was the confidence interval around the mean effect? Was the effect statistically significant?
n. Considering the information in Figure 1, answer the following questions:

    *   In which study was the effect size the largest? Was this effect size statistically significant?

    *   Were effect sizes nonsignificant in any studies?

    *   Were there any studies were the effect size was in the opposite direction from what was anticipated?

o. Were subgroup analyses undertaken? If yes, what were the key findings?
p. Did the researchers undertake a GRADE-type evaluation to assess confidence in the findings?

Questions for Discussion

a. Was the size of the sample (studies and participants) sufficiently large to draw conclusions about the overall intervention effects?
b. What other subgroups might have been interesting to examine (assume there was sufficient information in the original studies)?
c. How would you assess the overall rigor of this systematic review?
d. Based on this review, what is the evidence regarding interventions for medication adherence among patients with coronary artery disease?
e. Comment on the authors' discussion about study limitations.
f. Comment on the authors' discussion of the implications of this review for clinical practice.

Exercise D.2: Study in Appendix H

Read the report on the metasynthesis by Carr and colleagues ("Patient information needs and breast reconstruction after mastectomy") in Appendix H on pages 185–197 and then answer the following questions:

Questions of Fact

a. What type of systematic review was this? Would it be characterized as aggregative or interpretive?
b. Whose approach was used in this review?
c. What was the purpose of this synthesis?
d. Did the report articulate inclusion and exclusion criteria for studies in the review?
e. What methods did the reviewers use to search for primary studies?
f. Did the authors present a flow chart showing the progression of potential studies through the identification and screening process?
g. Where were the studies in the review conducted?
h. Were the studies from a single qualitative transition or multiple traditions?
i. How many mothers who had breast reconstruction participated in the primary studies that were included in the review?
j. How many themes were identified in this meta-synthesis? What were those themes?
k. Was Carr and colleagues' synthesis supported through the inclusion of raw data from the primary studies?

Questions for Discussion

a. Was the size of the sample sufficiently large to conduct a meaningful metasynthesis? Comment on the extent to which the diversity of the sample enhanced or weakened the metasynthesis.
b. Did the analysis and integration appear reasonable and thorough?
c. Were primary studies adequately described?
d. How would you assess the overall rigor of this metasynthesis?
e. Based on this metasynthesis, what is the evidence regarding the experiences of women who had breast reconstruction? How did the experiences of those with immediate reconstruction differ from those who delayed reconstruction?

Putting Research Evidence Into Practice: Evidence-Based Practice and Practice-Based Evidence

A. FILL IN THE BLANKS

How many terms have you learned in this chapter? Fill in the blanks in the sentences below to find out.

1. The _____ Collaboration, with centers in dozens of countries, has played a crucial role in promoting evidence-based practice (EBP).

2. _____ translation is a term related to EBP that is often associated with efforts to enhance systematic change in clinical practice.

3. Resources for EBP include various types of evidence that has been _____ by experts.

4. A clinical practice _____, based on rigorous systematic evidence, is an important tool for evidence-based care.

5. EBP _____, such as the one called PARiHS, are a resource to guide clinicians in planning and implementing an EBP project.

6. Some EBP models distinguish a knowledge-focused and problem-focused _____ for an EBP effort.

7. In the 5As scheme for an EBP effort, the first step is to _____ well-worded clinical questions.

8. In the 5As EBP scheme, Step 5 is to _____ the outcomes of the practice change.

9. In the "Appraise" step in the 5As scheme, the question about _____ concerns how much evidence there is.

10. In the "Appraise" step in the 5As scheme, the question about _____ concerns of evidence concerns the degree to which similar findings have been found across studies.

11. _____ is the degree to which research evidence can be applied to individuals, small groups, or local contexts.

110

12. _____-centered research focuses on the development of evidence that is meaningful and valuable to clients.

13. Information about _____ treatment effects from randomized controlled trials (RCTs) can be misleading if there is great diversity in response to an intervention.

14. When responses to an intervention vary, this is called _____ of treatment effects (HTE).

15. _____ effectiveness research involves comparing the effects of alternative interventions.

16. A(n) _____ clinical trial has features that are designed to enhance the generalizability and relevance of evidence about an intervention.

17. __ __ __ __ __ __-2 is the acronym for a tool used to score the location of a trial on the pragmatic-explanatory continuum.

18. If researchers want to test the hypothesis that men and women have different responses to an intervention, they would undertake a(n) _____ analysis.

19. When researchers undertake multiple subgroup analyses, there is a strong risk of a(n) _____ error.

20. The proper analysis for testing subgroup effects is to test for a(n) _____ with the treatment variable.

B. MATCHING EXERCISES

1. Match each of the statements in Set B with the appropriate phrase in Set A. Indicate the letter(s) corresponding to your response next to each of the statements in Set B.

SET A

a. Research utilization (RU)
b. Evidence-based practice (EBP)
c. Neither RU nor EBP
d. Both RU and EBP

SET B   RESPONSES

1. Has been easily and universally achieved in nursing   _____
2. Evidence hierarchies were developed within this context.   _____
3. Is useful only to nurses in academic environments   _____
4. Integrates research findings with clinical expertise and
   client inputs   _____
5. Always begins with a knowledge-focused trigger   _____
6. Uses evidence from research to suggest practice improvements   _____

C. STUDY QUESTIONS

1. Think about a nursing procedure that you have learned. What is the basis for this procedure? Examine whether the procedure is based on scientific evidence indicating that the procedure is effective. If it is not based on scientific evidence, on what is it based, and why do you think scientific evidence was not used?

2. Identify the factors in your own clinical setting that you think facilitate or inhibit research utilization and EBP (or, in an educational setting, the factors that promote or inhibit a climate in which EBP is valued).

3. Read one of the following articles and identify the steps of the Iowa model (or an alternative model of EBP) that are represented in the projects described.

    • *Blair, K., Eccleston, S., Binder, H., & McCarthy, M. (2017). Improving the patient experience by implementing an ICU diary for those at risk of post-intensive care syndrome. *Journal of Patient Experience*, *4*, 4–9.

    • Lemus, L., McMullin, B., & Balinowski, H. (2018). Don't ignore my snore: Reducing perioperative complications of obstructive sleep apnea. *Journal of Perianesthesia Nursing*, *33*, 338–345.

    • Wonder, A., Martin, E., & Jackson, K. (2017). Supporting and empowering direct-care nurses to promote EBP: An example of evidence-based policy development, education, and practice change. *Worldviews on Evidence-Based Nursing*, *14*, 336–338.

4. Read the following open-access journal article that reports a comparative effectiveness study conducted by an interdisciplinary team that included nurse researchers (a link is provided in the Internet resources section on **thePoint**). To what extent were the six "defining characteristics" of comparative effectiveness research (CER), as described in Chapter 18, embodied in the study?

    • Glass, N., Remy, M., Mayo-Wilson, L., Kohil, A., Sommer, M., Turner, R., & Perrin, N. (2020). Comparative effectiveness of an economic empowerment program on adolescent economic assets, education and health in a humanitarian settings. *BMC Public Health*, *20*, 170.

5. Read one of the following open-access journal articles that report an RCT. Were subgroup analyses performed? If no, should they have been? If yes, evaluate the extent to which the subgroup analyses conformed to the advice provided in the textbook.

    • George, A., Dahlen, H., Blinkhorn, A., Ajwani, S., Bhole, S., Ellis, S., . . . Johnson, M. (2018). Evaluation of a midwifery initiated oral health-dental service program to improve oral health and birth outcomes for pregnant women: A multi-centre randomised controlled trial. *International Journal of Nursing Studies*, *82*, 49–57.

    • Neil-Sztramko, S., Smith-Turchyn, J., Richardson, J., & Dobbins, M. (2020). Impact of a knowledge translation intervention on physical activity and mobility in older adults (the Move4Age study): Randomized controlled trial. *Journal of Medical Internet Research*, *22*(2), e15125.

---

*A link to this open-access article is provided in the Internet Resources for this chapter on thePoint website.

- Sandlund, C., Hetta, J., Nilsson, G., Ekstedt, M., & Westman, J. (2018). Impact of group treatment for insomnia on daytime symptomatology: Analyses from a randomized controlled trial in primary care. *International Journal of Nursing Studies*, 85, 126–135.

D. APPLICATION EXERCISES

Exercise D.1: Study in Appendix C

Read the abstract and introduction to the report by Saqe-Rockoff and colleagues ("Improving thermoregulation for trauma patients in the emergency department") in Appendix C on pages 135–141 and then answer the following questions:

Questions of Fact
a. What was the purpose of this EBP project?
b. What was the setting for implementing this project?
c. Which EBP model was used as a framework for this project?
d. Did the project have a problem-focused or knowledge-focused trigger?
e. Who were the team members in this study, and what were their affiliations?
f. What did the report say about their evidence searching efforts? Did the authors discuss efforts to appraise the evidence?
g. Was a pilot study undertaken?
h. What were the components of the EBP intervention—what changes were implemented?
i. Did this project involve an evaluation of the project's success? What outcomes were monitored?
j. What were the main findings from the evaluation of the practice changes?

Questions for Discussion
What are some of the praiseworthy aspects of this project? What could the team members have done differently to improve the project?

Exercise D.2: Study in Appendix A

Read the report by Stephens and colleagues ("Smartphone technology and text messaging for weight loss in young adults") in Appendix A. Then, answer the following questions:

Questions of Fact
a. Were stakeholders involved in the development of the intervention?
b. Is this study an example of comparative effectiveness research (CER)?
c. Was this trial pragmatic?
d. Did the researchers conduct any subgroup analyses?
e. Did the researchers discuss the study's generalizability?
f. Did the researchers discuss the study's applicability?

Questions for Discussion
a. Comment on the degree to which the study had the six characteristics of CER.
b. What subgroup analyses might be undertaken with the data from this study, using variables that the researchers measured?

Smartphone Technology and Text Messaging for Weight Loss in Young Adults
A Randomized Controlled Trial

Janna D. Stephens, PhD, RN; Allison M. Yager, BS; Jerilyn Allen, RN, ScD, FAAN

Background: Using smartphone technology and text messaging for health is a growing field. This type of technology is well integrated into the lives of young adults. However, few studies have tested the effect of this type of technology to promote weight loss in young adults **Objective:** The purpose of this study is to test the effectiveness of a behaviorally based smartphone application for weight loss combined with text messaging from a health coach on weight, body mass index (BMI), and waist circumference in young adults as compared with a control condition. **Methods:** Sixty-two young adults, aged 18 to 25 years, were randomized to receive (1) a smartphone application + health coach intervention and counseling sessions or (2) control condition with a counseling session. All outcome measures were tested at baseline and 3 months. These included weight, BMI, waist circumference, dietary habits, physical activity habits, and self-efficacy for healthy eating and physical activity. **Results:** The sample was 71% female and 39% white, with an average age of 20 years and average BMI of 28.5 kg/m^2. Participants in the smartphone + health coach group lost significantly more weight ($P = .026$) and had a significant reduction in both BMI ($P = .024$) and waist circumference ($P < .01$) compared with controls. **Conclusions:** The results of this weight loss trial support the use of smartphone technology and feedback from a health coach on improving weight in a group of diverse young adults.

KEY WORDS: self-efficacy, text messaging, weight loss, young adult

Overweight and obesity are major public health concerns in the United States. According to data published in 2014 by the National Health and Nutrition Examination Survey, more than one-half of US adults (60.3%) aged 20 to 39 years are overweight or obese with a body mass index (BMI) of 25 kg/m^2 or greater.[1] Weight gain is specifically a concern in college-aged individuals. Although the common theory that college freshman gain 15 lb has been disproven on most accounts,[2] studies have shown that many students do in fact gain weight.[3,4] A survey conducted in 2014 by the American College Health Association reported that more than 34% of undergraduate students are overweight or obese, and this number increases to 40% when surveying graduate students.[5] Being overweight greatly increases one's risk for stroke, heart disease, type 2 diabetes, and some forms of cancer.[6] Therefore, interventions to combat weight gain during these years are needed for healthy outcomes later in life.

The behaviors of college-aged individuals put them at risk for weight gain. Specifically, poor eating habits, decreased physical activity, decreased fruit and vegetable consumption, and increased alcohol consumption all contribute to weight gain.[7,8] The American College Health Association reports that 65% of students consume less than 2 servings of fruit/vegetables combined per day and that more than 50% of students report consuming alcohol in the past 9 days.[5] Of those consuming alcohol, 24% of students reported having 7 or more drinks the last time they drank.[5]

Technology is well integrated into the lives of young adults. Currently, 85% of young adults, aged 18 to 29 years, own a smartphone. Among those young adults owning a smartphone, 100% use their smartphone to send and receive text messages.[9] In addition, 77% of

Janna D. Stephens, PhD, RN
Assistant Professor, College of Nursing, Ohio State University, Columbus

Allison M. Yager, BS
BSN Student, School of Nursing, Johns Hopkins University, Baltimore, Maryland.

Jerilyn Allen, RN, ScD, FAAN
Professor, School of Nursing, Johns Hopkins University, Baltimore, Maryland.

Research in this publication was supported by the National Institute of Nursing Research of the National Institute of Health under award numbers 1T32NR012704 (Cardiovascular Research Training Grant) and F31NR013811 (National Research Service Award). The content is solely the responsibility of the authors and does not necessarily represent the official views of the National Institutes of Health.

The authors have no conflicts of interest to disclose.

Correspondence
Janna D. Stephens, PhD, RN, 5910 Kyles Station Rd, Hamilton OH 45011 (Jsteph22@jhu.edu).

DOI: 10.1097/JCN.0000000000000307

115

young adults have used their smartphone to look up health information.[9] A recent focus group study conducted by the first author identified that young adults are interested in using smartphone technology for weight loss; however, they know very little about the availability of different applications to assist with weight loss.[10]

Interventions for weight loss in this population have proven to be successful using various strategies. One study used technology and showed greater weight loss in a group that received a social networking site and text messages (−2.4 kg) compared with a social networking site alone (−0.63 kg).[11] Another study using the Internet reported increased fruit and vegetable consumption, although no differences in weight were noted.[12]

Smartphone technology can provide many tools to help one lose weight. However, there is limited knowledge on the use of smartphone technology for weight loss in young adults. Therefore, the purpose of this study is to test the effectiveness of a behaviorally based smartphone application combined with text messaging from a health coach on weight, BMI, and waist circumference in young adults as compared with a control condition.

Methods

The Young Adult Weight Loss Study was a randomized, controlled trial in which participants were randomly assigned to intervention or control. Assessments were completed at baseline and 3 months between 2014 and 2015. All participants provided informed written consent at baseline. The protocol was approved by the Johns Hopkins University Institutional Review Board. Study data were collected via paper/pencil questionnaires and a Web-based program for dietary recall. The Research Electronic Data Capture (REDCap), a secure, Web-based application, was used to store data.

Setting and Participants

Participants were recruited in and around the Johns Hopkins University campuses using many strategies including posters/flyers, Facebook, e-mail announcements, and word of mouth. Individuals between 18 and 25 years of age with a BMI between 25 and 40 kg/m^2 who owned an iPhone or Android phone were eligible to participate. Participants were not required to be a college undergraduate or graduate student. Interested individuals contacted the primary investigator to set up a telephone screening; if the individual qualified, they were asked to set up a baseline visit. Participants were excluded if they were currently participating in another structured weight loss program, were taking weight loss medications, were diagnosed with type I diabetes, or were currently pregnant or planning to become pregnant in the next 3 months. Individuals were also excluded if they currently exercised more than 150 min/wk at moderate intensity or have had symptoms of dis-

ordered eating in the previous 6 months. Symptoms of disordered eating were defined as answering yes to any question assessing binging/purging, laxative/diet pill use, and treatment for an eating disorder from the Eating Attitudes Test-26 (EAT-26) questionnaire.[13] Randomization to smartphone + health coach or control by blocks of 4 occurred after data were collected at the baseline visit. All participants received a $25 gift card for participation.

Outcome Measures

Data on the outcome measures were collected on all participants at baseline and 3 months. Body weight was measured using the Tanita BS-549 scale with the participant in light clothing. Height was measured using a wall stick measurement. Body mass index was then calculated using weight in kilograms/height in meters squared. Waist circumference was measured twice and then averaged according to the obesity guidelines.[14]

Physical activity was evaluated with the Godin Leisure-Time Exercise Questionnaire. The survey is self-administered and assesses strenuous, moderate, and mild activity over a 7-day period.[15] This survey method has been proven to be both valid and reliable in adults, with test-retest scores ranging from 0.74 to 0.81.[16] Nutrition data were collected using the National Cancer Institute's Automated Self-Administered 24-hour Recall (ASA-24). The ASA-24 is a Web-based, ASA 24-hour recall of foods and was filled out on the participant's computer. The ASA-24 provides analysis on calories, nutrients, and food group estimates.[17] It has been proven to be valid in an adult population, with the ASA-24 performing very close (87% matching) to standardized interviewer-administered 24-hour food recalls.[17] Information obtained from the ASA-24 included caloric intake, food pyramid equivalents, and nutrients from all foods reported according to the Food and Nutrient Database for Dietary Studies.[17]

Self-efficacy for healthy eating and exercise were evaluated with 2 questionnaires. Both of the self-efficacy scales were self-administered by the participant. The Self-Efficacy for Healthy Eating is a 13-item questionnaire that explores a person's belief in their ability to make better food choices in given situations. A reliability coefficient of 0.87 indicated high internal consistency on the scale tested in a group of adults, ages 19 to 64 years.[18] Self-efficacy for physical activity was assessed using a 14-item questionnaire called the Self-Efficacy for Exercise Scale. This questionnaire assesses individuals' belief in their ability to exercise in given situations. This scale was determined to be reliable and valid in a population of adults, with an internal consistency of 0.90 and a test-retest correlation of 0.67.[19]

Interventions

The behavioral intervention was based on self-efficacy theory, a construct of social cognitive theory,

Reprinted with permission from Stephens, J., et al. (2017). Smartphone technology and text messaging for weight loss in young adults: A randomized clinical trial. *Journal of Cardiovascular Nursing, 32,* 39–46.

which was used in our previous pilot study that focused on smartphone applications for weight loss in adults.[20] The self-efficacy theory states that there are 4 ways to increase one's self-efficacy: mastery experience, social modeling, social support, and verbal persuasion.[21] These 4 mechanisms were built into the intervention, which focused on increasing the participant's self-efficacy to achieve better health outcomes related to weight loss. The goals for both groups were to lose 1 to 2 lb per week and increase participation in physical activity. Participants were encouraged to exercise at least 150 minutes per week at moderate intensity, which would meet the Physical Activity Guidelines for Americans.[22] Both groups received a 1-time counseling session before randomization. This was a 20-minute session that discussed healthy eating, limiting alcohol and sugar-sweetened beverages, and increasing physical activity. After this session, participants were randomized to 1 of 2 groups, control or smartphone + health coach (intervention) for the 3-month study period.

Smartphone + Health Coach Group

Participants in this group were given an additional 30- to 40-minute counseling session on energy balance, nutrient density of foods, sugar-sweetened beverage consumption, and physical activity; therefore, they had 2 sessions total during their baseline visit. Participants were encouraged to identify specific goals that their health coach could help them achieve.

Participants were also guided to download and use the Lose it! application. This application is a free, commercially available smartphone application that is focused on nutrition and physical activity self-monitoring. Participants were encouraged to log all food and exercise into the daily log in the application. They were instructed to follow the caloric budget set by the application using the Mifflin equation. The application also offered social networking through a "friend" feature, which allowed individuals to view peer weight loss and physical activity participation and also allowed the interaction between peers. Participants were encouraged to use this feature.

Individualized text messages were delivered to the participant's smartphone from a health coach. The participants were asked to not text their health coach back. Based on data from a focus group study conducted by the first author, the participants could choose any frequency of messages they wanted to receive from a health coach, anywhere from 1 time per week up to 3 times per day.[9] The smartphone application provided the health coach with the ability to monitor and track all participant progress on a real-time basis and text messages focused on current diet or physical activity status (see Table 1). Texts were sent from the health coach's cell phone at the specified time and frequency of the participant.

TABLE 1   Example Text Messages

Nutrition/Exercise Focus	Example Text Message
Physical activity guidelines for Americans	I noticed you came very close to meeting your goal of 150 minutes of exercise last week. Great job! Let's work hard to meet that 150-minute goal this week
Physical activity social support	Working out with a group can be fun and motivating! Reach out to friends today and do something you all enjoy!
Breakfast consumption	Did you know that people who skip breakfast tend to snack more during the day? Try eating a balanced breakfast each morning!
Nutrient density/sugar-sweetened beverages	Drinking your calories does not provide a nutrient-rich diet! Keep up the good work of drinking zero-calorie beverages!

Control Group

The control group was asked to not use any smartphone applications focused on weight loss for the duration of the study. They received the Lose It! application with a training session at their 3-month visit.

Statistical Analysis

The study was powered to detect statistically significant differences in weight loss between the 2 groups. Using an effect size of 0.8, calculated from a similar study,[10] an α of 0.05, and a power of 80%, the sample size was determined to be 51. The sample size was increased by 15% to allow for attrition, to give a total sample size of 60, or 30 per group. Group differences in baseline sociodemographic and anthropometric characteristics were examined using Wilcoxon rank-sum tests and χ^2 or Fisher exact tests. The primary outcomes were changes from baseline to 3 months in weight in kilograms, BMI, and waist circumference in centimeters. Secondary outcomes were changes in diet, physical activity, and self-efficacy for diet and physical activity. A completers analysis was performed using generalized linear models, which were used to test for group differences, time effects, and interactions between group*time. All statistical analyses were done using Statistical Analysis System (SAS).

Results

Baseline Characteristics

Baseline characteristics of participants by group are shown in Table 2. Of the 62 participants enrolled, 71% were female, 33.8% were Asian, and 12.9% were African American. The overall median age was 20.0

Reprinted with permission from Stephens, J., et al. (2017). Smartphone technology and text messaging for weight loss in young adults: A randomized clinical trial. *Journal of Cardiovascular Nursing, 32,* 39–46.

TABLE 2 **Baseline Sample Characteristics by Treatment Group**

Characteristics	Total	Control	Smartphone + Health Coach	P
n	62	31	31	
Age, median (range), y	20.0 (18.0–25.0)	20.0 (18.0–24.0)	20.0 (18.0–25.0)	1
Race, n (%)				.7917
White	24 (38.7)	12 (38.7)	12 (38.7)	
Black	8 (12.9)	5 (16.1)	3 (9.7)	
Asian	21 (33.8)	9 (29.0)	12 (38.7)	
Other	9 (14.5)	5 (16.1)	4 (12.9)	
Sex, n (%)				.6322
Male	18 (29.0)	8 (25.8)	10 (32.3)	
Female	44 (71.0)	22 (71.0)	21 (67.7)	
BMI, median (range), kg/m^2	28.5 (25.0–40.4)	26.6 (25.0–39.7)	29.0 (25.2–40.4)	.0898
Waist circumference, median (range), cm	93.8 (81.0–120.0)	93.5 (81.0–120.0)	95.8 (82.5–120.0)	.294
Type of smartphone				.3493
iPhone	49 (79.0)	23 (74.2)	26 (83.9)	
Android phone	13 (21.0)	8 (25.8)	5 (16.1)	

Abbreviation: BMI, body mass index.

(18.0–25.0) years and median BMI was 28.5 (25.0–40.4) kg/m^2. Although the sample included both non–college and college students, only 10% of study participants were not current undergraduate or graduate students. There were no significant differences in baseline characteristics between the 2 groups.

Recruitment and Retention

The Figure is the CONSORT diagram reporting the participant flow through the study. We assessed 87 individuals for eligibility.

A total of 66 individuals met the criteria to participate. Of those, 4 (6%) declined to participate. The primary reason for refusal was lack of interest in participating in a study for 3 months. A total of 62 individuals were randomized to 1 of the 2 groups, which represented 71% of those who originally expressed interest in participating.

Fifty-nine (95%) returned at 3 months for follow-up measurements. Retention rates were similar in the 2 groups, 97% in the control group and 94% in the intervention group.

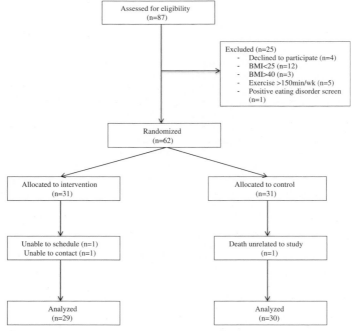

FIGURE. *Study flow diagram.*

Reprinted with permission from Stephens, J., et al. (2017). Smartphone technology and text messaging for weight loss in young adults: A randomized clinical trial. *Journal of Cardiovascular Nursing, 32,* 39–46.

Weight, Body Mass Index, and Wait Circumference

Changes from baseline to 3 months can be found in Table 3. The control group gained a slight amount of weight (0.3 kg) from baseline to 3 months, whereas participants in the smartphone + health coach group lost a significant amount (-1.8 kg, $P < .01$); the difference in weight change between groups was statistically significant ($P = .026$). The smartphone group also had a significant decrease in BMI ($P < .01$) and waist circumference ($P < .01$). The differences in BMI and waist circumference changes between groups were also statistically significant ($P = .024$ for BMI, $P < .01$ for waist circumference). Seven (24%) participants in the smartphone group who completed the study lost enough weight to change their weight status; 5 (17%) moved into the normal weight category and 2 (7%) went from the obese category to overweight.

Self-reported Behaviors

Changes in self-reported behaviors can also be found in Table 3. The smartphone + health coach group improved significantly in healthy eating self-efficacy ($P = .032$). They also improved in overall physical activity performed ($P < .01$); however, the differences were not significant when compared with the control group. Although both groups showed improvement in self-efficacy for physical activity, neither change was statistically significant. A comparison of degree of change between groups was also performed (group × time interaction with all subjects) adjusting for self-efficacy for healthy eating and exercise. When adjusting for self-efficacy for healthy eating, the data show

that it is a slight mediator for change in weight with a P value shifting from $P = .026$ for nonadjusted to $P = .052$ when adjusted. Tests were also run for BMI and waist circumference, but there was no shift in P value, suggesting that self-efficacy for healthy eating does not entirely account for the treatment group effect.

A total of 37 (63%) participants completed the diet questionnaire at follow-up, 22 (73%) control and 15 (52%) smartphone + health coach. Table 4 displays the results from the ASA-24. The smartphone group consumed significantly more fiber than the control group did at follow-up ($P = .049$). There were no additional significant differences between the 2 groups at follow-up. However, participants in the smartphone group consumed slightly more protein, more vegetables, more fruit, fewer total carbohydrates, and fewer added sugars than did participants in the control arm.

Application Use and Text Messaging

The number of text messages sent varied from 1 per day to 3 times per day. No participants requested less than 1 message per day. Overall, 22 (71%) participants requested 3 messages per day, 4 (13%) requested 2 per day, and 5 (16%) requested 1 per day. All text messages were delivered to participants successfully; no error messages were received and all messages were labeled as delivered. Also, no issues were reported by participants.

All participants assigned to the smartphone group logged exercise and diet. Over the 3-month period, 6 (21%) participants logged exercise on more than 50% of days and 18 (62%) logged diet on more than 50% of days. Of those participants who logged on

TABLE 3 Preintervention and Postintervention Measurements of Body Size and Self-reported Behaviors

	Control			Smartphone + Health Coach			
	Pre	Post	P^a	Pre	Post	P^b	P^c
Body size							
Weight, median (range), kg	75.8 (63.0–103.7)	77.3 (66.0–106.2)	.764	82.8 (61–117.5)	80.1 (57.1–120.7)	<.01	.026
BMI, median (range), kg/m²	27.9 (25.0–39.7)	27.6 (25.1–37.7)	.811	29.8 (25.5–40.2)	28.4 (24.7–41.3)	<.01	.024
Waist circumference, median (range), cm	93.3 (81–120)	92.3 (81–117)	.964	95.8 (82.5–120)	92.3 (77–122)	<.01	<.01
Self-reported behaviors							
Self-efficacy (healthy eating), raw score (range)	102 (60–130)	109 (77–130)	.273	100 (66–120)	106 (73–128)	.032	.190
Self-efficacy (exercise), raw score (range)	87.5 (54–131)	92 (42–124)	.258	86 (25–127)	97 (30–140)	.151	.541
Physical activity, 7-day recall, raw score (range)	34 (3–108.5)	36 (6.0–92)	.099	32 (0–72)	43 (15–81)	<.01	.503

Variables summarized as median (range) and compared from pre-post using Wilcoxon rank-sum test; between-group interaction tested using repeated-measures analysis of variance.
Abbreviation: BMI, body mass index.
[a]Comparison of post versus pre in the control group (group effect in generalized linear model for control only).
[b]Comparison of post versus pre in the smartphone group (group effect in generalized linear model for treated only).
[c]Comparison of degree of change between groups (group × time interaction with all subjects).

TABLE 4   Diet Quality of Study Participants During Follow-Up

Diet Parameter, Median (Range)	Total Study Population (N = 37)	Control (n = 22)	Smartphone + Health Coach (n = 15)	P
Calories	1356.7 (586–3288)	1282.2 (831–3288)	1670.5 (586–2689)	.221
Protein	61.1 (24.2–137.5)	58.7 (24.2–110.3)	78.5 (28.3–137.5)	.080
Total fat	47.7 (14.0–129.9)	44.8 (22.2–129.9)	53.7 (14.0–111.5)	.394
Total carbs	175.9 (73.3–453.7)	176.7 (73.3–453.7)	170.0 (85.9–312.0)	.816
Total sugar	61.8 (10.7–180.7)	60.5 (14.8–180.7)	65.0 (10.7–163.3)	.378
Total fiber	14.6 (2.1–61.7)	13.0 (2.1–61.7)	18.4 (7.2–31.7)	.049
Water	1638.8 (717–4277)	1541.3 (851–4277)	1684.1 (717–3869)	.816
Total sodium	2781.4 (1223–4784)	2720.3 (1272–4542)	2792.9 (1223–4784)	.631
Saturated fat	14.6 (2.6–43.9)	13.3 (6.6–43.9)	18.2 (2.6–41.2)	.506
Total vegetables	1.1 (0.0–6.1)	1.0 (0.0–6.1)	1.2 (0.5–4.2)	.193
Total fruit	0.7 (0.0–5.0)	0.5 (0.0–5.0)	0.9 (0.0–4.0)	.219
Total dairy	1.1 (0.0–5.2)	0.9 (0.0–5.2)	1.4 (0.0–2.9)	.768
Added sugars	7.1 (0.0–28.6)	8.2 (0.7–28.6)	5.6 (0.0–23.6)	.077

Continuous variables summarized as median (range) and compared between groups using Wilcoxon rank-sum test.

more than 50% of days, 3 (50%) logged physical activity on more than 75% of days and 7 (38%) logged diet on more than 75% of days. Table 5 displays the significant relationship between number of physical activity days logged and weight loss (0.03 kg weight loss per additional day of physical activity [PA] logging; $P = .026$). The 6 participants who logged PA more than 50% of the time lost 1.57 kg more than those who did not. When the threshold was reduced to 25% days logged, the 9 participants logging PA 25% or more of the time lost 1.43 kg more than those logging PA less than 25% of the time. The same directional trends were observed with increased logging frequency for food as well, but these were not significant ($P = .226$), possibly because of overall good compliance with food logging.

Discussion

To date, to the authors' knowledge, this is the first trial focused on young adults that used both individualized text messages and a smartphone application for weight loss. This trial showed that the use of a smartphone application combined with individualized text messages is successful in helping individuals to lose weight. Individuals in the smartphone group lost significantly more weight, had a significant decrease in BMI, and significantly decreased their waist circumference compared with the control group. However,

many individuals did not meet the recommended goal in the study to lose 1 to 2 lb per week. The mean weight loss in the smartphone + health coach group was 4 lb over the 3-month trial. These results are promising when examining other similar research. Although studies using technology or text messaging have seen improvements in weight, many did not report any significant improvements when compared with a control condition.[23,24] It is possible that the combination of a smartphone application with text messaging led to significant improvements in body weight in this group of young adults.

It is noteworthy that self-efficacy increased significantly for healthy eating ($P = .03$) in the smartphone + health coach group and both groups experienced an increase in self-efficacy for exercise, although this was not significant. It is possible that there were differences in self-efficacy between men and women or based on racial category in this study; however, these differences were not tested. Recent studies conducted in college-aged individuals reported implications for testing the differences in self-efficacy between men and women and also indicate possible racial differences in self-efficacy for improving certain health behaviors. A study published in 2015 by Bruce et al[25] reported significantly lower self-efficacy for changing sugar-sweetened beverage consumption in African American college men compared with white college men. In addition, a study examining

TABLE 5   Relationships Between Logging Consistency and Weight Change

	n/N	B	95% CI	P
No. days logged (PA)	—	−0.03[a]	−0.05 to −0.01	.026
Logging >50% PA	6/29	−1.57[b]	−3.31 to 0.17	.089
No. days logged (food)	—	−0.02[a]	−0.04 to 0.01	.226
Logging >50% food	18/29	−0.70[b]	−2.24 to 0.74	.375

Abbreviation: CI, confidence interval.
[a]Expected weight change per additional day of logging.
[b]Expected weight change for more than 50% logging versus less than 50% logging.

Reprinted with permission from Stephens, J., et al. (2017). Smartphone technology and text messaging for weight loss in young adults: A randomized clinical trial. *Journal of Cardiovascular Nursing, 32*, 39–46.

What's New and Important

- This is the first study to examine use of smartphone technology and text messaging for weight loss in young adults.
- This study shows that using smartphone technology and text messaging can help young adults lose weight.
- Increased logging of physical activity on a smartphone led to increases in weight loss.

Korean college students reported that self-efficacy for physical activity is a significant predictor of physical activity in Korean men but not in Korean women.[26] Future studies should include analyses on differences in self-efficacy but should also examine other components of social cognitive theory, such as social support or outcome expectations, which are known predictors of behaviors.[21]

An increase in logging into the smartphone application for both physical activity and diet led to better outcomes with weight loss. It is therefore important that accountability be a focus in future interventions. Accountability in this study was exhibited through the behavior of logging into an application; however, accountability could be achieved many different ways in upcoming trials. In trials that use technology, increasing compliance and accountability with smartphone logging could be achieved through a counselor stressing the importance of logging during a session or more frequent reminders could be sent to participant phones.

There are several strengths to note in this study. Strengths of the study include the randomized design powered to detect significant differences between groups, use of a commercially available smartphone application, and an attrition rate of only 5%. In addition, the study population was diverse: 38 (62%) participants were from a minority group and 21 (33%) identified as Asian and 8 (13%) identified as African American.

Study limitations include the small sample size and limited generalizability of the study population in that most were attending college at a single university on the east coast. Also, the study was of short duration (3 months) with no extended follow-up. Finally, it cannot be determined whether differences between groups were a result of the health coach text messaging or the smartphone application.

Conclusion

This randomized controlled trial using a smartphone application for weight loss combined with individualized text messages has provided valuable information that the combination of self-monitoring via an application and feedback from a health coach is successful in helping young adults lose weight. The study had a meaningful impact on weight, BMI, and waist circumference. In future trials, a sample that includes equal amounts of individuals attending college and those not attending college could strengthen the generalizability of the results. Smartphone technology seems to be an appropriate resource to use when working with the young adult population and it has the potential to greatly impact the serious public health problem of obesity.

REFERENCES

1. Ogden CL, Carroll MD, Kit BK, Flegal KM. Prevalence of childhood and adult obesity in the United States, 2011–2012. *JAMA.* 2014;311(8):806–814.
2. Holm-Denoma JM, Joiner TE, Vohs KD, Heatherton TF. The "freshman fifteen" (the "freshman five" actually): predictors and possible explanations. *Health Psychol.* 2008; 27(supplement 1):S3–S9.
3. Economos CD, Hildebrandt ML, Hyatt RR. College freshman stress and weight change: differences by gender. *Am J Health Behav.* 2008;32(1):16–25.
4. Gropper SS, Newton A, Harrington P, Simmons KP, Connell LJ, Ulrich P. Body composition changes during the first two years of university. *Prev Med.* 2011;52(1):20–22.
5. American College Health Association. *American College Health Association- National College Health Assessment II: Undergraduate Students Reference Group Executive Summary Spring 2014.* Hanover, MD: American College Health Association; 2014.
6. Burton BT, Foster WR, Hirsch J, Van Itallie TB. Health implications of obesity: an NIH consensus development conference. *Int J Obes.* 1985;9:155–169.
7. Kasparek DG, Corwin SJ, Valois RF, Sargent RG, Morris RL. Selected health behaviors that influence college freshman weight change. *J Am Coll Health.* 2008;56(4):437–444.
8. Lloyd-Richardson EE, Lucero ML, DiBello JR, Jacobson AE, Wing RR. The relationship between alcohol use, eating habits and weight change in college freshmen. *Eat Behav.* 2008; 9(4):504–508.
9. Smith A. U.S. smartphone use in 2015. April 1, 2015. http://www.pewinternet.org/2015/04/01/us-smartphone-use-in-2015/. Accessed April 20, 2015.
10. Stephens J, Moscou-Jackson G, Allen JK. Young adults, technology, and weight loss: a focus group study. *J Obes.* 2015;2015:379769.
11. Napolitano MA, Hayes S, Bennett GG, Ives AK, Foster GD. Using Facebook and text messaging to deliver a weight loss program to college students. *Obesity (Silver Spring).* 2013; 21(1):25–31.
12. Lachausse RG. My student body: effects of an internet-based prevention program to decrease obesity among college students. *J Am Coll Health.* 2012;60(4):324–330. doi:10.1080/07448481.2011.623333.
13. Garner DM, Olmsted MP, Bohr Y, Garfinkel PE. The eating attitudes test: psychometric features and clinical correlates. *Psychol Med.* 1982;12(4):871–878.
14. National Heart, Lung and Blood Institute. *Guidelines on Overweight and Obesity: Electronic Textbook.* Bethesda, MD: National Institutes of Health.
15. Godin G, Shephard RJ. Godin Leisure-Time Exercise Questionnaire. *Med Sci Sports Exerc.* 1997;26(suppl 6):S36–S38.
16. Jacobs DR Jr, Ainsworth BE, Hartman TJ, Leon AS. A simultaneous evaluation of 10 commonly used physical activity questionnaires. *Med Sci Sports Exerc.* 1993;25(1):81–91.

Reprinted with permission from Stephens, J., et al. (2017). Smartphone technology and text messaging for weight loss in young adults: A randomized clinical trial. *Journal of Cardiovascular Nursing, 32,* 39–46.

17. Kirkpatrick SI, Subar AF, Douglass D, et al. Performance of the Automated Self-Administered 24-hour Recall relative to a measure of true intakes and to an interviewer-administered 24-h recall. *Am J Clin Nutr.* 2014;100(1):233–240.

18. Schouwstra SJ. The Nutrition Efficacy Scale: development and construct validation using the deductive design. *UvA-Dare.* 2014;7:78–117.

19. Wilson M, Allen DD, Li JC. Improving measurement in health education and health behavior research using item response modeling: comparison with the classical test theory approach. *Health Educ Res.* 2006;21(suppl 1):i19–i32.

20. US Department of Health and Human Services. Physical activity guidelines for Americans, 2008. http://health.gov/paguidelines. Accessed April 20, 2015.

21. Glanz K, Rimer BK, Viswanath K. *Health Behavior and Health Education.* 4th ed. San Francisco, CA: Jossey-Bass; 2008.

22. Allen JK, Stephens J, Dennison Himmelfarb CR, Stewart KJ, Hauck S. Randomized controlled pilot study testing use of smartphone technology for obesity treatment. In: *J Obes,* vol. 2013;2013:151597.

23. Zuercher JL. *Developing Strategies for Helping Women Improve Weight-Related Health Behaviors.* Chapel Hill, NC: University of North Carolina at Chapel Hill; 2009.

24. Hebden L, Cook A, van der Ploeg HP, King L, Bauman A, Allman-Farinelli M. A mobile health intervention for weight management among young adults: a pilot randomized controlled trial. *J Hum Nutr Diet.* 2014;27(4):322–332.

25. Bruce MA, Beech BM, Thorpe RJ Jr, Griffith DM. Racial disparities in sugar-sweetened beverage consumption change efficacy among male first-year college students [published online ahead of print August 15, 2015]. In: *Am J Mens Health.* pii:1557988315599825.

26. Choi JY, Chang AK, Choi EJ. Sex differences in social cognitive factors and physical activity in Korean college students. *J Phys Ther Sci.* 2015;27(6):1659–1664.

Reprinted with permission from Stephens, J., et al. (2017). Smartphone technology and text messaging for weight loss in young adults: A randomized clinical trial. *Journal of Cardiovascular Nursing, 32,* 39–46.

An Ethnography of Parents' Perceptions of Patient Safety in the Neonatal Intensive Care Unit

Madelene J. Ottosen, PhD, MSN, RN; Joan Engebretson, DrPH, AHN-BC, RN, FAAN;
Jason Etchegaray, PhD; Cody Arnold, MD, MS; Eric J. Thomas, MD, MPH

ABSTRACT
Background: Parents of neonates are integral components of patient safety in the neonatal intensive care unit (NICU), yet their views are often not considered. By understanding how parents perceive patient safety in the NICU, clinicians can identify appropriate parent-centered strategies to involve them in promoting safe care for their infants.
Purpose: To determine how parents of neonates conceptualize patient safety in the NICU.
Methods: We conducted qualitative interviews with 22 English-speaking parents of neonates from the NICU and observations of various parent interactions within the NICU over several months. Data were analyzed using thematic content analysis. Findings were critically reviewed through peer debriefing.
Findings: Parents perceived safe care through their observations of clinicians being present, intentional, and respectful when adhering to safety practices, interacting with their infant, and communicating with parents in the NICU. They described partnering with clinicians to promote safe care for their infants and factors impacting that partnership. We cultivated a conceptual model highlighting how parent-clinician partnerships can be a core element to promoting NICU patient safety.
Implications for Practice: Parents' observations of clinician behavior affect their perceptions of safe care for their infants. Assessing what parents observe can be essential to building a partnership of trust between clinicians and parents and promoting safer care in the NICU.
Implications for Research: Uncertainty remains about how to measure parent perceptions of safe care, the level at which the clinician-parent partnership affects patient safety, and whether parents' presence and involvement with their infants in the NICU improve patient safety.
Key Words: neonatal intensive care, parent engagement, parent roles, partnership, patient safety

BACKGROUND AND SIGNIFICANCE

The unique complexities of the neonatal intensive care unit (NICU) environment can pose threats to

Author Affiliations: *Department of Research, Cizik School of Nursing, The University of Texas Health Science Center at Houston (Drs Ottosen and Engebretson); Senior Biobehavioral Scientist, RAND Corporation, Santa Monica, California (Dr Etchegaray); Department of Neonatology, McGovern Medical School, The University of Texas Health Science Center at Houston (Dr Arnold); and Department of Internal Medicine, The University of Texas-Memorial Hermann Center for Healthcare Quality and Safety, McGovern Medical School, The University of Texas Health Science Center at Houston (Dr Thomas).*

This research was supported in part through a grant from the Agency for Healthcare Research and Quality, R03HS022944, Parent perceptions in NICU safety culture: Parent-Centered Safety Culture Tool, and a grant from the Agency for Healthcare Research and Quality, 1P30HS024459-01, caregiver innovations to reduce harm in neonatal intensive care.

No conflicts of interest exist for any of the coauthors.

Supplemental digital content is available for this article. Direct URL citation appears in the printed text and is provided in the HTML and PDF versions of this article on the journal's Web site (www.advancesinneonatalcare.org).

Correspondence: *Madelene J. Ottosen, PhD, MSN, RN, Cizik School of Nursing, The University of Texas Health Science Center at Houston, 6901 Bertner Ave, Ste #567E, Houston, TX 77030 (Madelene.j.ottosen@uth.tmc.edu).*

DOI: 10.1097/ANC.0000000000000657

patient safety.[1,2] Medical errors, adverse events, and preventable harms are higher in neonates than full-term infants involving as many as 74 events per 100 hospitalized infants within NICUs.[2,3] Strategies to address these errors in the NICU include teamwork and leadership training, improved order-entry processes for providers, and development of reliable measures evaluating the culture of patient safety.[1,2] Building and evaluating a culture of patient safety involve understanding the shared knowledge, attitudes, perceptions, behaviors, and beliefs of the individuals and groups within an organization.[4] Assessments of these dimensions are often obtained solely from clinicians and staff members of the healthcare team.[5] Within the NICU, parents constitute an integral component of patient safety culture, yet their views are often not considered.

Increasingly, healthcare systems are involving patients and families as partners, not just recipients of healthcare.[6] Parents' and caregivers' values and beliefs sometimes differ from those of clinicians regarding the care of infants in the NICU[7]; thus, engaging as partners with the healthcare team can be challenging for parents. Parents often struggle

123

with anxiety, stress, depression, confusion, and difficulty coping, and sometimes hide behind feelings of uncertainty.[8,9] While parents desire to be involved in their infants' care, they are often unsure how to be effective parents in the NICU environment.[8] By gaining a better understanding of how parents experience the culture of the NICU, providers can identify appropriate parent-centered strategies to involve them as partners in care. Similarly, determining parents' perceptions about patient safety can help healthcare providers understand how to engage them in safety promotion activities that parents find meaningful and appropriate. Patient safety is defined as "the freedom from accidental or preventable injury produced by healthcare as well as the practices that create a safe environment of care."[10] The Agency for Healthcare Research and Quality identified a major gap in understanding how patients and families want to be engaged in patient safety and cited the need for patient and family input in assessing patient safety within healthcare environments.[11] Therefore, understanding how parents of neonates perceive patient safety and how they conceptualize their role in supporting patient safety in the NICU is both timely and necessary. The aims of this study were to determine how parents of neonates conceptualize patient safety within the NICU and how they perceive their roles in contributing to the safe care of their infants in the NICU. The purpose of this article is to describe a conceptual model derived from the findings that depicts the how parents conceptualize patient safety and how they see their role as safety advocates in the NICU setting.

> ## What This Study Adds
> - Parents as partners of NICU patient safety conceptual model.
> - Identified patient safety behaviors important to parents of neonates in the NICU including how clinicians adhere to safety practices, communicate with parents about their infants, and interact with infants in the NICU.
> - Caregiver presence, intention, and respect are key concepts in building parent-clinician partnerships.

METHODS

Design

Using a medically focused ethnographic approach,[12] we conducted interviews and field observations to understand NICU parents' views and practices related to patient safety. Ethnography involves the study of culture or the beliefs, values, behaviors, and language of a group of people to understand how they assign meaning to the cultural norms and behaviors within an environment.[12,13] This method is particularly important in understanding the relationship between differing "cultural systems," such as clinicians and patients.[12-15]

Setting

This study was conducted in a 128-bed level IV NICU within a large academic hospital in Texas that serves as a regional neonatal care center for high-risk neonates, admitting 1200 infants annually, and is staffed by more than 350 specialty clinicians, including physicians, nurses, respiratory therapists, nutritionists, and pharmacists. The NICU comprises 2 distinct units, a level III-IV unit with 8 open pods of 8 to 10 infant beds on 1 floor and a level II unit with 6 pods of 8 private rooms on the floor above.

Procedures

The study was approved by The University of Texas Health Science Center at Houston Committee for the Protection of Human Subjects. Participants received a copy of the signed consent document and a $50 gift card for participating. We obtained a purposive sampling of participants and field observations representing NICU cultural norms, environment, and participant characteristics.[15-17] Field observations were conducted across day and night shifts, on weekdays, and weekends to witness parent interactions during rounds, with clinicians, while at their infant's bedside, and during educational sessions. Participants were identified during field observations and in consultation with nurse clinicians who identified parents who were present in the NICU regularly and comfortable speaking up about issues with their infants. Parents were invited to participate while they were in the NICU by the lead author who described the purpose, procedures, risks and benefits, and voluntary nature of study participation. If they agreed, parents were given the option of when and where they would like to be interviewed and whether they preferred to be interviewed one-on-one, with their partner, or with another parent. Most parents chose to be interviewed with their partner in a separate conference room adjacent to the NICU.

Sampling Selection

Parents were purposively selected to match the age, ethnicity, parity, and infant's gestational age representative of the parents in the NICU. Parents were eligible to participate if their primary language was English and if their infants were considered stable and had been in the NICU for at least 3 weeks. Three parents of infants who graduated from the NICU 2 years prior agreed to participate as a NICU parent advisory board. These parents participated in a group interview for this study and provided feedback on the development of the interview guide.

Reprinted with permission from Ottosen, M., et al. (2019). An ethnography of parents' perceptions of patient safety in the neonatal intensive care unit. *Advances in Neonatal Care, 19*, 500–508.

Participants were enrolled until saturation in the depth and breadth of the interview content was reached, as evidenced by redundancy in the thematic content of responses.[17,18]

Field Observations

Concurrent with the interview period (January to November 2014), field observations in the NICU were conducted across all shifts and days to observe encounters of parents interacting and communicating with their infants, their families, NICU clinicians, and other parents, and NICU staff interacting and communicating with and about parents and families of neonatal infants. These observations included any parent or staff interaction not just of the participants involved in interviews. Notes of field observations and informal conversations were collected by lead author and provided relevant contextual information and exemplars that were used during data collection and incorporated into the analysis.[19]

Interviews

Parents chose to be interviewed one-on-one, with their partner, or in a group with 1 to 2 other parents. Interviews were conducted with parents in the NICU by lead author using a semistructured interview guide (see Supplemental Digital Content Appendix A, available at: http://links.lww.com/ANC/A51) developed in consultation with the other coauthors to address the themes and topics of interest. Three NICU clinicians (2 neonatologists and 1 neonatal nursing director) and the NICU parent advisory board reviewed the interview guide to ensure that the questions were clinically relevant and in language comfortable to parents. During this process, parents stated that the term "safe care" was preferable to the term "patient safety," so it was used in the interviews. Interview questions were open-ended and asked parents to describe their overall experience in the NICU, their perceptions of their interaction and communications with the NICU team, their involvement as parents in the NICU, and how they view overall safety in the NICU. Interviews were digitally recorded, transcribed into Word documents, and downloaded to a secure password-protected network drive along with field notes.

Data Analysis

Analysis involved organizing, connecting, and corroborating or legitimating the data in an iterative process that culminated in an accurate representation of the participants' accounts.[19-21] Throughout data collection, we verified and clarified the interpretations of the participants' comments and behaviors during interviews and informal conversations. We analyzed transcripts of interviews and field notes using a qualitative data management system, ATLAS.ti software GmbH (v. 7; Berlin, Germany), in which we applied codes to quotations, phrases, and observations to represent the meaning expressed. Codes are "short phrases or words which assign summative, salient, essence-capturing attributes for a portion of language-based or visual data."[21] The lead author initially coded the data and reviewed the codes with 2 coauthors to reach consensus on interpreted findings. Thematic results and exemplars were presented by lead author at a peer debriefing of 4 nurse colleagues with NICU and/or qualitative experience to validate the congruency and clarity of the data supporting the findings.[13]

RESULTS

More than 150 hours of observations and informal conversations with parents of neonates and clinical staff were conducted in the NICU in addition to individual or group interviews with 22 parents of NICU infants. Three parents declined interviews due to time constraints. Parent participants reflected the diversity and overall demographics of parents in this NICU (Table 1).

TABLE 1. Demographics of Parent Informants (N = 22)	
Category	n (%)
Gender	
Female	18 (82%)
Male	4 (18%)
Marital status	
Married	15 (68%)
Single	7 (32%)
Age, y	
18-30	10 (45%)
31-45	12 (55%)
Race	
African American	9 (41%)
Hispanic	6 (27%)
White	3 (14%)
Asian/Pacific Islander	2 (9%)
Other	2 (9%)
Parity of mother (n = 18)[a]	
1 live birth	11 (61%)[a]
2 live births	7 (38%)[a]
4 live births	1 (0.10%)[a]
	Mean (Range)
Infant's gestational age at birth, wk	27.3 (22-37)
Infant's length of stay at interview, d	105 (21-365)
[a]Based on number of deliveries represented n = 18	

Reprinted with permission from Ottosen, M., et al. (2019). An ethnography of parents' perceptions of patient safety in the neonatal intensive care unit. *Advances in Neonatal Care, 19,* 500–508.

Parents as Partners With Clinicians to Promote Safe Care

Central to parents' perceptions of safety was their desire to feel engaged with clinicians in promoting safe care for their infants. Their perception of engagement was precipitated by clinicians being present, intentional, and respectful while communicating with them, interacting with their infant, and adhering to practices of safe care in the NICU. Presence was described by parents as having clinicians especially bedside nurses watching the infants and aware of their needs,

> the fact that they're very responsive and very aware and observant. Those are all things that make you feel comfortable and That made me feel good, but even though the nurses are in charge of other babies, they're still always looking out to see what they can do and what, how they can help.

Intentional was described as focused attention in performing duties, "The ones (nurses) that have true passion are the ones... that stay focused on what they're doing. Finish that up before they try to do anything else." Respect was described as being treated as important, listening to parents' concerns, and responding to them, "For me it was more of him (doctor) stopping, taking the time, not acting rushed or like he had more important things to do. He genuinely seemed concerned and genuinely wanted to answer our questions."

Parents of neonates in our study recognized specific parenting roles for protecting their infants, which they believed they shared with clinicians. From the data, these roles were described as Caregiver, Guardian, Advocate, Decision maker, and Learner. Definitions and exemplars for each role are listed in Table 2. Parents were aware that clinicians were primarily responsible for these roles during the initial phases of their infant's care in the NICU. However, as a strong partnership between clinicians and parents formed and their infants progressed, these parents recognized their need to assume more responsibility to protect and care for their infant. As 1 mother of a very preterm infant stated,

> I'm the mom. I have to take care of the baby. Just like, if you have kids, they don't necessarily have to be in the NICU, but if something's wrong, you're going to fix it, or at least try. And so that's the same situation ... we have to look at it, not—like, these are professionals and I have to take a backseat to what they say. You know, because at the end of the day, this is your child and so you have to just treat it that way.

Parents required varying degrees of time and support to gain confidence in these roles. One mother sought the help of a counselor to help her cope with her parental role in the NICU,

> At the beginning, it's surreal ... you never know the NICU until you actually live in it. And then overtime, it becomes—it's familiar. And so I think the best thing is for them (parents of neonates) to be involved. And like my counselor told me to be an advocate. Like, stay involved and know everything that's going on, and everything that's happening.

TABLE 2. Definitions and Exemplars of Parent Roles to Promote Safe Care

Role	Definition	Exemplar
Advocate	Speak up for my infant's needs to the healthcare team in the NICU.	"It definitely is frustrating when a nurse is trying to tell you something different. And **I'm trying to educate you about my baby** so I can leave and be comfortable."
Caregiver	Recognize and provide the activities of care that my infant needs.	"Once they get into the crib, there are certain milestones that they have to hit before we take them upstairs. And then we'll get a chance to interact with the babies a little bit more, **get used to being around them and identifying what their needs are.** So when we get them home it'll be, you know, easier."
Decision maker	Help make decisions about my infant's care.	"(Mom was told) We're gonna go through the weekend and if it's still bad by Monday, we'll give her the medicine." And my thing was why? Why are we waiting until Monday? It's not like it's going to change. **This is something you already know, so let's just be proactive. So I don't want to wait until Monday.**
Guardian	Protect my infant from uncertain harms and ensure he or she is in a safe environment.	"**You (as the mom) want to know** who's coming in the room, who's going to touch him, or if somebody's looking at him, like who are you? Who you with?"
Learner	Learn how to provide individualized care for my infant's needs.	"**My responsibilities while I'm in here, basically just to try my best to know her needs.** So when I go home, her needs—her concern—what to look for—what not to look for .... I tell nurses all the time, **What you tell me (about my baby) is gold.**"

Reprinted with permission from Ottosen, M., et al. (2019). An ethnography of parents' perceptions of patient safety in the neonatal intensive care unit. *Advances in Neonatal Care, 19*, 500–508.

Contributing Factors to Parent-Clinician Partnership

Several individual and unit "contributing factors" (see Figure 1) emerged throughout the data that influenced the partnerships between parents and clinicians in promoting safe care. Examples of individual factors affecting parent participation in the NICU included their emotional recovery from delivery, having other children at home, and having to return to work. One mother, who lives 8 hours from the NICU, states, "just being separated from my husband…. It's a lot of issues, I guess, and factors for me, you know, being a parent of a child in the NICU." Individual factors impacting clinician participation with parents involved clinician attitudes about and toward the parents' role in the NICU. A parent, struggling with depression because of the multiple surgical procedures of her extremely low birth-weight infant, felt overwhelmed by seeing her infant in the NICU. She called the unit for an update and overheard the nurse say,

> the mom is right here at (one of the parent rooms). I don't understand why she doesn't just come over here and check on her and…this poor girl (infant), they only come in and see her for, like, five minutes and they leave.

Unfortunately, overhearing these words left this mother feeling more distressed and less willing to engage with her clinicians.

Unit factors also impact the parent-clinician partnership such as the transitions in care that occur with rotating clinicians and movement of infants within the unit, varying communication practices used by clinicians, and the type of teamwork among clinicians. These factors influence the formation of the clinician-parent partnership, parents' perceptions of clinicians' safety promotion behaviors, and parents' adoption of roles to promote safe care throughout the NICU experience.

Parent-Perceived Safety Behaviors Exhibited by NICU Staff

These parents perceived their infant's care as safe when observing NICU clinicians performing 3 types of behaviors: (1) adherence to safety and infection control practices, (2) interactions with their infant, and (3) communication with parents. Parents described the importance of clinicians/staff who were present to them and their infants, intentional in their actions, and respectful toward parents and infants while performing these behaviors.

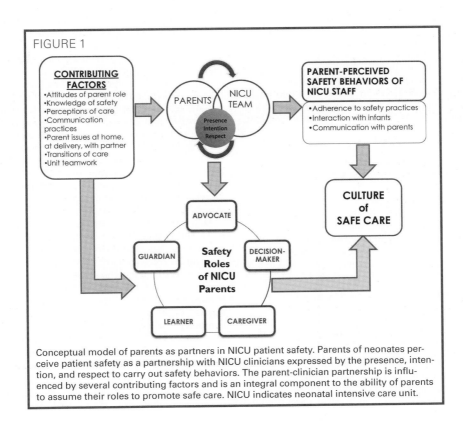

FIGURE 1

Conceptual model of parents as partners in NICU patient safety. Parents of neonates perceive patient safety as a partnership with NICU clinicians expressed by the presence, intention, and respect to carry out safety behaviors. The parent-clinician partnership is influenced by several contributing factors and is an integral component to the ability of parents to assume their roles to promote safe care. NICU indicates neonatal intensive care unit.

Reprinted with permission from Ottosen, M., et al. (2019). An ethnography of parents' perceptions of patient safety in the neonatal intensive care unit. *Advances in Neonatal Care, 19*, 500–508.

Adherence to Safety Practices

When asked about patient safety in the NICU, parents first described the security procedures to enter the unit. Having someone present at the front desk at all times strictly adhering to visitation policies assured parents that their infant was safe when they left the NICU. Being able to authorize the persons who were allowed to see their infant in the NICU gave parents added feelings of security, as 1 parent expressed, "Because you hear so much on the news nowadays where people come in and try to take babies … when I leave here, I feel safe and secure that (baby) is secure."

Parents were comforted when observing clinicians intently following safety procedures and routines that stressed infection control, such as handwashing, using bedside hand sanitizers, wearing gloves during procedures, keeping the environment and equipment clean around the infants, and making sure that visitors—including the parents themselves—were free from illness. Even rules about who could visit were important to parents, one of whom noted, "They eliminated multiple visitors for a little bit here whenever the RSV (Respiratory Syncytial Virus) and all that stuff was going around real bad …. Yes, that did make me feel safe and feel better."

Conversely, parents felt that safety was threatened when they witnessed unit practices that seemed incongruent with infection control procedures. A parent described her concern over a new infant admitted to the middle of the NICU pod. Red tape had been placed on the floor in a 3- to 4-ft perimeter around the infant's isolette. While respecting another family's right to privacy about their infant's condition, a parent of an infant in the same pod of the NICU expressed uncertainty whether the safety measures taken would adequately protect her infant:

> They have like the biohazard things you put stuff in, this and … all kinds of little stuff so I'm just thinking like if they have all of that, then that baby shouldn't be in the middle...of the (other) kids.

Interactions With Infants

Most parents also described safe care as the presence of a nurse watching over their infant, quickly and intentionally responding to emergent needs, and respectfully interacting with their infant as a parent would interact (ie, in the same manner as that exhibited by a parent). One parent reflected,

> They still keep a close eye on him even when I'm there with him …. And because they know the baby very well … it's like me being there. And so they told the doctors, 'Well, I don't think he likes this' and stuff like that. And it's the same thing I think.

Parents felt safe knowing that nurses were physically present in the unit, near their infant, to respond to their physical and comfort needs, especially when they could not be in the unit. Most parents could give examples of when nurses responded quickly to emergencies with their infant or other infants in the NICU. They felt confident when clinicians calmly responded to emergencies and worked as a team, often surprised at the number of clinicians responding to assist. Parents were sensitive to the intention of the nurse when interacting with their infant. It was important to parents to see nurses respond to alarms after having looked at their infant first and not just silencing alarms. One parent noted,

> I've seen them … if the heart rate is going up or down, they'll stand … there for a while and see if it will change. And if not, then they'll go in and stimulate the baby …. I mean, just like that example of my son. He was already extubated. But if the nurse had not paid attention to his desatting and just turned him up and didn't hear him—he was crying—he had a voice—she would not be able to intervene in time.

Seeing nurses interacting with their infants in a personal way by talking to them, patting them, and treating them like their own infants made parents feel safe. This parent described, "I love that they talk to him and not just go in there and startle him and then just do what they have to do. He's a little person, okay?" Another parent stated, "Even though he was in the hospital and those nurses (were) paid to take good care of those babies, I felt like, there is another mom for him there that was not me … I love that."

When asked about issues of unsafe care, many parents found it difficult to relay any negative issues and instead responded with compliments for the care their infants received in the NICU. A few parents stated that they "never felt unsafe" or "saw anything that made (them) question the safety of (their) child." Parents felt that their infants were safer with the nurses they had developed a relationship with or chosen to be primary nurses for their infant. After being in the NICU for several weeks, parents learned from the staff that they could choose the nurse(s) they were most comfortable with to be the primary nurse(s). Parents felt a connection with their nurses based on how the nurses interacted with their infant, especially during the most critical times of their care.

Despite their overall contentment with care, when given time to think, most parents could recall at least 1 situation that gave them concern about the care their infant received. Parents were concerned when they observed nurses who seemed inattentive to the needs of the infants, even if the inattention was toward another infant. Parents also felt unsafe when nurses appeared more concerned with completing computer work or were preoccupied with admitting an infant to the NICU rather than responding to the immediate needs of their infant. A parent cited her concerns upon a new admission,

> Didn't you notice that when they're admitting someone, they don't handle … like, this alarm had been going off for two minutes already, and nobody

Reprinted with permission from Ottosen, M., et al. (2019). An ethnography of parents' perceptions of patient safety in the neonatal intensive care unit. *Advances in Neonatal Care, 19*, 500–508.

would pay attention? When the pod is full, it's good because there won't be any admissions. But if it's not, and there's an admission, I'm concerned for my baby.

Communication With Parents

The types and manner of communication that parents experienced with clinicians were an important aspect of safety. Parents appreciated clinicians inviting them to rounds, asking about their preferences in their infant's care, and getting their feedback about their infant's responses to care. Regular and honest information from clinicians about what would take place, why, and what to expect, even if by phone, made parents feel more like partners. Even when adverse events occurred, such as when an infant whose parents were Jehovah's Witness received a blood transfusion without the parents' permission, parents felt respected by clinicians intentionally providing an environment for them to verbalize their concerns and being responsive in planning how to prevent future occurrences. Another parent echoed the importance of staff nurses intentionally encouraging her to speak up when her child experienced a delay in treatment,

> They gave us that background and made us feel comfortable the first few weeks in the NICU. So even though it was uncomfortable talking about a negative incident, it was easier to do so with that kind of network in place.

Parents were not always confident raising concerns, but when they did speak up, they felt reassured when the staff addressed their concerns,

> So I asked the nurse, "Is it normal for him, for his head to be like this and his body to be kind of slightly turned?" She (the nurse) said, "No, let me turn him completely so he can breathe a little bit better." And she (the nurse) went over and adjusted his little breathing thing, and he was good to go.

Parents were concerned about safety when they experienced or heard about clinicians who did not respect the warnings raised by them or other parents. A parent gave this example:

> I did speak to a mom ... scheduled to go home on a Sunday, and Saturday her baby was crying and crying and crying, and she asked the nurse, "You know what's wrong with him?" And she (the day shift nurse) was like, "Oh, you know, babies cry." And she went to her baby, and said, "No, because he never just cries like this."... then she said the night shift nurse came, and she said, "Something's wrong with him. He's crying." And I think they called someone and did an x-ray. They came to find out he had NEC (necrotizing enterocolitis).

A Conceptual Model of Parents as Partners in Patient Safety in the NICU

These findings led to construction of a conceptual model that highlights the importance of clinician behaviors in forming parents' perceptions of safe care in the NICU, how these behaviors influence parent-clinician partnerships, and how parents interpret and participate in promoting patient safety in the NICU (see Figure 1). This model posits that a positive neonatal patient safety culture is achieved through effective clinician-parent partnerships, which develop over time through mutual respect, intention, and presence and a shared commitment to adopt behaviors of safe care. Parents in our study perceived patient safety in the NICU through their observations of clinicians' behaviors adhering to safety practices, communicating with them, and interacting with their infants. We contend that parents share roles with clinicians in promoting safe care that are modeled and empowered through the partnership they develop with clinicians.

To determine whether the model resonated with parents of neonates, we presented and discussed the findings of this conceptual model to 6 members of the study site's NICU parent advisory council. These parents agreed that the model was congruent with their perceptions of clinicians' behaviors to support patient safety, the types of roles they experienced as parents in the NICU, and the dynamic of a parent-clinician partnership to achieve safe care in the NICU.

DISCUSSION

Parents of neonates perceive safe care through the actions of clinicians and want to be involved as partners in promoting safe care for their infants in the NICU. Parents identified positive and negative instances of communications with clinicians or interactions with their infant, which led to their overall perceptions of safe care. Engaging parents to share concerns about what they observe signals an intentional and respectful desire to collaborate or partner with parents in caring for their infant. Parent-clinician partnerships employ the clinician's expertise while maintaining the unique role of the parents in advocating for their infant. When clinicians intentionally responded to infants' needs and were respectful to parent input, parents felt more confident caring for their infant and more comfortable reporting issues of concern.

Parents were astute in identifying breaches of safety, mistakes, and problems in care. Previous studies have shown that a lack of teamwork and poor communication are often causes of reported adverse events in the NICU.[22] Given the number of clinicians involved in caring for NICU infants, the parents remain the one constant caregiver at the bedside. Listening to parents' concerns, engaging them in decisions about their infant's care, and asking for their feedback[23] are ways bedside clinicians can engage parents to promote safer care in the NICU. In addition, by debriefing with parents after adverse

Reprinted with permission from Ottosen, M., et al. (2019). An ethnography of parents' perceptions of patient safety in the neonatal intensive care unit. *Advances in Neonatal Care, 19*, 500–508.

events, we can learn how to calm anxiety and better support parents to prevent and heal from unexpected events such as unplanned extubations.

When parents are uncomfortable communicating with clinicians about their infant or unable to be present or interact with their infant regularly, clinicians need to respectfully seek understanding of the circumstances that NICU parents may be experiencing. As seen in our sample, feelings of guilt, inability to cope, or fear of uncertainty may preclude parents from participating in their roles as parents.[8] Parents may also struggle to speak up about concerns when they perceive dissonance between their trust of the clinicians caring for their infant and observances of problems in their infant's care or how their communication will be perceived by clinicians.[24] Building open and transparent relationships between clinicians and parents consisting of mutual trust and respect is an important step toward developing a culture of safety in the NICU.

Our findings compliment and expand the limited number of qualitative studies describing parent perceptions of patient safety. In a study by Lyndon et al,[25] parents of infants in the NICU described the importance of clinicians "watching over my baby" as a central to their views of patient safety. Participants described concern over the skill level of new nurses, nurses' availability to hold or feed their infant, and nurses' unfamiliarity with their infant.[25] In our sample, parents viewed clinicians' presence and intention in caring for their infant as central to patient safety and raised similar concerns when bedside nurses seemed unskilled or unfamiliar with their infant. Mazor et al[23] reported that parents perceived errors in the care of their children when clinicians did not listen to their concerns about their children or did not pay close enough attention to their children's problems. The value parents place on skilled nurses being present with their infants and having intentional and respectful communication with clinicians to promote safe care is evident. These findings expand our knowledge about parents' perceptions of safety by including an ethnically diverse population of parents and proposing that an effective partnership between clinicians and parents is essential to promote safe care for infants in the NICU.

The clinician-parent partnership is based on the concepts of presence, intention, and respect, described as integral components to the nurse-patient relationship, central to Jean Watson's Theory of Human Caring.[26] The caring relationship includes, in part, respect for the person, defined as "honoring his/her needs, wishes, routines and rituals," having "authentic presence defined as honoring/connecting human to human," and "intention for doing for another and being with another who is in need."[26] We further define intention as purposeful attention leading to an action or behavior. Further exploration of these concepts is needed within the context of safety culture.

This study had several strengths and limitations. A primary strength was the ethnic diversity of our parent population, with 68% of parents classified as African American or Hispanic. The study was

Summary of Recommendations for Practice and Research	
What we know:	• Parents of neonates view safety through the behaviors of clinicians, adherence to safety practices, communication with parents, and interaction with their infants.
	• Parents form a partnership with clinicians supported by mutual presence, intention, and respect in their behaviors to promote patient safety over time.
	• As the partnership and their experience in the NICU develop, parents assume specific roles in promoting patient safety.
What needs to be studied:	• Measures of parent perceptions of patient safety in the NICU.
	• The influence of partnerships or relationships between parents and clinicians on NICU patient safety culture.
	• Relationship of parents' presence and involvement with their infants in the NICU on patient safety.
	• Differences in maternal and paternal observations and contributions in promoting patient safety
What we can do today:	• NICU clinicians should ask parents to share their concerns about their infant's care.
	• Bedside nurses need to listen and respond intentionally and respectfully to parent input.
	• Empower parents to activate their parental roles in the NICU as soon as possible.
	• Mentor clinician colleagues to perform effective communication strategies with parents.

Reprinted with permission from Ottosen, M., et al. (2019). An ethnography of parents' perceptions of patient safety in the neonatal intensive care unit. *Advances in Neonatal Care, 19*, 500–508.

limited in several ways. First, we excluded non–English-speaking parents owing to language limitations of the investigator and the lack of translators and therefore do not have their perspectives. Second, since excluded parents of infants spending less than 3 weeks in the NICU, we did not capture the perceptions of parents with less time in the NICU. Third, we obtained these findings from parents in a single NICU within a large academic institution. Previous studies have shown a wide variation in safety culture across NICUs[21]; therefore, parents in smaller, community-based NICUs may have different perceptions. Despite the limitations, these findings may be applicable to other settings and situations. We recommend replication studies be conducted with parents in other NICUs to continue to refine this emerging conceptual model.

Given this model, additional research questions remain, such as whether differences in safety culture across NICUs are related to differences in the level of partnerships between parents and clinicians and how to measure parents' perceptions of safe care in the NICU. Likewise, it is uncertain whether parents' presence and involvement with their infants in the NICU or their ability to enact their parental roles affects their infant's patient safety. It is also unclear whether fathers and mothers view patient safety initiatives differently. Fathers often perceive barriers being involved with their infant in the NICU,[27] yet when allowed to provide skin-to-skin contact or feed their infants in the NICU, they increase bonding with their infant.[28] Fathers or parent partners may play an integral role in patient safety during the initial NICU period when mothers are still recovering from delivery and less able to be present with their infants. Understanding the complexities parents of neonates face being present with their infants throughout the NICU hospitalization may illuminate important care strategies and health policy considerations, such as improved family leave policies and/or additional compensation to aid in childcare of siblings.

These findings pose important clinical implications. Assessing what parents observe can be essential to building a partnership of trust between clinicians and parents and promoting safer NICU care. Neonatal intensive care unit clinicians should ask parents to share their concerns, listen and respond intentionally and respectfully to parent input, empower parents to activate their parental roles in the NICU as soon as possible, and mentor clinician colleagues in effective communication strategies with parents. These actions would alleviate parents' fears and concerns and empower parents to be integral partners in promoting safe care for their infants. In conclusion, creating a normative culture whereby all clinicians are able to engage with parents of neonates as partners in patient safety may be the essential goal for achieving safe care in the NICU.

References

1. Raju T, Suresh G, Higgins R. Patient safety in the context of neonatal intensive care: research and educational opportunities. *Pediatr Res.* 2011;70:109-115.
2. Samra H, McGrath J, Rollins W. Patient safety in the NICU: a comprehensive review. *J Perinat Neonatal Nurs.* 2011;25:123-132.
3. Sharek PJ, Horbar JD, Mason W, et al. Adverse events in the neonatal intensive care unit: development, testing, and findings of an NICU–focused trigger tool to identify harm in North American NICUs. *Pediatrics.* 2006;118:1332-1340.
4. Sexton JB, Helmreich RL, Neilands TB, et al. The Safety Attitudes Questionnaire: psychometric properties, benchmarking data, and emerging research. *BMC Health Serv Res.* 2006;6:44.
5. Sammer CE, Lykens K, Singh KP, Mains DA, Lackan NA. What is patient safety culture? A review of the literature. *J Nurs Scholarsh.* 2010;42:156-165.
6. Conway J, Johnson B, Edgman-Levitan S, et al. *Partnering With Patients and Families to Design a Patient- and Family–Centered Health Care System: A Roadmap for the Future.* Boston, MA: Institute for Healthcare Improvement; 2006. http://www.ihi.org/resources/Pages/Publications/PartneringwithPatientsandFamilies.aspx. Accessed March 1, 2015.
7. Latour JM, Hazelzet JA, Duivenvoorden HJ, Goudoever JB. Perceptions of parents, nurses, and physicians on neonatal intensive care practices. *J Pediatr.* 2010;157:1-18.
8. Ricciardelli R. Unconditional love in the neonatal intensive care unit. *J Neonatal Nurs.* 2012;18;94-97.
9. Weiss S, Goldlust E, Vaucher YE. Improving parent satisfaction: an intervention to increase neonatal parent-provider communication. *J Perinatol.* 2010;30:425-430.
10. Agency for Healthcare Research and Quality. *Funding Opportunity Announcement Guidance.* Rockville, MD: Agency for Healthcare Research and Quality; 2019. https://www.ahrq.gov/funding/policies/foaguidance/index.html. Accessed February 2, 2019.
11. Carmen KL, Dardess P, Maurer M, et al. Patient and family engagement: a framework for understanding the elements and developing interventions and policies. *Health Aff (Millwood).* 2013;32:223-231.
12. Engebretson J. Clinically applied medical ethnography: relevance to cultural competence in patient care. *Nurs Clin North Am.* 2011;46(2):145-154.
13. Green J, Thorogood N. *Qualitative Methods for Health Research.* 3rd ed. Thousand Oaks, CA: Sage Publications; 2013.
14. Chrisman N, Johnson T. Clinically applied anthropology. In: *Handbook of Medical Anthropology: Contemporary Theory and Method.* New York, NY: Praeger Publishers; 1990.
15. Miller WL, Crabtree BF. Clinical research: a multimethod typology. In: Crabtree B, Miller WL, eds. *Doing Qualitative Research.* 2nd ed. Thousand Oaks, CA: Sage Publications; 1999.
16. Mayan MJ. *Essentials of Qualitative Inquiry.* Walnut Creek, CA: Left Coast Press; 2009.
17. Kuzel AJ. Sampling in qualitative inquiry. In: Crabtree B, Miller WL, eds. *Doing Qualitative Research.* 2nd ed. Thousand Oaks, CA: Sage Publications; 1999.
18. Richards L, Morse JM. *Readme First for a User's Guide to Qualitative Methods.* 2nd ed. Thousand Oaks, CA: Sage Publications; 2007.
19. Spradley JP. *Participant Observation.* 1st ed. Belmont, CA: Wadsworth; 1980.
20. Mason J. *Qualitative Researching.* 2nd ed. Thousand Oaks, CA: Sage Publications; 2002.
21. Saldana J. *The Coding Manual for Qualitative Researchers.* 1st ed. Thousand Oaks, CA: Sage Publications; 2012.
22. Profit J, Etchegaray J, Petersen L, et al. Neonatal intensive care unit safety culture varies widely. *Arch Dis Child Fetal Neonatal Ed.* 2012;97:120-126.
23. Mazor KM, Goff SL, Dodd KS, Velten SJ, Walsh KE. Parent perceptions of medical errors. *J Patient Saf.* 2010;6:102-107.
24. Lyndon A, Wisner K, Holschuh C, Fagan KM, Franck LS. Parents' perspectives on navigating the role of speaking up in the NICU. *J Obstet Gynecol Neonatal Nurs.* 2017;46(5):716-726.
25. Lyndon A, Jacobson CH, Fagan KM, Wisner K, Franck LS. Parents' perspectives on safety in neonatal intensive care: a mixed-methods study. *BMJ Qual Saf.* 2014;23:902-909.
26. Watson J. *Core Concepts of Jean Watson's Theory of Human Caring/Caring Science.* 2010. Boulder, CO: Watson Caring Science Institute. https://www.watsoncaringscience.org/files/PDF/watsons-theory-of-human-caring-core-concepts-and-evolution-to-caritas-processes-handout.pdf. Accessed February 2, 2019.
27. Feeley N, Waitzer E, Sherrard K, Boisvert L, Zelkowitz P. Fathers' perceptions of the barriers and facilitators to their involvement with their newborn hospitalised in the neonatal intensive care unit. *J Clin Nurs.* 2013;22:521-530.
28. Noergaard B, Ammentorp J, Garne E, Fenger-Gron J, Kofoed P. Father's stress in neonatal intensive care unit. *Adv Neonatal Care.* 2018;18(5):413-422.

Reprinted with permission from Ottosen, M., et al. (2019). An ethnography of parents' perceptions of patient safety in the neonatal intensive care unit. *Advances in Neonatal Care, 19,* 500–508.

Appendix A

INTERVIEW GUIDE (Group or Individual)

Thank you for agreeing to talk with me today. As I mentioned I will be recording this interview. I will also take notes while we talk so that if I can jot down questions or important points I want to remember.

- Tell me about your experience in the neonatal ICU, how has it been for you?

  - Tell me about what brought your baby to the NICU.
    (Include if this information is not addressed after the first question.)
  - *How long has your baby been in the NICU?*
  - *Was your baby delivered here at Memorial Hermann?*

- How would you describe the NICU to your friends and family?

- How have your views of the NICU changed over time? How are they different from when your baby was first admitted?

- What do you know or what have you heard about hospitals making the quality of care better and safer for patients?

- Are there any particular issues with patient safety that you have heard about?

  - Where have you heard it? Or where did find that information?
  - If they haven't heard of anything, mention our purpose is to identify what parents observe and experience which can impact the quality of care in the NICU. Things like the good communication, teamwork among hospital staff and doctors and consistent handwashing are ways we can improve patient care.

- We are interested in understanding what parents know about the quality and safety of the care that babies receive in the NICU. Since you have been here can you tell me what comes to mind when you think about what is done to provide good quality care and promote patient safety for the babies in the NICU.

  - Tell me about a time in the NICU when you felt the care was safe.

    - What did you observe or hear that made it seem safe?

  - Tell me about a time when you felt or heard about something that was unsafe
    - What types of things did you observe or hear that made it seem unsafe?

  - If you noticed a questionable behavior or incident what do you think you would do or what do you think other parent's might do?
    Tell me what you think would encourage parents to speak up about a questionable incident?
  - What would prevent a parent from speaking up about this type of incident?

Reprinted with permission from Ottosen, M., et al. (2019). An ethnography of parents' perceptions of patient safety in the neonatal intensive care unit. *Advances in Neonatal Care, 19*, 500–508.

- Do you know who the persons are that provide care for your baby?

  - Can you name the differing roles of the caregivers/providers that help take care of your baby?
  - Do you have a primary caregiver ie primary nurse or primary doctor responsible for your baby?

- Tell me how the hospital staff talk with you about your baby.

  - How do you think the hospital staff talk with each other in general?
  - How do you think the physicians, nurses and other healthcare providers in the NICU function as team in providing care to your baby?

- Tell me what it is like when you ask questions about your baby.
  - Are your questions answered so that you understand?
  - How do people respond?
    What are the positive responses like?
  - What are the negative responses like?
    Who provides you the best information to your questions?
  - Does everyone?

- How involved do feel in the care of your baby?

  - Tell me what your role as a parent is while your baby is in the NICU.
  - What should the role of parents be?
  - What makes that difficult?

- What thoughts or ideas to suggest how the quality of care might be better in the NICU: environment, communication among providers, communication between providers and parents?

- What would you want to tell the doctors and nurses about your child's care that would help them take better care of their patients and families in the NICU?

- How should we involve parents in learning how to improve the care of babies in the NICU?

- How would you want to share your concerns about the care your baby has received in the NICU? When would be the best time?

Thank you so much for your time. Do you have any you would like to tell me that I didn't ask you about?

Reprinted with permission from Ottosen, M., et al. (2019). An ethnography of parents' perceptions of patient safety in the neonatal intensive care unit. *Advances in Neonatal Care, 19*, 500–508.

Improving Thermoregulation for Trauma Patients in the Emergency Department: An Evidence-Based Practice Project

Ada Saqe-Rockoff, MSN, RN, AG-CNS, CEN ■ Finn D. Schubert, MPH ■ Amanda Ciardiello, RN, BSN, CEN ■ Elizabeth Douglas, RN, BSN, CCRN

ABSTRACT

Extensive evidence exists on the association between hypothermia and increased morbidity and mortality in trauma patients. Gaps in practice related to temperature assessment have been identified in literature, along with limited personnel knowledge regarding management of patients with accidental hypothermia. An interdisciplinary team identified gaps in practice in our institution regarding temperature assessment and documentation of rewarming and initiated an evidence-based practice project to change practice at our institution. The goals were to decrease time to temperature assessment, increase core temperature assessment, and increase implementation of appropriate rewarming methods. This project used the Iowa Model of Evidence-Based Practice to provide a framework for execution and evaluation. We conducted a literature review to address all aspects of hypothermia, including incidence, associated and contributing factors, prevention, recognition, and treatment. This evidence-based knowledge was then applied to clinical practice through staff education and training, equipment availability, and environmental adjustments. More patients with hypothermia and hyperthermia were identified in 2017, as compared with 2016. There was a significant increase in core temperature assessment from 4% in 2016 to 23% in 2017 ($p < .001$). Blanket use in normothermic patients increased in 2017 ($p = .002$). This project is an example of how nurses can utilize an evidence-based practice model to translate research into clinical practice. Best practice interventions regarding temperature assessment and rewarming measures for trauma patients can be successfully implemented with negligible cost. Further research should be dedicated to examine barriers to implementation and adherence to evidence-based practice interventions.

Key Words

Hypothermia, Nursing, Thermoregulation, Trauma

Unintentional injuries are the fourth highest cause of death for Americans and lead to an estimated 28.1 million visits to emergency departments (EDs) yearly (Heron, 2016). Many trauma patients are hypothermic, defined as body temperature of less than 36°C (96.8°F; Block, Lilienthal, Cullen, & White, 2012). Hypothermia has been reported in as many as two-thirds of all trauma patients, of this, 9% present with body temperatures of 33°C (91.4°F) or lower (Farkash et al., 2002).

Extensive evidence exists on the association between hypothermia and increased morbidity and mortality for trauma patients (Balvers et al., 2016; Ireland, Endacott, Cameron, Fitzgerald, & Paul, 2011; Keane, 2016; Langhelle, Lockey, Harris, & Davies, 2010; Simmons, Pittet, & Pierce, 2014; van der Ploeg, Goslings, Walpoth, & Bierens, 2010; Zafren & Mechem, 2017). Along with metabolic acidosis and coagulopathy, hypothermia is a factor in the "triad of death," a cycle that can decrease the success of resuscitation efforts (Keane, 2016; Simmons et al., 2014). Hypothermia leads to peripheral vasoconstriction, followed by lactate buildup and acidosis (Keane, 2016). In addition, hypothermia leads to a decrease in thrombin production, inhibition of fibrinogen synthesis, and impaired platelet aggregation and adhesion. These deleterious effects are seen starting at body temperatures of 36°C (96.8°F) and progressively worsen with further temperature drops (Martini, 2009; Mitrophanov, Rosendaal, & Reifman, 2013; Wolberg, Meng, Monroe, & Hoffman, 2004). Hypothermia increases risk for arrhythmias, which are frequently unresponsive to cardioactive drugs, electrical pacing, and defibrillation (Soar et al., 2010). Other associated complications include multiorgan failure, pulmonary edema, hypoglycemia, hyperkalemia, and infection (American College

Author Affiliations: Departments of Nursing (Mss Saqe-Rockoff, Ciardiello, and Douglas) and Clinical Research (Mr Schubert), NYU Langone Hospital – Brooklyn, Brooklyn, New York.

All of the authors have nothing to declare.

Correspondence: Finn D. Schubert, MPH, Clinical Research Office, NYU Langone Hospital – Brooklyn, 150 55th St, Brooklyn, NY 11220 (finn.schubert@nyumc.org).

DOI: 10.1097/JTN.0000000000000336

Reprinted with permission from Saqe-Rockoff, A., et al. (2018). Improving thermoregulation for trauma patients in the emergency department: An evidence-based practice project. *Journal of Trauma Nursing, 25*, 14–20.

of Surgeons Committee on Trauma, Simon, & Hunt, 2014; Keane, 2016; van der Ploeg et al., 2010). Large multicenter studies have identified hypothermia as a significant and independent predictor of mortality (Balvers et al., 2016; Ireland et al., 2011), making patient temperature an important modifiable risk factor in the ED for mortality among trauma patients. For example, one study found that hypothermic trauma patients who had further temperature drop in the ED had a 50% mortality versus 29.9% mortality among those who did not have further temperature drop (Ireland et al., 2011).

Fortunately, hypothermia is arguably the easiest factor of the triad of death to address (Keane, 2016). Various modalities are available for temperature assessment and detection of hypothermia, such as oral, tympanic, rectal, and bladder thermometers (van der Ploeg et al., 2010). There exist a multitude of rewarming methods with varying degrees of efficacy, including warmed intravenous fluids, warmed blankets, forced-air warming blankets, bladder irrigation, gastric irrigation, and arteriovenous bypass (Paal et al., 2016; van der Ploeg et al., 2010). Trauma nurses should be encouraged to take ownership of vital sign assessment, including early temperature evaluation (Keane, 2016), and initiate appropriate steps for rewarming. Gaps in practice related to temperature assessment have been identified in the literature, along with limited personnel knowledge regarding management of patients with accidental hypothermia (van der Ploeg et al., 2010). At our own institution, an interdisciplinary team identified gaps in practice regarding temperature assessment and documentation of rewarming and initiated an evidence-based practice (EBP) project to change practice.

METHODS

Context

NYU Langone Hospital—Brooklyn (formerly NYU Lutheran Medical Center) is a 450-bed teaching facility located in southwest Brooklyn, New York City. It is a Level I trauma center with more than 75,000 annual ED visits. In 2016, 2,383 trauma cases were evaluated at NYU Langone Hospital—Brooklyn (NYU Langone Medical Center, 2016). The year 2016 marked several milestones for NYU Langone Hospital—Brooklyn, including its first year as part of the NYU Langone Health System, and the launch of a new electronic medical record (EMR).

Approach

Our project utilized the Iowa Model of Evidence-Based Practice to provide a framework for execution and evaluation (Brown, 2014). Thermoregulation in trauma patients was a problem-focused trigger. It was determined that the trigger is of high priority to the ED and trauma program, which facilitated organizational engagement.

An interdisciplinary team formed that was charged with developing and implementing EBP change. Relevant publications were gathered and evaluated for reliability, validity, and bias. The team found sufficient research with consistent findings to warrant a practice change. The changes were piloted for a 3-month period to assess for feasibility and any improvement in outcomes.

The clinical nurse specialist (CNS) conducted a systematic search on PubMed for articles pertaining to temperature assessment, incidence, and implications of hypothermia on trauma patients, rewarming methods, and prior EBP projects on thermoregulation for trauma patients. Evidence-based practice interventions were derived from the best available clinical evidence with a focus on clinical expertise and patient values and expectations (Melnyk & Fineout-Overholt, 2014).

Block et al. (2012) developed and implemented a nurse-led, evidence-based protocol to improve temperature control in hypothermic trauma patients. The team sought to expand on its project and conduct a literature review to address all aspects including incidence of hypothermia, associated and contributing factors, prevention, recognition, and treatment. The evidence-based knowledge was then applied to clinical practice through staff education and training, equipment availability, and environmental adjustments. The project's goals were to decrease time to temperature assessment, increase core temperature assessment, and increase implementation of appropriate rewarming methods.

PRACTICE CHANGES

Warmed Blankets

Prevention of hypothermia or further heat loss in trauma patients is a primary concern. Impaired homeostasis, prehospital exposure, and resuscitation efforts can all lead to hypothermia in trauma patients (Keane, 2016). Trauma patients are also fully exposed in the early stages of assessment as part of the primary survey (Emergency Nurses Association, 2014). Warmed blankets are not adequately utilized during trauma evaluation as the team needs access to the patient for acquiring intravenous access, performing a Focused Assessment with Sonography in Trauma, and other assessments and interventions. The team encouraged the use of warm blankets for all patients when exposure was not necessary for medical interventions.

Trauma Bay Temperature

In preparation for the EBP changes, the CNS discussed with leadership from point of care, pharmacy, and central processing whether a room temperature of 80°F would negatively impact equipment and supplies located in the trauma bay. It was determined that temperature change would not disrupt normal storage and function of equipment.

Reprinted with permission from Saqe-Rockoff, A., et al. (2018). Improving thermoregulation for trauma patients in the emergency department: An evidence-based practice project. *Journal of Trauma Nursing, 25,* 14–20.

With collaboration from the engineering department, the trauma bay ambient temperature was set to the recommended 80°F (Block et al., 2012; Zafren & Mechem, 2017). Staff were educated about the importance of keeping the trauma bay doors closed at all times to maintain the temperature. In order for the trauma doors to remain closed at all times, extensive reinforcement was required with staff of all disciplines, including nursing, nursing assistants, physicians, and environmental services. Education on the importance of hypothermia prevention for the exposed, critical patient was conducted frequently through huddles. Regular reminders were provided to the staff to ensure that the trauma bay doors remained closed.

Temperature Assessment

Prior studies have shown a pervasive lack of temperature assessment in trauma patients (Block et al., 2012; Ireland et al., 2006; Langhelle et al., 2010). The use of peripheral thermometers to expedite temperature assessment has been promoted in some works (Block et al., 2012; Keane, 2016). However, a systematic review and meta-analysis found that peripheral thermometers lack clinically acceptable accuracy. Their use is discouraged when accurate body temperature measurement will influence clinical decision, such as in postoperative, injured, or critically ill patients (Niven et al., 2015). Huddles were held to raise awareness about the significance of accidental hypothermia on trauma patients. The need for patient temperature assessment on arrival was reinforced, with an emphasis on core temperature evaluation.

Appropriate Escalation of Rewarming Measures

Rewarming measures available and a clear pathway of escalation based on the patient's temperature were outlined. Nursing staff competencies for use of the rapid infuser with automatic fluid warming are maintained through yearly competency training. More invasive core rewarming measures, such as warm irrigation of the bladder, stomach, or pleural space, are to be implemented by physicians in rare scenarios of severe hypothermia that require aggressive rewarming (van der Ploeg et al., 2010; Zafren & Mechem, 2017). The importance of follow-up temperature assessment was also stressed, because trauma patients have been shown to have further temperature drop during resuscitation (Block et al., 2012; van der Ploeg et al., 2010).

Educational Interventions

A thermoregulation checklist was adapted from a previous work (Block et al., 2012) in collaboration with ED management, ED nurse educator, and the manager of the surgical intensive care unit (Figure 1). Final feedback and adjustments were provided by staff nurses. Huddles were conducted by the CNS multiple times per day for 1 week before launching the checklist. All ED nurses received a mass e-mail outlining the EBP project and checklist. After go-live, weekly huddles were conducted with staff of all shifts. During huddles, the checklist was disseminated with education and rationale for each field. Experienced and motivated staff nurses were approached to serve as champions. The champions were asked to promote

Patient label

Trauma bay external temperature _____ F/C (80F)

Patient Temp on Arrival _____ F/C Time: _____ Source: _____

(Rectal temp for Level 1, environmental exposure, AMS, Provider/RN discretion)

Patient Temp at end of trauma _____ F/C Time: _____ Source: _____

Normothermia 96.8-98.9F		Mild Hypothermia 95-96.8F		Moderate – Severe Hypothermia <94.9F
Interventions				
☐ Warm Blankets	☐	IVF & Blood through fluid warmer	☐	IVF and Blood through fluid Warmer
☐ All blood products through fluid warmer	☐	Bair Hugger	☐	Bair Hugger
			☐	RT for warm oxygen therapy
Monitoring				
☐ Temp Q30min x2 Then per protocol	☐	Gaymar Continuous Temperature	☐	Gaymar Continuous Temperature
	☐	Temp documentation in Epic Q15min	☐	Temp documentation in Epic Q15min
		Return to Normothermia when temp >96.8F ⬅		Return to Mild Hypothermia when temp >94.9F ⬅

Figure 1. Hypothermia checklist for all level 1 and level 2 trauma activations. Adapted from "Evidence-Based Thermoregulation for Adult Trauma Patients," by J. Block, M. Lilienthal, L. Cullen, and A. White, 2012, *Critical Care Nursing Quarterly*, 35(1), pp. 50–63. doi:10.1097/cnq.0b013e31823d3e9b. Reprinted with permission from the authors.

Reprinted with permission from Saqe-Rockoff, A., et al. (2018). Improving thermoregulation for trauma patients in the emergency department: An evidence-based practice project. *Journal of Trauma Nursing, 25*, 14–20.

the checklist and thermoregulation interventions to their peers, as well as periodically checking implementation of rewarming measures. Random trauma charts were audited by the CNS with verbal or e-mail feedback provided to the staff. The thermoregulation checklist outlined expectations for assessment and interventions of trauma patients.

Evaluation

The impact of the interventions was assessed by review of all charts for Level 1 and Level 2 trauma activations from January to March 2017. Trauma activations from January to March of 2016 were also reviewed and entered in REDCap, a secure data collection portal (Harris et al., 2009), to serve as a comparison group in understanding the impact of the intervention. The CNS verified every 20th record against the EMR to ensure the accuracy of collected data. All completed checklists were collected and reviewed. Compliance with temperature assessment and documentation, rewarming methods implemented, and trauma bay temperature were reviewed. Findings postintervention were compared with trauma patients from the same time period in 2016.

Data analysis included descriptive statistics for all variables and assessment of differences between the pre- and postintervention time frames using the χ^2 test, Fisher exact test, and Student t test as appropriate. All data analysis was completed in R version 3.3.3 (R Core Team, 2016) using RStudio version 1.0.136 (RStudio Team, 2015). Analysis also included assessment of certain variables collected only in the postintervention time period, such as trauma bay temperature and adherence to the new protocols. Informal feedback was collected from the staff during the project.

RESULTS

During the period of January–March 2017, there were 193 trauma activations. Of these activations, 82 (41%) had a completed checklist; however, we were able to analyze data for all trauma activations using data from the chart. More patients with hypothermia and hyperthermia were identified in 2017 than those in 2016. There was a significant increase in core temperature assessment from 4% in 2016 to 23% in 2017 ($p < .001$). Blanket use in normothermic patients increased in 2017 ($p = .002$) (Table 1).

Our institution did not have continuous temperature monitoring of the trauma bay preintervention. On the day that trauma bay temperature was adjusted (January 2017), the thermostat setting and thermometer reading were 70°F. After the intervention, trauma bay ambient temperature was monitored and recorded in the checklist during trauma activations. The CNS monitored and trended the bay temperature over the course of 3 months of the project (Figure 2). Over the period of 3 months, there was a steady increase in the average temperature of the trauma bay.

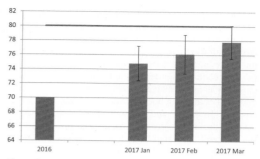

Figure 2. Changes in trauma bay ambient temperature over time. Error bars represent standard deviation.

Another goal of this project was to increase compliance with temperature assessment during trauma evaluations. While the number of temperatures taken within 9 minutes of activation dropped between 2016 and 2017, the overall number of temperatures taken within 19 or fewer minutes increased slightly from 81.4% to 83.9% (Table 2). Of note, the previous EMR made it easier to backdate all trauma documentation, which may have made the times to first temperature in 2016 appear shorter than they were in practice. Core temperature assessment increased from 4.9 % in 2016 to 24.4% in 2017 ($p < .001$) (Table 1).

Over the two 3-month periods reviewed for this project, there were a total of 10 hypothermic patients. Indoor exposure was the most common mechanism associated with hypothermia and was a factor in all three cases of severe hypothermia. All hypothermic patients were identified from rectal temperatures. Alcohol ingestion was identified in 40% of hypothermic patients (Table 3).

DISCUSSION

Various sources provide a range of temperature cutoffs for hypothermia (Block et al., 2012; Keane, 2016; Langhelle et al., 2010; Niven et al., 2015; van der Ploeg et al., 2010). To create a process with standardized interventions, the team set the hypothermia cutoff at 96.8°F (Langhelle et al., 2010; Niven et al., 2015). While this cutoff is higher than some found in the literature, hypothermia has been associated with progressively worsening coagulopathy starting at 96.8°F (Mitrophanov et al., 2013; van der Ploeg et al., 2010; Zafren & Mechem, 2017).

One project goal was to improve time to first temperature. Previous articles have recommended use of peripheral thermometers because of the ease of obtaining a temperature reading (Block et al., 2012; Keane, 2016). Oral thermometers are accurate in confirming normothermia but lack accuracy in hypothermic patients and are subject to interference from head and face temperature (Paal et al., 2016). A systematic review and meta-analysis found that peripheral thermometers lack clinically acceptable

Reprinted with permission from Saqe-Rockoff, A., et al. (2018). Improving thermoregulation for trauma patients in the emergency department: An evidence-based practice project. *Journal of Trauma Nursing, 25,* 14–20.

TABLE 1 Patient Characteristics and Main Results			
	2016 *n = 271*	**2017** *n = 202*	*p*
Characteristics			
Age in years (median, IQR)	52.4 (28.2, 74.9)	68.6 (45.1, 81.8)	<.001
Sex			.278
Male	163 (60.1)	110 (54.7)	
Female	108 (39.9)	91 (45.3)	
Temperature category			.006
Hyperthermia	6 (2.2)	13 (6.4)	
Normothermia	261 (96.3)	179 (88.6)	
Mild hypothermia	0 (0)	4 (2.0)	
Moderate-severe hypothermia	2 (0.7)	4 (2.0)	
Missing	2 (0.7)	2 (1.0)	
Temperature source			<.001
Oral	174 (64.2)	142 (70.3)	
Rectal	7 (2.6)	43 (21.3)	
Tympanic	2 (0.7)	1 (0.5)	
Axillary	9 (3.3)	4 (2.0)	
Missing	70 (29.2)	12 (5.9)	
Warming measures			
Normothermia	n = 261	n = 179	
Blankets	208 (79.7)	163 (91.1)	.002
Mild hypothermia	No patients	n = 4	N/A
Blankets		4 (100)	
Warm IV fluids		0 (0)	
Moderate-severe hypothermia	n = 2	n = 4	
Blankets	1 (50)	2 (50)	1.0
Bair hugger	2 (100)	3 (75)	1.0
Warm IV fluids	1 (50)	3 (75)	1.0
Checklist completed	–	82 (40%)	

Note. IQR = interquartile range; IV = intravenous.

accuracy. Their use was discouraged in critical or injured patients and any scenario where accurate body temperature would influence decisions (Niven et al., 2015). Of note, all cases of hypothermia were detected with core temperature readings. One patient in 2016 had an initial oral temperature of 97.0°F and a rectal temperature of 87.9°F. Increased use of rectal thermometers in 2017 may have contributed to the increased identification of hypothermia, allowing earlier implementation of rewarming modalities and prevention of further heat loss for these trauma patients (Table 2).

Increasing the ambient temperature was met with the most staff resistance. Block et al. (2012) reported similar difficulties in implementing warming of the environment, although they did not include data on their progress. Frequent reminders to the staff and adjustments to the trauma bay thermostat and closing of the doors were required. Although there was a steady increase in trauma bay temperature in January through March 2017, compliance with maintaining the 80°F temperature remained inconsistent, and in May 2017, after the evaluation period presented in this article, a lockbox was placed over

TABLE 2 Time to First Temperature, by Year		
Time to Temperature	2016 n (%)	2017 n (%)
0-9 min	188 (69.9)	116 (60.1)
10-19 min	31 (11.5)	46 (23.8)
20-29 min	21 (7.8)	13 (6.7)
30+ min	29 (10.7)	18 (9.3)

the thermostat to ensure consistency. For the following 2 weeks, daily checks of the trauma bay temperatures revealed a consistent temperature of 80°F.

Nurses often identify lack of education, access to information, and time for implementing EBP as barriers to implementing change (Melnyk, Fineout-Overholt, Gallagher-Ford, & Kaplan, 2012). Compliance with EBP interventions can still remain low even after removing barriers. Research has identified that staff attitude and beliefs regarding whether EBP improves patient care can differ (Warren et al., 2016). Further research should be dedicated to examine barriers to culture and behavior changes necessary for implementing EBP.

During the evaluation period, overall compliance with checklist completion was 40%. The checklist served as a reminder to the staff to maintain the trauma bay at 80°F, assess patient temperature on arrival, and to prioritize core temperature evaluation and implementation of rewarming techniques. The trauma registrars will continue to complete 100% chart review and provide feedback to the ED when trauma patients do not have temperature assessment within 30 minutes.

Contextual elements that may have contributed to the success of our EBP include elements regarding our institution's support of nursing research. Over the past year, our institution has seen a substantial increase in nursing staff and better patient ratios, which allows for more time for staff education and implementation of EBP interventions. Nurses are also able to work with a research consultant, who provides support regarding project design, evaluation, and statistics.

Concurrently, recent changes at our facility made certain aspects of evaluation more difficult. Conversion to a new EMR system may have contributed to the failure to see improvement in time to first documented temperature. Furthermore, the new trauma documentation does not contain reminders for required fields and consists of multiple separate sections that require additional steps and time for documentation With documentation becoming more time consuming, temperature assessment time may be reflected as completed at a later time.

Limitations

This was a single-center EBP project in an urban Level 1 trauma center. Because of the small number of hypothermic patients, our project was unable to determine changes in patient outcomes from our interventions (Table 3).

Although this evaluation used a comparison group comprising the same months of patient admissions, enabling us to control for obvious seasonal effects related to the incidence of hypothermia, the evaluation may have been vulnerable to secular effects related to other hospital initiatives or broader changes in the health care landscape between the pre- and postintervention data. One important hospital-wide effect was the launch of a new EMR system in August 2016, which changed many workflows and made it more difficult to backdate temperatures in the system, reducing the validity of the time to temperature comparison.

CONCLUSIONS

This project is an example of how nurses can utilize an EBP model to translate research into clinical practice and demonstrated that best practice interventions regarding temperature assessment and rewarming measures for trauma patients can be successfully implemented with negligible cost. Implementation of EBP projects requires extensive staff education to facilitate cultural and behavioral changes. Further research should examine barriers to implementation and adherence to EBP interventions. Further steps for this project may include review of more trauma patient records to determine efficiency of rewarming methods and any changes in patient outcomes associated with these interventions.

TABLE 3 Characteristics of Hypothermic Patients	
Mechanism of Trauma	N = 10
Indoor exposure	
Fall	5
Hanging	1
Self-inflicted wrist laceration	1
Outside exposure	
Assault	1
Fall	1
Submersion	
Accidental fall in river	1
Source of temperature	
Rectal	10 (100%)
Alcohol consumption	4 (40%)

Reprinted with permission from Saqe-Rockoff, A., et al. (2018). Improving thermoregulation for trauma patients in the emergency department: An evidence-based practice project. *Journal of Trauma Nursing, 25,* 14–20.

Acknowledgments

The authors thank the NYU Langone Hospital—Brooklyn ED nurses for their hard work and dedication to improving patient care and Kathy Peterson, RN, MSN, CEN, and Staci Mandola, RN, BSN, for their leadership and support.

KEY POINTS

- Hypothermia is a high impact presentation that requires vigilance.
- Critical and trauma patients should have core temperature assessment to ensure optimal detection of abnormal temperatures.
- Extensive education is required to successfully implement evidence-based interventions and achieve practice change.

REFERENCES

American College of Surgeons Committee on Trauma, Simon, R., & Hunt, J. (2014). *Hypothermia.* Retrieved from https://www.facs.org/~/media/files/quality%20programs/trauma/publications/hypothermia%20poster.ashx

Balvers, K., Van der Horst, M., Graumans, M., Boer, C., Binnekade, J. M., Goslings, J. C., & Juffermans, N. P. (2016). Hypothermia as a predictor for mortality in trauma patients at admittance to the intensive care unit. *Journal of Emergencies, Trauma, and Shock, 9*(3), 97–102. doi:10.4103/0974-2700.185276

Block, J., Lilienthal, M., Cullen, L., & White, A. (2012). Evidence-based thermoregulation for adult trauma patients. *Critical Care Nursing Quarterly, 35*(1), 50–63. doi:10.1097/cnq.0b013e31823d3e9b

Brown, C. G. (2014). The Iowa model of evidence-based practice to promote quality care: An illustrated example in oncology nursing. *Clinical Journal of Oncology Nursing, 18*(2), 157–159. doi:10.1188/14.cjon.157-159

Emergency Nurses Association. (2014). *Trauma nursing core course provider manual, 7th edition.* Des Plaines, IL: Emergency Nurses Association.

Farkash, U., Lynn, M., Scope, A., Maor, R., Turchin, N., Sverdlik, B., & Eldad, A. (2002). Does prehospital fluid administration impact core body temperature and coagulation functions in combat casualties? *Injury, 33*(2), 103–110. doi:10.1016/s0020-1383(01)00149-8

Harris, P. A., Taylor, R., Thielke, R., Payne, J., Gonzalez, N., & Conde, J. G. (2009). Research electronic data capture (REDCap)—A metadata-driven methodology and workflow process for providing translational research informatics support. *Journal of Biomedical Informatics, 42*(2), 377–381. doi:10.1016/j.jbi.2008.08.010

Heron, M. (2016). *Deaths: Leading causes for 2014, National vital statistics reports* (Vol. 65, no. 5). Hyattsville, MD: National Center for Health Statistics.

Ireland, S., Endacott, R., Cameron, P., Fitzgerald, M., & Paul, E. (2011). The incidence and significance of accidental hypothermia in major trauma—A prospective observational study. *Resuscitation, 82*(3), 300–306. doi:10.1016/j.resuscitation.2010.10.016

Ireland, S., Murdoch, K., Ormrod, P., Saliba, E., Endacott, R., Fitzgerald, M., & Cameron, P. (2006). Nursing and medical staff knowledge regarding the monitoring and management of accidental or exposure hypothermia in adult major trauma patients. *International Journal of Nursing Practice, 12*(6), 308–318. doi:10.1111/j.1440-172x.2006.00589.x

Keane, M. (2016). Triad of death: The importance of temperature monitoring in trauma patients. *Emergency Nurse, 24*(5), 19–23. doi:10.7748/en.2016.e1569

Langhelle, A., Lockey, D., Harris, T., & Davies, G. (2010). Body temperature of trauma patients on admission to hospital: A comparison of anaesthetised and non-anaesthetised patients. *Emergency Medicine Journal, 29*(3), 239–242. doi:10.1136/emj.2009.086967

Martini, W. Z. (2009). Coagulopathy by hypothermia and acidosis: Mechanisms of thrombin generation and fibrinogen availability. *The Journal of Trauma: Injury, Infection, and Critical Care, 67*(1), 202–209. doi:10.1097/ta.0b013e3181a602a7

Melnyk, B. M., & Fineout-Overholt, E. (2014). *Evidence-based practice in nursing & healthcare: A guide to best practice* (3rd ed.). Philadelphia, PA: Lippincott Williams & Wilkins.

Melnyk, B. M., Fineout-Overholt, E., Gallagher-Ford, L., & Kaplan, L. (2012). The state of evidence-based practice in US nurses. *JONA: The Journal of Nursing Administration, 42*(9), 410–417. doi:10.1097/nna.0b013e3182664e0a

Mitrophanov, A. Y., Rosendaal, F. R., & Reifman, J. (2013). Computational analysis of the effects of reduced temperature on thrombin generation. *Anesthesia & Analgesia, 117*(3), 565–574. doi:10.1213/ane.0b013e31829c3b22

Niven, D. J., Gaudet, J. E., Laupland, K. B., Mrklas, K. J., Roberts, D. J., & Stelfox, H. T. (2015). Accuracy of peripheral thermometers for estimating temperature. *Annals of Internal Medicine, 163*(10), 768. doi:10.7326/m15-1150

NYU Langone Medical Center. (2016). *Above & beyond: 2016 annual report.* Retrieved from http://nyulangone.org/files/publication_issues/nyu-langone-institutional-annual-report-2016.pdf

Paal, P., Gordon, L., Strapazzon, G., Brodmann Maeder, M., Putzer, G., Walpoth, B., ... Brugger, H. (2016). Accidental hypothermia—an update. *Scandinavian Journal of Trauma, Resuscitation and Emergency Medicine, 24*, 111. doi:10.1186/s13049-016-0303-7

R Core Team. (2016). *R: A language and environment for statistical computing.* Vienna, Austria: R Foundation for Statistical Computing. Retrieved from https://www.R-project.org/

RStudio Team. (2015). *RStudio: Integrated development for R.* Boston, MA: RStudio, Inc. Retrieved from http://www.rstudio.com/

Simmons, J. W., Pittet, J.-F., & Pierce, B. (2014). Trauma-induced coagulopathy. *Current Anesthesiology Reports, 4*(3), 189–199. doi:10.1007/s40140-014-0063-8

Soar, J., Perkins, G. D., Abbas, G., Alfonzo, A., Barelli, A., Bierens, J. J., ... Nolan, J. P. (2010). European resuscitation council guidelines for resuscitation 2010 section 8. Cardiac arrest in special circumstances: Electrolyte abnormalities, poisoning, drowning, accidental hypothermia, hyperthermia, asthma, anaphylaxis, cardiac surgery, trauma, pregnancy, electrocution. *Resuscitation, 81*(10), 1400–1433. doi:10.1016/j.resuscitation.2010.08.015

van der Ploeg, G. J., Goslings, J. C., Walpoth, B. H., & Bierens, J. J. (2010). Accidental hypothermia: Rewarming treatments, complications and outcomes from one university medical centre. *Resuscitation, 81*(11), 1550–1555. doi:10.1016/j.resuscitation.2010.05.023

Warren, J. I., McLaughlin, M., Bardsley, J., Eich, J., Esche, C. A., Kropkowski, L., & Risch, S. (2016). The strengths and challenges of implementing EBP in healthcare systems. *Worldviews on Evidence-Based Nursing, 13*(1), 15–24. doi:10.1111/wvn.12149

Wolberg, A. S., Meng, Z. H., Monroe, D. M., & Hoffman, M. (2004). A systematic evaluation of the effect of temperature on coagulation enzyme activity and platelet function. *The Journal of Trauma: Injury, Infection, and Critical Care, 56*(6), 1221–1228. doi:10.1097/01.ta.0000064328.97941.fc

Zafren, K., & Mechem, C. C. (2017). *Accidental hypothermia in adults.* Retrieved from https://www.uptodate.com/contents/accidental-hypothermia-in-adults

For 6 additional continuing education articles related to hypothermia, go to NursingCenter.com/CE.

Reprinted with permission from Saqe-Rockoff, A., et al. (2018). Improving thermoregulation for trauma patients in the emergency department: An evidence-based practice project. *Journal of Trauma Nursing, 25*, 14–20.

Fatigue in the Presence of Coronary Heart Disease

Ann L. Eckhardt ▼ Holli A. DeVon ▼ Mariann R. Piano ▼ Catherine J. Ryan ▼ Julie J. Zerwic

Background: Fatigue is a prevalent and disabling symptom associated with many acute and chronic conditions, including acute myocardial infarction and chronic heart failure. Fatigue has not been explored in patients with stable coronary heart disease (CHD).

Objectives: The purpose of this partially mixed sequential dominant status study was to (a) describe fatigue in patients with stable CHD; (b) determine if specific demographic (gender, age, education, income), physiological (hypertension, hyperlipidemia), or psychological (depressive symptoms) variables were correlated with fatigue; and (c) determine if fatigue was associated with health-related quality of life. The theory of unpleasant symptoms was used as a conceptual framework.

Methods: Patients ($N = 102$) attending two cardiology clinics completed the Fatigue Symptom Inventory, Patient Health Questionnaire-9, and Medical Outcomes Study Short Form-36 to measure fatigue, depressive symptoms, and health-related quality of life. Thirteen patients whose interference from fatigue was low, moderate, or high participated in qualitative interviews.

Results: Forty percent of the sample reported fatigue more than 3 days of the week lasting more than one half of the day. Lower interference from fatigue was reported on standardized measures compared with qualitative interviews. Compared with men, women reported a higher fatigue intensity ($p = .003$) and more interference from fatigue ($p = .007$). In regression analyses, depressive symptoms were the sole predictor of fatigue intensity and interference.

Discussion: Patients with stable CHD reported clinically relevant levels of fatigue. Patients with stable CHD may discount fatigue as they adapt to their symptoms. Relying solely on standardized measures may provide an incomplete picture of fatigue burden in patients with stable CHD.

Key Words: coronary heart disease & fatigue & mixed methods

Fatigue is often defined as the subjective sensation of extreme and persistent exhaustion, tiredness, and lack of energy (Aaronson et al., 1999; Dittner, Wessely, & Brown, 2004; Ream & Richardson, 1996). Similar to other symptoms such as pain, fatigue is multidimensional, is influenced by physical and psychosocial factors, and shares common features with some mood and anxiety disorders (Aaronson et al., 1999; American Psychiatric Association, 2013). In patients with coronary heart disease (CHD), fatigue is a prevalent and debilitating symptom associated with poor quality of life and reduced physical activity (Pragodopol & Ryan, 2013).

CHD, also referred to as ischemic heart disease and acute coronary syndrome (ACS), encompasses conditions that arise because of atherosclerosis and a reduction in coronary artery blood flow (American Heart Association, 2013). Emerging evidence indicates that new onset or elevated levels of fatigue may be associated with an impending ACS event or may indi-

cate worsening or progressive CHD. Among patients ($N = 256$, mean age = 67 years) presenting to the emergency department for ACS, patients reported that "unusual fatigue" was one of the three most prevalent symptoms that propelled them to seek care (DeVon, Ryan, Ochs, & Shapiro, 2008). In a large prospective longitudinal study enrolling only men ($N = 5,216$, mean age = 59 years), Ekmann, Osler, and Avlund (2012) found that fatigue was associated with first hospitalization for nonfatal ischemic heart disease (hazard ratio [HR] = 1.98, 95% CI [1.09, 3.61]) and all-cause mortality (HR = 3.99, 95% CI [2.27, 7.02]). After adjusting for smoking and alcohol consumption, fatigue remained the only significant predictor of first hospitalization for nonfatal ischemic heart disease in men. In a large study enrolling women and men ($N = 11,795$, mean age = 57 years), Lindeberg, Rosvall, and Östergren (2012) found that exhaustion predicted cardiac events in both men (HR = 1.49, 95% CI [1.06, 2.11]) and women (HR = 1.78, 95% CI [1.23, 2.58]). After adjusting for depression and anxiety, the association between exhaustion and CHD was strengthened in men (HR = 1.62, 95% CI [1.05, 2.50]) but was no longer statistically significant in women.

Fennessy et al. (2010) found that both men and women reported moderate-to-high levels of fatigue at the time of acute myocardial infarction (AMI). Women reported significantly less fatigue 30 days after AMI, whereas men did not report

Ann L. Eckhardt, PhD, RN, is Assistant Professor, School of Nursing, Illinois Wesleyan University, Bloomington.

Holli A. DeVon, PhD, RN, is Associate Professor; **Mariann R. Piano, PhD, RN,** is Professor and Department Head; **Catherine J. Ryan, PhD, RN,** is Clinical Assistant Professor; and **Julie J. Zerwic, PhD, RN,** is Professor and Executive Associate Dean, Department of Biobehavioral Health Science, College of Nursing, University of Illinois at Chicago.

DOI: 10.1097/NNR.0000000000000019

Reprinted with permission from Eckhardt, A., et al. (2014). Fatigue in the presence of coronary heart disease. *Nursing Research, 63,* 83–93.

a change. Using quantitative coronary artery angiography, Zimmerman-Viehoff and colleagues (2013) examined the relationship between vital exhaustion (Maastricht questionnaire) and progression of coronary artery atherosclerosis in women ($N = 103$, mean age = 55 years) who had experienced an acute coronary event. Vital exhaustion significantly correlated with coronary artery diameter, with women having the highest vital exhaustion scores (46-57) showing the most pronounced coronary artery diameter narrowing ($M = 0.21$ mm, 95% CI [0.15, 0.27]) compared with intermediate vital exhaustion scores (43-45; coronary artery diameter, $M = 0.11$ mm, 95% CI [0.05, 0.17]). Women with vital exhaustion scores in low (score: 20-34) and lower intermediate (score: 35-42) range had no significant change in coronary artery diameter. These findings indicate that women with the highest level of vital exhaustion had the fastest coronary artery atherosclerosis progression.

Considering that fatigue may be an indicator of new onset or progressive CHD, it is important to determine the severity and characteristics of fatigue in a stable CHD population. Stable CHD is defined as patients who have been diagnosed with CHD but have not experienced a worsening of symptoms, symptoms at rest, or an episode of ACS for at least 60 days (Goblirsch et al., 2013). Therefore, the purpose of this partially mixed sequential dominant status study was to

1. describe fatigue (intensity, distress, timing, and quality) in patients with stable CHD;

2. determine if specific demographic (gender, age, education, income), physiological (hypertension, hyperlipidemia), or psychological (depressive symptoms) variables were correlated with fatigue; and

3. determine if fatigue was associated with health-related quality of life (HRQoL).

ORGANIZING FRAMEWORK

The organizing framework for this study was derived from the theory of unpleasant symptoms, which includes physiological, psychological, and situational factors that influence the symptom experience and describes symptoms in terms of intensity, distress, timing, and quality (Lenz, Pugh, Milligan, Gift, & Suppe, 1997). Although not consistent across all CHD studies, others have reported that fatigue is associated with gender, age, HRQoL, medication type, smoking status, pain, and depressed mood (DeVon et al., 2008; Ekmann et al., 2012; Fink et al., 2012; Fink, Sullivan, Zerwic, & Piano, 2009; Hägglund, Boman, Stenlund, Lundman, & Brulin, 2008; McSweeney & Crane, 2000; Shaffer et al., 2012). Figure 1 depicts the conceptualization of the theory of unpleasant symptoms for the current study as adapted by the authors.

In the theory of unpleasant symptoms, gender and age are considered situational factors, whereas depressed mood is categorized as a psychological factor. The symptom experience was examined using the Fatigue Symptom Inventory (FSI; Hann et al., 1998). The average of the first three FSI questions was used to evaluate symptom (fatigue) intensity.

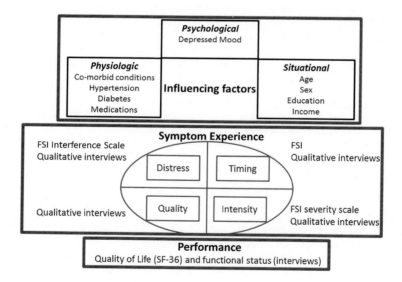

FIGURE 1 Organizing framework based on the theory of unpleasant symptoms used to understand fatigue in the presence of coronary heart disease.

Reprinted with permission from Eckhardt, A., et al. (2014). Fatigue in the presence of coronary heart disease. *Nursing Research, 63,* 83–93.

The FSI-Interference Scale was used to determine symptom (fatigue) distress. The distress dimension within the theory of unpleasant symptoms refers to the degree to which a person is bothered by the symptom and the symptom interferes with activities of daily living. The FSI has several items, which corresponded to the timing of fatigue (time of day, number of days per week fatigue occurs, and pattern of fatigue). The Short Form-36 (McHorney, Ware, & Raczek, 1993), a measure of HRQoL, was used as a reflection of performance. Qualitative interviews were completed to obtain a comprehensive description of fatigue and add descriptive depth to each of the dimensions within the theory of unpleasant symptoms.

METHODS

Research Design

The study was conducted using a partially mixed sequential dominant status design, whereby the main study design was quantitative (QUAN) followed by a qualitative (qual) component (QUAN → qual). In a partially mixed sequential dominant status design, the qualitative and quantitative elements are deployed one after the other with one method being emphasized over the other (Leech & Onwuegbuzie, 2009). This mixed-methods design was chosen to achieve complementarity, which seeks to achieve convergence between quantitative and qualitative findings and to provide descriptive depth through qualitative interviews (Greene, 2007). The cross-sectional quantitative data were collected first, and participants for the qualitative component were recruited from this sample. Integration of qualitative and quantitative data occurred at the data analysis and discussion stages.

Sample and Setting

One hundred and two participants with stable CHD were recruited from two cardiology clinics during routine cardiovascular appointments. One clinic served primarily minority, urban patients ($n = 51$), and one served predominantly Caucasian patients from a small city in a rural setting ($n = 51$). Eligibility was determined by review of medical records. Inclusion criteria included a diagnosis of stable CHD, the ability to speak and read English and living independently. Exclusion criteria included heart failure with reduced ejection fraction (ejection fraction < 40%), terminal illness with prediction of less than 6 months to live, myocardial infarction or coronary artery bypass grafting in the past 2 months, unstable angina, symptoms due to worsening or exacerbation of cardiac disease, and hemodialysis. These exclusion criteria were chosen to eliminate patients with a recent acute event, those with new or worsening symptoms of CHD, and those with comorbid conditions known to be associated with significant fatigue. The institutional review boards at both sites approved the study. All participants provided written informed consent.

Quantitative Measurement

Fatigue Fatigue was measured using the FSI, a 14-item self-report instrument measuring fatigue intensity, duration, and interference with activities of daily living over the past week (Hann et al., 1998). The FSI has been used to measure fatigue in patients with AMI (Fennessy et al., 2010; Fink et al., 2010) and patients with heart failure (Fink et al., 2009). Similar to others, the first three items of the FSI were used to measure fatigue intensity/severity (Donovan, Jacobsen, Small, Munster, & Andrykowski, 2008). Questions 5–11, which are referred to as the FSI-Interference Scale, were used to measure the degree to which fatigue has interfered with patients' daily activities in the past week. Each question on the FSI is answered using an 11-point Likert-type scale (0 = *not at all fatigued/no interference* to 10 = *as fatigued as I could be/extreme interference*). Interference in physical, cognitive, and emotional aspects of daily living are measured using the interference scale. Questions 1–3 and 5–11 were summed and then divided by the total number of items (3 and 7, respectively) to generate the intensity fatigue score and FSI-Interference Scale score, yielding scores ranging from 0 to 10. Higher scores reflect higher intensity of fatigue and more interference because of fatigue. The FSI-Interference Scale has excellent reliability as estimated by coefficient alphas ranging from 0.93 to 0.95 (Hann, Denniston, & Baker, 2000; Hann et al., 1998). Using the SF-36 vitality subscale as a comparison, Donovan et al. determined that an intensity score of ≥3 was reflective of clinically meaningful fatigue. In the current sample, reliability was strong for the FSI-Interference Scale ($\alpha = 0.93$) and the FSI intensity score ($\alpha = 0.86$).

Depressive Symptoms Depressive symptoms were measured using the Patient Health Questionnaire-9 (PHQ-9), which has been used in prior studies with cardiovascular patients (Fink et al., 2012; Lee, Lennie, Heo, & Moser, 2012). The PHQ is a nine-item self-report instrument with a 4-point Likert-type scale (0 = *not at all*; 1 = *several days*; 2 = *more than half the days*; 3 = *nearly every day*) for each question and was developed using the Diagnostic and Statistical Manual for Mental Disorders' criteria for major depression (American Psychiatric Association, 2013; Kroenke, Spitzer, & Williams, 2001). Scores of ≥10 indicate moderate/severe depressive symptoms; scores between 5 and 9 indicate minor depression. Using a structured mental health professional interview as the criterion standard, the sensitivity and specificity of the PHQ-9 (score ≥ 10) was 88% for detecting major depression (Kroenke et al., 2001). In this study, a score of ≥5 was used as the cutoff for the presence of depressive symptoms.

HRQoL HRQoL includes physical and mental health perceptions of positive and negative aspects of life (Centers for Disease Control and Prevention, 2012). The SF-36 has been extensively used to measure HRQoL and has established reliability and validity in numerous populations (McHorney et al.,

Reprinted with permission from Eckhardt, A., et al. (2014). Fatigue in the presence of coronary heart disease. *Nursing Research*, 63, 83–93.

1993), including CHD populations (Fink et al., 2009; Hägglund et al., 2008). The SF-36 is a 36-item questionnaire that consists of eight subscales designed to measure quality of life in the domains of physical and mental functioning. The eight subscales are physical functioning, physical role limitation, emotional role limitation, vitality, mental health, social functioning, pain, and general health. The SF-36 generates eight subscale scores and two summary scores (physical component score and mental component score). Raw scores are standardized to range from 0 to 100, with lower scores indicating a lower level of functioning. Within the current study, reliability was good (α = .79–.88) for seven of the eight subscales, with a lower reliability for the general health subscale (α = .69).

Quantitative Analysis

Data were analyzed using the Statistical Package for the Social Sciences (Statistics for Windows, Version 19.0, IBM, Armonk, NY). A nominal alpha level of <.05 was designated for statistical significance. Chi-squared tests for independence and independent samples t tests were used to analyze demographic data and fatigue stratified by gender. Pearson's correlation and Spearman's rho were used to identify factors associated with fatigue. Multiple regression was used to identify predictors of fatigue.

Qualitative Measurement

Using scores from the FSI-Interference Scale, participants were identified as experiencing high ($\geq$2.5), moderate (1.15–2.4), or low (1.14) levels of interference from fatigue (Fink et al., 2010). Participants from each fatigue level were selected for the qualitative interview. Participants for the qualitative arm were interviewed within 3-5 weeks of enrollment. This time frame was selected to prevent potential recall bias and reduce the likelihood of participants experiencing cardiovascular events. Purposive sampling was used to achieve heterogeneity of the sample and to increase transferability of findings.

The principal investigator or research assistant completed all interviews, which lasted approximately 30 minutes. The principal investigator reviewed interviews completed by the research assistant to ensure consistency between interviewers. A semistructured interview guide was used to collect data. Questions included, "Describe a typical day," "What time of day do you feel most fatigued?" and "Describe your fatigue." Additional questions and probes were used to enhance the quality of the data. Field notes and an audit trail were maintained throughout data collection to ensure confirmability. Data saturation was reached after completing 13 interviews.

Qualitative Analysis

Interviews were digitally recorded and transcribed verbatim. Transcripts were imported into NVivo 9 (QSR International,

Burlington, MA) for coding and analysis. Transcripts were reviewed for accuracy by checking transcripts against the digitally recorded interview. Narrative analysis, which considers the potential for stories to give meaning to the data (Onwuegbuzie & Combs, 2010), was used as the primary analytic technique. Using the theory of unpleasant symptoms; themes of situational, psychological, and physiological factors; symptom description (timing, intensity, distress, quality); and performance (HRQoL) were analyzed. As data were coded, emerging themes were added, including an overall definition of fatigue, the worst part of being fatigued and aggravating/alleviating factors. To avoid biasing results, interviews were initially analyzed without regard to fatigue group. After all interview analyses were complete, within- and between-group analyses were done by comparing interviews from each group to determine similarities and differences between groups.

Mixed-Methods Analysis

After qualitative and quantitative analyses were complete, data were compared to determine patterns, enhance description, and address any discrepancies. Qualitative data were used to expand the overall depth of quantitative findings and provide a more thorough description of fatigue. If discrepancies were found, the authors reviewed discrepant data to determine if narrative data were revealing a concept not included on the standard instruments. Discrepancies in mixed-methods findings are generative, as they lead to further analysis and future research directions (Greene, 2007).

RESULTS

Demographic Characteristics

The mean age of participants (N = 102) was 65 years (SD = 11 years, range: 34-86 years). Most were men, non-Hispanic White, married, and had a high school education or greater (Table 1). The qualitative sample included nine men and four women (mean age = 67 years, SD = 12 years, range: 50-85 years); five participants reported low interference from fatigue, four reported moderate interference, and four reported high interference (Table 1).

Fatigue Intensity/Severity

Quantitative Analysis Women reported significantly higher levels of fatigue intensity (M = 4.38, SD = 2.16) than men (M = 3.43, SD = 2.16; t = 2.27, p = .003). Fifty-seven percent of men and 78.4% of women had clinically meaningful fatigue as indicated by an intensity score of $\geq$3. Fatigue intensity was significantly correlated with PHQ-9 score, smoking history, and income (Table 2). In a regression model, PHQ-9 (depressive symptoms) was the only predictor of fatigue intensity (Table 3).

Reprinted with permission from Eckhardt, A., et al. (2014). Fatigue in the presence of coronary heart disease. *Nursing Research, 63*, 83–93.

TABLE 1. Demographic and Clinical Characteristics of the Sample

Variable	Total sample (N = 102)		Qualitative sample (n = 13)	
	N	%	n	%
Gender				
Men	65	63.7	9	69.2
Women	37	36.3	4	30.8
Race/ethnicity				
Non-Hispanic White	57	55.9	9	69.2
Black	36	35.3	4	30.8
Hispanic	4	3.9	0	0
Asian	2	2.0	0	0
Other	3	2.9	0	0
Marital status				
Married/long-term committed	60	58.8	10	76.9
Divorced/separated	23	22.5	1	7.7
Widowed	10	9.8	2	15.4
Single	9	8.8	0	0
Education				
Less than 12 years	17	16.8	2	15.4
High school diploma	38	37.3	4	30.8
Some college/associate degree	20	19.6	3	23.1
Baccalaureate degree	13	12.7	3	23.1
Graduate degree	13	12.7	1	7.7
Employment				
Full/part-time work	27	26.5	5	38.5
Retired	53	52.0	6	46.2
Disabled/unemployed/medical leave	18	17.6	1	7.7
Homemaker	2	2.0	0	0
Comorbid conditions				
Type 2 diabetes	40	39.2	5	38.5
Depression	12	11.8	2	15.4
Hypertension	91	89.2	11	84.6
Hyperlipidemia	95	93.1	12	92.3
Prior myocardial infarction	34	33.3	4	30.8
Prior percutaneous coronary intervention	79	77.5	11	84.6
Prior coronary artery bypass graft	24	23.5	3	23.1

Continues

TABLE 1. Continued

Variable	Total sample (N = 102)		Qualitative sample (n = 13)	
	N	%	n	%
Medications				
Aspirin	88	86.3	13	100
Ace inhibitor	60	58.8	9	69.2
Beta blocker	75	73.5	11	84.6
Lipid-lowering agent	88	86.3	13	100

Qualitative Analysis Participants in the qualitative arm of the study reported varying degrees of fatigue intensity. Some participants reported not recognizing fatigue until they "hit a wall" and did not want to do anything else. Others reported noticing a change from the past, stating, "I'd be able to doze off sitting up. I didn't used to be able to do that" (58-year-old woman, low fatigue interference) and "I'm more tireder (*sic*) this year than I was a year ago" (50-year-old man, high fatigue interference). One participant mentioned that she noticed an overall slowing down, "since I was sick." Most participants indicated a general slowing down but could not relate the change to any specific event. Of note, one participant stated, "I just get tired. Some

TABLE 2. Correlations: Fatigue Intensity and Interference With Demographic and Clinical Variables

Variable	Fatigue intensity		Fatigue interference	
	r	p	r	p
Age	−.08	.43	−.24	.02
Gender	.24	.02	.22	.02
PHQ-9 (depressive symptoms)	.56	<.0001	.66	<.0001
Income	−.20	.05	−.16	.12
Race	.09	.39	.09	.37
Education	−.16	.12	−.16	.12
Smoking history	.20	.05	.19	.06
Diabetes	.00	.99	−.03	.76
Hypertension	−.02	.82	−.13	.21
Myocardial infarction	−.13	.19	−.04	.67
PCI	.04	.71	.02	.81
Coronary artery bypass graft	.06	.540	.01	.93

Note. PHQ = Patient Health Questionnaire; PCI = percutaneous coronary intervention.

TABLE 3. Regression of Fatigue Intensity on Gender, Age, Income, History of Smoking, and Depressive Symptoms

Model	Predictors	b	t	p
1	Gender	.05	0.62	.54
	Income	.01	0.07	.99
	History of smoking	.04	0.41	.68
	PHQ-9	.54	5.80	<.0001
2	Gender	.05	0.60	.55
	Age	.03	0.38	.70
	PHQ-9	.55	6.15	<.0001

Note. PHQ = Patient Health Questionnaire. Model 1 variables were those correlated with fatigue intensity; $R^2 = .32$, adjusted $R^2 = .30$, SE = 1.73, $F_{2, 99} = 22.92$, and $p < .0001$. Model 2 variables were those hypothesized to be related to fatigue intensity; $R^2 = .32$, adjusted $R^2 = .30$, SE = 1.74, $F_{5, 96} = 15.20$, and $p < .0001$.

days I almost start crawling" (81-year-old man, low fatigue interference). This participant reported no interference from fatigue (score of 0 on FSI-Interference Scale), rated his worst fatigue severity as a 4 on an 11-point Likert scale, and consistently scored ≥50 (range: 0–100) on all HRQoL subscales. This incongruent finding may represent an accommodation to decreased physical capacity because of CHD.

Fatigue Interference

Quantitative Analysis Women reported significantly more interference from fatigue ($M = 3.28$, $SD = 2.71$; $t = 2.74$, $p = .007$) than men ($M = 1.99$, $SD = 2.03$). The FSI-Interference Scale score was significantly correlated with age and PHQ-9 score (Table 2). Depressive symptoms were the only predictor of interference from fatigue in a regression model (Table 4).

Qualitative Analysis A common theme was a general slowing down. "I have like a certain amount of energy in my bank account in the morning, and it just kind of gradually depletes during the day, and when it's gone, it's gone" (62-year-old man, moderate fatigue interference). Other participants reported rearranging their activities around the time of worst fatigue. "Then I arrange my day so that I can take my walk, come back and take a nap, and be fresh for the appointment. And that's the way I handle it" (81-year-old woman, high fatigue interference). Other descriptors of symptom distress included: "I remember I taught Grapes of Wrath. And ma would say, 'I'm sick tired,' you know.... You're almost sick, you're so tired" (74-year-old woman, moderate fatigue interference). Some participants described their distress in terms of activity, "like you want to lie down and take a nap" (50-year-old man, moderate fatigue interference). Participants who reported the lowest FSI-Interference Scale scores reported fewer instances of

daily fatigue but still reported having days when they were exhausted.

Timing of Fatigue

Quantitative Results Fatigue intensity was significantly correlated with the number of days per week participants experienced fatigue ($r = .63$, $p < .0001$) and the portion of the day participants felt fatigue ($r = .66$, $p < .0001$). Participants reported being fatigued a mean of 3.43 ($SD = 2.38$) days per week.

Qualitative Results Reports of the timing of fatigue varied. Some people reported fatigue every day at the same time: "Here lately it's been pretty much every day.... I get up and get [spouse] out to work...it feels like I'm drained" (85-year-old man, high fatigue interference). Other participants reported that fatigue only affected them after being busy and finally sitting down for the day, whereas some stated that there was no pattern. Two participants reported no fatigue on their quantitative measures, but they reported slowing down and needing more frequent breaks. One participant reported, "I take a nap...but as far as fatigue; I've got a lot of energy" (53-year-old man, low fatigue interference). Participants often did not relate slowing down, taking more frequent breaks, or needing naps to fatigue.

Quality of Fatigue

Qualitative Analysis The quality dimension of the theory of unpleasant symptoms refers to the symptom description, how the symptom manifests, or alleviating factors. Descriptors of fatigue included "I get winded a lot quicker," "going at a slower pace," and "a little aggravated and drained." Participants often reported that sitting down and resting was an alleviating factor. Many participants reported that simply going slower was helpful,

TABLE 4. Regression of Fatigue Interference on Gender, Age, and Depressive Symptoms

Model	Predictors	b	t	p
1	Gender	.07	0.90	.37
	Age	-.12	-1.54	.13
	PHQ-9	.61	7.56	<.0001
2	Gender	.07	0.90	.37
	Age	-.12	-1.54	.13
	PHQ-9	.61	7.56	<.0001

Note. PHQ = Patient Health Questionnaire. Model 1 variables were those correlated with fatigue interference; $R^2 = .46$, adjusted $R^2 = .43$, SE = 12.49, $F_{5, 96} = 16.07$, and $p < .0001$. Model 2 variables were those hypothesized to be related to fatigue interference; $R^2 = .45$, adjusted $R^2 = .42$, SE = 12.59, $F_{3, 98} = 19.60$, and $p < .0001$.

Reprinted with permission from Eckhardt, A., et al. (2014). Fatigue in the presence of coronary heart disease. *Nursing Research, 63*, 83–93.

"so instead of working three hours, I should work two and then leave it" (79-year-old woman, low fatigue interference).

All participants in the qualitative arm were asked to define fatigue. Definitions included "being completely wore (*sic*) out," "different kind of fatigue," "bone weary," and "low energy, low mental processing." Participants often described it as being different than the feeling after a long day at work, "I've done a hard day's work before and not quite feel, wouldn't be the same.... I really don't know how to explain it...just more or less completely exhausted" (85-year-old man, high fatigue interference). Although the descriptions and definitions varied, it was obvious that fatigue was a physically and mentally taxing symptom that was affecting the individuals' daily lives. Definitions of fatigue did not vary whether participants experienced high, moderate, or low interference from fatigue.

HRQoL and Fatigue

Quantitative Analysis Fatigue intensity and interference from fatigue were negatively correlated with each of the SF-36 subscales that measure HRQoL (Table 5). Participants who reported more fatigue intensity and more interference from fatigue reported significantly worse scores on all eight subscales.

Qualitative Analysis Overall, participants reported that fatigue did not affect their enjoyment of life. Some participants reported feelings of jealousy when they saw people who were older doing things more easily than they could themselves: "I get jealous. Sometimes I'll see people in their 70s and 80s, and they're walking fast, like there's nothing wrong with them. They're full of piss and vinegar. It's like, 'wow I'm only 52'" (52-year old-man, high fatigue interference). Others reported finding ways to adapt to the fatigue by "unconsciously" planning their outings around times of worst fatigue.

TABLE 5. Correlations: Fatigue Intensity and Interference With Health-Related Quality of Life

HR-QoL[a]	Fatigue intensity	Fatigue interference
Physical functioning	−.54*	−.60*
Role limitation physical	−.50*	−.54*
Role limitation emotional	−.44*	−.53*
Vitality	−.65*	−.75*
Mental health	−.47*	−.60*
Social functioning	−.55*	−.65*
Pain	−.51*	−.52*
General health	−.53*	−.66*

Note. HR-QoL = health-related quality of life.
[a]HR-QoL variables are subscales from the SF-36.
*$p < .01$.

INTEGRATED ANALYSIS

There was concordance of findings between quantitative and qualitative measures on timing and distress dimensions of the theory of unpleasant symptoms. Table 6 summarizes the integrated analysis.

Participants with the highest FSI-Interference Scale scores tended to report the most difficulty with fatigue during qualitative interviews, with one exception: An 81-year-old man categorized as having low fatigue interference reported high fatigue during the interview. On the day of his interview, he reported he was "feeling pretty good" but described how bad he felt on his high fatigue days. It is possible that, when he completed the FSI, he was having a good day and did not answer the questions based on how he felt at any time other than the present.

Although participants during the qualitative interviews did not always acknowledge fatigue, they reported a general slowing, an increased frequency of breaks, and an overall tailoring of their lifestyle to avoid fatigue. All interviewed participants who reported low fatigue interference ($n = 5$) reported needing additional breaks. Neither the FSI fatigue severity score or interference score captured this phenomenon; therefore, without the addition of the qualitative component, important information might have been lost. The use of a partially mixed sequential dominant status design in which qualitative data enhance and expand data acquired through validated quantitative tools provided a deeper and contextualized picture of fatigue in patients with CHD.

DISCUSSION

A key finding of the study was that more than 50% of stable male and female participants with CHD reported clinically meaningful fatigue that occurred on an average of 3.43 days of the week. This indicates that patients with stable CHD experience a high degree of fatigue. Women ($M = 3.28$, $SD = 2.71$), but not men ($M = 1.99$, $SD = 2.03$), reported higher interference with activities because of fatigue than those reported by cancer patients undergoing active treatment ($M = 2.3$, $SD = 2.2$; Hann et al., 1998) and patients with reduced ejection fraction heart failure ($M = 2.9$, $SD = 2.7$; Fink et al., 2009).

The presence of depressive symptoms was the only predictor of fatigue intensity and interference among the potential contributors to fatigue. Interestingly, in the univariate analysis, women reported significantly greater fatigue intensity and interference compared with men; however, after controlling for depressive symptoms, there were no gender differences, indicating that depressed mood was a dominant factor. Finally, fatigue intensity and interference were correlated with poor HRQoL. Patients with higher PHQ-9 scores (depressive symptoms) reported more interference from fatigue and fatigue intensity. On the basis of the regression analysis, 45%

Reprinted with permission from Eckhardt, A., et al. (2014). Fatigue in the presence of coronary heart disease. *Nursing Research, 63*, 83–93.

TABLE 6. Integrated Data Analysis

Fatigue dimension	Quantitative data (select)	Qualitative data (select)	Integrated analysis
Frequency and pattern	• 9.8% reported no fatigue in the past week • 47% reported fatigue 1–3 days in the past week • 43% reported fatigue ≥4 days in the past week • 20% reported fatigue worse in the morning • 21% reported fatigue worse in the afternoon • 28% reported fatigue worse in the evening • 23% reported no consistent pattern	• "Here lately it's been pretty much every day…" (high fatigue) • "…as far as fatigue, I've got a lot of energy." (low fatigue) • "…don't happen every day." (low fatigue) • "…sometimes in the afternoon, I'll get a little tired, and I'll lay down for a little bit. But most of the time it's more evenings…" (moderate fatigue) • "In the morning. And I usually have to end up stopping what I'm doing, getting up, and moving around." (moderate fatigue) • "It's no certain time. It varies." (high fatigue)	• Quantitative reports of frequency of fatigue correlated with qualitative comments such as "lots or energy" or "every day" • No consistent pattern of fatigue identified in qualitative or quantitative results
Distress	• 72% reported fatigue interfered with general activity • Nearly 65% reported that fatigue interfered with normal work activity, enjoyment of life, and mood. • Over 50% reported interference with relationships and ability to concentrate.	• "I felt that my medical condition had finally turned a corner, and so now I'm going to try to become more active…and then you find out you can't…" (low fatigue) • "I find myself nodding off…. Nobody saw me, did they? And it's embarrassing." (moderate fatigue)	• Even those participants who reported low fatigue on standardized instruments noted fatigue affecting daily life. • Standard instruments failed to capture the lifestyle tailoring that patients with stable CHD reported. • Providers need to ask more detailed questions about fatigue to determine if patients are compensating for the symptom.
Intensity	• Mean score of 5.44 (SD = 2.64) on the rating of most fatigue (range: 0–10) • Mean score of 3.71 (SD = 2.23) on the rating of average fatigue (range: 0–10) • Mean score of 2.17 (SD = 2.14) on the rating of least fatigue (range: 0–10)	• "I've been awful tired, and that usually is not me." (high fatigue) • "…you don't realize you were fatigued until…trying to go out and hanging on the cart keeping you up." (low fatigue)	• Rating of average fatigue intensity indicative of clinically meaningful fatigue • Qualitative reports of fatigue intensity did not differ significantly between high, moderate, and low fatigue groups.

Continues

Reprinted with permission from Eckhardt, A., et al. (2014). Fatigue in the presence of coronary heart disease. *Nursing Research, 63*, 83–93.

TABLE 6. Continued

Fatigue dimension	Quantitative data (select)	Qualitative data (select)	Integrated analysis
Performance	• Participants classified as high fatigue using the FSI composite reported lower quality of life.	• "I'm going in there and get something done and get it done. Now you just kind of stretch it out." (moderate fatigue) • "…you just learn to accept it." (moderate fatigue) • "I've got a lot to do, but just don't get it done…when you're feeling tired, you ain't got no business on a ladder." (high fatigue) • "I think that's what's the hardest on a guy that's like me…being shut down from what you used to be doing." (high fatigue) • "I can get out of the notion of going somewhere a lot easier." (low fatigue)	• Consistent qualitative reports of adapting to fatigue and changing lifestyle to accommodate restrictions • Overall, patients reported that they adapted and did not allow fatigue to dictate the quality of life they lived. • It appears that patients with stable CHD adapt to a decreased functional capacity over time and do not allow quality of life to be dictated by the symptoms they experience.
(health-related quality of life)	• FSI scores were correlated with all of the SF-36 subscales.		

of fatigue interference scores were explained by the presence of depressive symptoms. Even participants categorized as having mild depressive symptoms reported higher levels of fatigue. The link between fatigue and depression has been documented in patients with cardiovascular disease (Evangelista et al., 2008; Fennessy et al., 2010; Fink et al., 2012). Others have also indicated a strong relationship between fatigue and depression among patients attending primary care clinics. Skapinakis, Lewis, and Mavreas (2004) conducted a secondary analysis of data from the World Health Organization longitudinal collaborative study of psychological problems in general healthcare. Individuals with depression at baseline were 4 times more likely to develop new unexplained fatigue at the 12-month follow-up. In patients with cardiovascular disease, depressed mood or depression often coexist, and it remains to be determined if depression is the cause or consequence of fatigue.

Younger age was associated with higher fatigue interference but not fatigue intensity. It is possible that younger individuals find that fatigue interferes with daily activities, whereas older individuals are not as active or adapt more readily to fatigue by altering their activities. Kop, Appels, Mendes de Leon, and Bar (1996) found that younger age and female gender were significant predictors of vital exhaustion in patients with CHD.

Similar to others, fatigue intensity and fatigue interference were negatively correlated with all eight SF-36 subscales (HRQoL). Pragodpol and Ryan (2013) examined 17 studies and found that fatigue was a predictor of diminished HRQoL in patients with newly diagnosed CHD. In another study of patients with confirmed CHD and chronic angina, a symptom cluster containing fatigue, dyspnea, and chest pain frequency was found to be predictive of lower HRQoL (Kimble et al., 2011). Staniute, Bunevicius, Brozaitiene, and Bunevicius (2013) determined that poor HRQoL was associated with greater fatigue and reduced exercise capacity independent of mental health and severity of CHD. The findings validate the critical impact that the symptom of fatigue has on HRQoL.

All qualitative participants who reported low interference from fatigue on their standardized instruments ($n = 5$) reported fatigue during the interview. These individuals reported low levels of fatigue interference and severity but described not doing as much, tailoring their lifestyle to prevent fatigue, and moving at a slower pace. Lifestyle alterations in response to fatigue have been described in the heart failure literature (Jones, McDermott, Nowels, Matlock, & Bekelman, 2012). In an interpretive study of 26 patients with heart failure, emergent themes included descriptions of patients adapting to being tired and identifying ways to proactively prevent fatigue by rescheduling their days (Jones et al., 2012). This adaptation may also have occurred with patients in this study. It remains unknown if measurement error or other factors explain differences between quantitative and qualitative reports of fatigue in this study.

Reprinted with permission from Eckhardt, A., et al. (2014). Fatigue in the presence of coronary heart disease. *Nursing Research*, 63, 83–93.

Strengths and Limitations

Although previous research has focused on determining if fatigue predicts CHD in healthy individuals and the prevalence of fatigue before and after AMI, this is the first study that specifically describes fatigue in a stable CHD population. This study is innovative in that the design included the use of mixed methods, which combined validated quantitative measures with in-depth qualitative interviews. The qualitative interviews complemented findings from the quantitative instruments and added rich descriptive details to the findings. Sampling an urban and rural population resulted in ethnic and geographic diversity, thus increasing the generalizability of findings. There were limitations to this study including the use of a convenience sample and the potential inclusion of patients with undiagnosed heart failure. Differences in reports of fatigue intensity between standardized instruments and interviews in the low fatigue group may indicate that the FSI-interference Scale is not as sensitive in individuals with lower interference from fatigue.

CONCLUSION

Fatigue was common in patients with stable CHD. Women experienced a greater burden from fatigue compared with men, and this was primarily because of the contribution of depressive symptoms. The use of mixed methods was beneficial to the study of fatigue in stable CHD and provided additional insight, especially in participants who reported low interference from fatigue. This study provides an important contribution to understanding fatigue as a possible symptom of stable CHD; however, these descriptive findings preclude determining if fatigue is an indicator of new onset or progressive CHD. Future research is needed to establish the mechanisms of fatigue in this population. In addition, longitudinal studies are essential to understand causal relationships between depression and fatigue. Further study is also needed to examine the effectiveness of interventions on reducing fatigue to improve HRQoL in patients with stable CHD.

Accepted for publication November 12, 2013.

The authors acknowledge that this research was supported in part by grants from the Midwest Nursing Research Society and Sigma Theta Tau International.

The authors have no conflicts of interest to disclose.

Corresponding author: Ann L. Eckhardt, PhD, RN, School of Nursing, Illinois Wesleyan University, P.O. Box 2900, Bloomington, IL 61702 (e-mail: aeckhard@iwu.edu).

REFERENCES

Aaronson, L. S., Teel, C. S., Cassmeyer, V., Neuberger, G. B., Pallikkathayil, L., Pierce, J., & Wingate, A. (1999). Defining and measuring fatigue. *Image: The Journal of Nursing Scholarship, 31*, 45-50.

American Heart Association. (2013). Coronary artery disease. Retrieved from http://www.heart.org/HEARTORG/Conditions/More/MyHeartandStrokeNews/Coronary-Artery-Disease—The-ABCs-of-CAD_UCM_436416_Article.jsp

American Psychiatric Association. (2013). *Diagnostic and statistical manual of mental disorders* (5th ed.). Arlington, VA: American Psychiatric Publishing.

Centers for Disease Control and Prevention. (2012). Health-related quality of life (HRQOL). Retrieved from http://www.cdc.gov/hrqol/

DeVon, H. A., Ryan, C. J., Ochs, A. L., & Shapiro, M. (2008). Symptoms across the continuum of acute coronary syndromes: Differences between women and men. *American Journal of Critical Care, 17*, 14-24.

Dittner, A. J., Wessely, S. C., & Brown, R. G. (2004). The assessment of fatigue: A practical guide for clinicians and researchers. *Journal of Psychosomatic Research, 56*, 157-170. doi:10.1016/S0022-3999(03)00371-4

Donovan, K. A., Jacobsen, P. B., Small, B. J., Munster, P. N., & Andrykowski, M. A. (2008). Identifying clinically meaningful fatigue with the fatigue symptom inventory. *Journal of Pain and Symptom Management, 36*, 480-487. doi:10.1016/j.jpainsymman.2007.11.013

Ekmann, A., Osler, M., & Avlund, K. (2012). The predictive value of fatigue for nonfatal ischemic heart disease and all-cause mortality. *Psychosomatic Medicine, 74*, 464-470. doi:10.1097/PSY.0b013e318258d294

Evangelista, L. S., Moser, D. K., Westlake, C., Pike, N., Ter-Galstanyan, A., & Dracup, K. (2008). Correlates of fatigue in patients with heart failure. *Progress in Cardiovascular Nursing, 23*, 12-17.doi:10.1111/j.1751-7117.2008.07275.x

Fennessy, M. M., Fink, A. M., Eckhardt, A. L., Jones, J., Kruse, D. K., VanderZwan, K. J., . . . Zerwic, J. J. (2010). Gender differences in fatigue associated with acute myocardial infarction. *Journal of Cardiopulmonary Rehabilitation and Prevention, 30*, 224-230. doi:10.1097/HCR.0b013e3181d0c493

Fink, A. M., Eckhardt, A. L., Fennessy, M. M., Jones, J., Kruse, D., VanderZwan, K. J., . . . Zerwic, J. J. (2010). Psychometric properties of three instruments to measure fatigue with myocardial infarction. *Western Journal of Nursing Research, 32*, 967-983. doi:10.1177/0193945910371320

Fink, A. M., Gonzalez, R. C., Lisowski, T., Pini, M., Fantuzzi, G., Levy, W. C., & Piano, M. R. (2012). Fatigue, inflammation, and projected mortality in heart failure. *Journal of Cardiac Failure, 18*, 711-716. http://dx.doi.org/10.1016/j.cardfail.2012.07.003

Fink, A. M., Sullivan, S. L., Zerwic, J. J., & Piano, M. R. (2009). Fatigue with systolic heart failure. *Journal of Cardiovascular Nursing, 24*, 410-417. doi:10.1097/JCN.0b013e3181ae1e84

Goblirsch, G., Bershow, S., Cummings, K., Hayes, R., Kokoszka, M., Lu, Y., Sanders, D., & Zarling, K. (2013). Stable coronary artery disease. Institute for Clinical Systems Improvement. Retrieved from https://www.icsi.org/_asset/t6bh6a/SCAD.pdf

Greene, J. C. (2007). *Mixed methods in social inquiry*. San Francisco, CA: Jossey-Bass.

Hägglund, L., Boman, K., Stenlund, H., Lundman, B., & Brunlin, C. (2008). Factors related to fatigue among older patients with heart failure in primary health care. *International Journal of Older People Nursing, 3*, 96-103.

Hann, D. M., Denniston, M. M., & Baker, F. (2000). Measurement of fatigue in cancer patients: Further validation of the fatigue symptom inventory. *Quality of Life Research, 9*, 847-854. doi:10.1023/A:1008900413113

Hann, D. M., Jacobsen, P. B., Azzarello, L. M., Martin, S. C., Curran, S. L., Fields, K. K., . . . Lyman, G. (1998). Measurement of fatigue in cancer patients: Development and validation of the Fatigue Symptom Inventory. *Quality of Life Research, 7*, 301-310. doi:10.1023/A:1024929829627

Jones, J., McDermott, C. M., Nowels, C. T., Matlock, D. D., & Bekelman, D. B. (2012). The experience of fatigue as a distressing symptom of heart failure. *Heart & Lung: The Journal of Acute and Critical Care, 41*, 484–491. doi:10.1016/j.hrtlng.2012.04.004

Kimble, L. P., Dunbar, S. B., Weintraub, W. S., McGuire, D. B., Manzo, S. F., & Strickland, O. L. (2011). Symptom clusters and health-related quality of life in people with chronic stable angina. *Journal of Advanced Nursing, 67*, 1000–1011. doi:10.1111/j.1365-2648.2010.05564.x

Kop, W. J., Appels, A. P. W. M., Mendes de Leon, C. F., & Bar, F. W. (1996). The relationship between severity of coronary artery disease and vital exhaustion. *Journal of Psychosomatic Research, 40*, 397–405.

Kroenke, K., Spitzer, R. L., & Williams, J. B. W. (2001). The PHQ-9: Validity of a brief depression severity measure. *Journal of General Internal Medicine, 16*, 606–613. doi:10.1046/j.1525-1497.2001.016009606.x

Lee, K. S., Lennie, T. A., Heo, S., & Moser, D. K. (2012). Association of physical versus affective depressive symptoms with cardiac event-free survival in patients with heart failure. *Psychosomatic Medicine, 74*, 452–458. doi:10.1097/psy.0b013e31824a0641

Leech, N. L., & Onwuegbuzie, A. J. (2009). A typology of mixed methods research designs. *Quality & Quantity, 43*, 265–275. doi:10.1007/s11135-007-9105-3

Lenz, E. R., Pugh, L. C., Milligan, R. A., Gift, A., & Suppe, F. (1997). The middle-range theory of unpleasant symptoms: An update. *Advances in Nursing Science, 19*, 14–27.

Lindeberg, S. I., Rosvall, M., & Östergren, P.-O. (2012). Exhaustion predicts coronary heart disease independently of symptoms of depression and anxiety in men but not in women. *Journal of Psychosomatic Research, 72*, 17–21. doi:10.1016/j.jpsychores.2011.09.001

McHorney, C. A., Ware, J. E., & Raczek, A. E. (1993). The MOS 36-item short-form health survey (SF-36): II. Psychometric and clinical tests of validity in measuring physical and mental health constructs. *Medical Care, 31*, 247–263.

McSweeney, J. C., & Crane, P. B. (2000). Challenging the rules: Womens prodromal and acute symptoms of myocardial infarction. *Research in Nursing & Health, 23*, 135–146. doi:10.1002/(SICI)1098-240X(200004)23:2<135::AID-NUR6>3.0.CO;2-1

Onwuegbuzie, A. J., & Combs, J. P. (2010). Emergent data analysis techniques in mixed methods research: A synthesis. In TashakkoriA.TeddlieC. (Eds.), *Handbook of mixed methods in social and behavioral research* (2nd ed., pp. 397–430). Los Angeles, CA: Sage.

Pragodpol, P., & Ryan, C. (2013). Critical review of factors predicting health-related quality of life in newly diagnosed coronary artery disease patients. *Journal of Cardiovascular Nursing, 28*, 277–284. doi:10.1097/JCN.0b013e31824af56e

Ream, E., & Richardson, A. (1996). Fatigue: A concept analysis. *International Journal of Nursing Studies, 33*, 519–529. doi:10.1016/0020-7489(96)00004-1

Shaffer, J. A., Davidson, K. W., Schwartz, J. E., Shimbo, D., Newman, J. D., Gurland, B. J., & Maurer, M. S. (2012). Prevalence and characteristics of anergia (lack of energy) in patients with acute coronary syndrome. *American Journal of Cardiology, 110*, 1213–1218. doi:10.1016/j.amjcard.2012.06.022

Skapinakis, P., Lewis, G., Mavreas, V. (2004). Temporal relations between unexplained fatigue and depression: Longitudinal data from an international study in primary care. *Psychosomatic Medicine, 66*, 330–335. doi:10.1097/01.psy.0000124757.10167.b1

Staniute, M., Bunevicius, A., Brozaitiene, J., & Bunevicius, R. (2013). Relationship of health-related quality of life with fatigue and exercise capacity in patients with coronary artery disease. *European Journal of Cardiovascular Nursing*. doi:10.1177/1474515113496942

Zimmermann-Viehoff, F., Wang, H. X., Kirkeeide, R., Schneiderman, N., Erdur, L., Deter, H. C., & Orth-Gomer, K. (2013). Womens exhaustion and coronary artery atherosclerosis progression: The Stockholm female coronary angiography study. *Psychosomatic Medicine, 75*, 478–485. doi:10.1097/PSY.0b013e3182928c28

Reprinted with permission from Eckhardt, A., et al. (2014). Fatigue in the presence of coronary heart disease. *Nursing Research, 63*, 83–93.

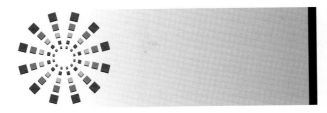

Ulrica Langegård, MSc, RN

Karin Ahlberg, PhD, RN

Thomas Björk-Eriksson, PhD, MD

Per Fransson, PhD, RN

Birgitta Johansson, PhD, RN

Emma Ohlsson-Nevo, PhD, RN

Petra Witt-Nyström, PhD, MD

Katarina Sjövall, PhD, RN

The Art of Living With Symptoms: A Qualitative Study Among Patients With Primary Brain Tumors Receiving Proton Beam Therapy

KEYWORDS

Symptom experience

Symptom management

Proton beam therapy

Brain tumor

Qualitative study

Background: Symptom management in conjunction with proton beam therapy (PBT) from patient's perspective has not been explored. Such knowledge is essential to optimize the care in this relatively new treatment modality. **Objective:** The aim of this study was to explore the process of symptom management in patients with brain tumor receiving PBT. **Methods:** Participants were 22 patients with primary brain tumor who received PBT, recruited in collaboration with a national center for proton therapy and 2 oncology clinics at 2 university hospitals in Sweden. Interviews using open-ended questions were conducted before, during, and/or after treatment. Verbatim interview transcripts were analyzed using classic Grounded Theory. **Results:** "The art of living with symptoms" emerged as the core concept. This encompassed 3 interconnected symptom management concepts: "Adapting to limited ability," "Learning about oneself," and "Creating new routines." These concepts were summarized in a substantive theoretical model of symptom management. Despite the struggle to manage symptoms, participants lived a satisfactory life. **Conclusions:** Symptom management in conjunction with PBT comprises a process of action, thoughts, and emotions. The concepts that emerged indicated patients' symptom

Author Affiliations: Institute of Health and Care Sciences, Sahlgrenska Academy, University of Gothenburg (Mrs Langegård and Dr Ahlberg); Department of Oncology, Institute of Clinical Sciences, Sahlgrenska Academy, University of Gothenburg, and Regional Cancer Center West, Gothenburg (Dr Björk-Eriksson); The Skandion Clinic, Uppsala (Drs Björk-Eriksson and Witt-Nyström); Department of Nursing, Umeå University, and Department of Cancercentrum, Norrlands University Hospital, Umeå (Dr Fransson); Experimental Oncology, Department of Immunology, Genetics and Pathology, Uppsala University, Uppsala University Hospital (Dr Johansson); University Healthcare Research Centre, Faculty of Medicine and Health, Örebro University (Dr Ohlsson-Nevo); Department of Immunology, Genetics and Pathology, Section of Oncology, Uppsala University (Dr Witt-Nyström); and Department of Oncology, Skåne University Hospital, and Department of Oncology, Lund University, Sweden (Dr Sjövall).

The authors have no conflicts of interest to disclose.

This work was supported by the Cancer Foundation in Sweden (grant nos. CAN2015/428 and CAN 2016/809).

Correspondence: Ulrica Langegård, MSc, RN, Institute of Health and Care Sciences, University of Gothenburg, Box 457, 405 30 Göteborg, Sweden (ulrica.langegard@gu.se).

This is an open-access article distributed under the terms of the Creative Commons Attribution-Non Commercial-No Derivatives License 4.0 (CCBY-NC-ND), where it is permissible to download and share the work provided it is properly cited. The work cannot be changed in any way or used commercially without permission from the journal.

Accepted for publication November 7, 2018.

DOI: 10.1097/NCC.0000000000000692

155

> management strategies were based on their own resources. **Implications for Practice:** It is important that PBT facilities develop an approach that facilitates the symptom management process based on patients' experiences of symptoms, as well as their actions and available resources.

Primary brain tumors (both benign and malignant) are predicted to occur in approximately 1400 adults in Sweden each year.[1] Brain tumors affect people of all ages but commonly occur in individuals older than 60 years. Radiotherapy is used to treat brain tumors, either as the primary treatment modality or as a supplement to surgery, and is often combined with chemotherapy.[2] Conventional photon radiotherapy treatment is associated with patient-reported acute and late symptoms.[3] Optimizing radiation parameters in terms of the lowest efficient total doses and (when possible) limiting radiation volume may improve outcomes and reduce neurotoxicity for patients with brain tumors.[4] Proton beam therapy (PBT) is a radiotherapy modality in which proton particles penetrate deep into the target and stop at a certain depth depending on their energy. This spares normal tissues beyond the target from unnecessary radiation, thereby reducing the risk for adverse effects in patients with brain tumors.[5] Proton beam therapy may reduce the risk of damage to healthy tissues; in some cases, the dose targeted at the tumor may be increased, meaning control over the tumor is also increased.[6] There is emerging evidence that PBT has lower toxicity in treating brain tumors and thereby achieves better patient-reported health-related quality of life (QoL) than conventional radiotherapy does.[7,8] However, most available literature is quantitative and is based on studies that used retrospective or cross-sectional designs.

The diagnosis of a primary brain tumor and the effects of treatment have a major impact on patients' QoL, particularly as treatment is often extensive.[9] In addition to suffering from treatment adverse effects, patients must manage fear and psychosocial distress associated with the disease. Symptoms may remain unnoticed and underdiagnosed but still have a major impact on daily life.[10] Debilitating symptoms may affect a patient's cognitive and physical abilities. Studies on symptom prevalence in connection with a brain tumor describe physical symptoms (fatigue, headache, double vision, nausea, vomiting, seizures, sleep disturbance), emotional symptoms (mood disturbances, depression, and anxiety), and neurocognitive symptoms (confusion, memory loss, speech difficulties, and decreased concentration).[2,11–13] The distinction between a cancer diagnosis and a benign tumor in the central nervous system when it comes to patient-related outcome before treatment, during treatment (surgery and/or radiotherapy and/or chemotherapy), and months after treatment may not be 2 distinct separate categories divided by the prognosis. However, little is known about how patients with brain tumors experience these symptoms and how they manage them during radiotherapy.

■ Symptom Experience and Management

In healthcare settings, the experience of symptoms is central to communication and dialogue about illness between patients and professionals. Various theories have been developed to explain the occurrence of symptoms and their relationships with other factors.[14,15] Symptoms generally become known through reports of the person experiencing those symptoms. The present study defines a symptom as "a subjective experience reflecting changes in the biopsychosocial functioning, sensations or cognition of an individual."[16] Both symptoms and signs disrupt patients' QoL, and they are important in evaluating a patient's health and illness. Symptom management aims to prevent or delay negative outcomes through biomedical, professional, and self-care strategies. A basic assumption is that all troublesome symptoms require management. Symptom management should influence or control the symptom experience, rather than only symptom outcomes.[16] It is well known that the burden of symptoms that affect QoL for patients with brain tumor undergoing PBT is significant.[17] Despite existing theories and models, there is a gap in the literature regarding symptom management from the perspective of patients with brain tumor receiving PBT.

No previous studies in the target patient population have explored the symptom management and the effects on patients' everyday life. Such knowledge is essential to enhance understanding of the experiences and needs of patients with brain tumors. Increased understanding in this area will inform new hypotheses for future research and identify practice issues that healthcare professionals should address in more depth. Therefore, the present qualitative study aimed to explore the process of symptom management in patients with brain tumor receiving PBT.

■ Methods

Study Design

This study used a prospective, longitudinal design and incorporated the procedures and principles of classic Grounded Theory (GT).[18] The approach described by Glaser and Strauss[18] was used to answer the research question "How do patients manage the symptoms they experience?" Data were collected through individual interviews with participating patients.

Methodology

Glaser and Strauss[18] and Glaser[19] stated that the constant comparative method is essential in GT analysis. Furthermore, Glaser and Strauss[18] presented GT as a method that aims to generate a substantive or formal theory. A substantive theory means that the result is applicable in a specific area, whereas a formal theory can be applied in different areas. Grounded Theory studies create concepts through constant comparative methods that include all parts of the data as well as interpreted emerged codes, categories, and main concerns to explore variations, similarities, and

Reprinted with permission from Langegard, U., et al. (2020). The art of living with symptoms: A qualitative study among patient with primary brain tumors receiving proton beam therapy. *Cancer Nursing*, 43(2), E79–E86.

differences. All extracted categories, concepts, and their indicators should be grounded in data. With this method, the analysis process proceeds as the researcher continuously writes theoretical drafts or memos.[18,19] Classic GT indicates that the researcher should include existing preunderstanding in parentheses, by raising consciousness about the preunderstanding and thereby controlling influence as far as possible. This study used a deductive/inductive approach that stressed the process rather than the meaning of the studied phenomenon. An inductive approach allows participants to describe their thoughts and actions in their own words, and at the same time a deductive approach focuses on finding new indicators for the concepts or main concern. We aimed to develop a substantive theoretical model based on empirical data to show the process of how patients with brain tumor receiving PBT managed their symptoms.

Setting

Interviews were conducted at the Skandion Clinic and 2 university hospitals in Sweden. The Skandion Clinic is the first Nordic clinic to offer PBT treatment, and patients travel to the clinic from all over Sweden. Patients are referred for PBT after preparation (including imaging and treatment planning) at their home university hospital. Most patients are unable to commute between their homes and the Skandion Clinic and therefore have to stay in a nearby patient hotel during treatment. Costs for the stay are covered by the national public health insurance system.

Participants

This study was a multicenter study, including participants who were referred for PBT from 1 of Sweden's 7 university hospitals. Participants were 22 adult patients with primary brain tumor who were receiving PBT. The patients were all selected for PBT and included into the Proton Radiotherapy for Primary Central Nervous System Tumours in Adults study[20] and subsequently into the current study owing to nonresectable brain tumors, substantial tumor volumes, and continuous tumor growth on repeated computed tomography scans before start of treatment. One patient declined to participate, with the explanation that she lacked time. Patients who agreed to participate provided written informed consent before the interview. Ten participants were interviewed during the treatment period. Another 12 were interviewed both before and immediately after the treatment period.

Ethical Consideration

The Ethics committee in Gothenburg, Sweden, no. 433-15, approved the study in July 2015. All participation in the study is based on informed consent.

Procedure

This study is a part of a larger multicenter study that is approved by the research committees at all involved hospitals. All patients were informed about the study and invited to participate via telephone by the first author (U.L.). Face-to-face interviews were conducted by the first author (28 interviews) and another experienced oncology nurse (6 interviews). Having 2 experienced nurses conducting the

interviews enabled inclusion of participants from all parts of Sweden. Five interviews were conducted by telephone when face-to-face interviews were not possible. To ensure dependability, interview techniques were discussed between the 2 interviewers according to the recommendations of Morse et al[21] about stepwise verification strategies. The same interview guide was used by the 2 interviewers. The interview guide was modified over time according to GT principles,[18] with changes based on identified concepts.

Data Collection

Interviews were conducted with the aim of exploring how participants managed their symptoms. In the first step of the recruitment process, participants were strategically selected to provide a broad perspective, with selection based on age, sex, and civil status (Table 1) and on how participants managed their symptoms. Most of included participants had malignant tumor at this stage of the sampling. After analyzing the initial interviews, we replaced the strategical sampling with theoretical sampling based on the emerging findings. In this second step, participants with benign tumors were primarily selected. This was done to gain variation of symptom management during the treatment period and also to confirm saturation. Recruitment of new participants and data collection concluded when saturation was reached, which was the point at which the most recent interviews did not seem to make a substantial contribution to the model that was successively generated from earlier data. Three participants were selected to confirm the extracted concepts, giving a total of 34 interviews.

Interviews started with the open-ended question, "Can you please tell me about your situation based on your current illness, including how you manage the symptoms you experience?" Follow-up questions were asked, such as "What does it mean to you in your daily life?" This resulted in a deeper narrative in

Table 1 • Participant's Demographic Information (n = 22)

Parameters	n
Gender	
Women	10
Men	12
Age, y	
26-35	5
36-45	4
46-55	8
56-65	1
66-75	4
Diagnosis	
Malignant brain tumor	14
Benign brain tumor	8
Civil status	
Married with children living at home	11
Single	6
Married	5
Education	
Elementary	3
Secondary	11
University	8

which participants reflected on how they managed their symptoms. Memos describing what was experienced were written immediately after the interviews. The interviews lasted 30 to 70 minutes. All interviews were performed in Swedish, as well as the data analysis. Translation to English was made when writing the manuscript. Manuscript was then reviewed by a professional translator.

Data Analysis

Interviews were transcribed verbatim and consecutively analyzed using the constant comparative method.[18] NVivo (version 11; QSR International, Melbourne, Australia) was used for categorizing the transcribed verbatim. The first step involved open coding. Data were examined line by line to identify each patient's description of their thought patterns, feelings, and actions related to the themes mentioned in the interviews. The derived codes were formulated in words used by the patients to maintain the semantics of the data. Codes were compared to verify their descriptive content and confirm they were grounded in the data. Indicators of symptom management were identified. Table 2 illustrates the analytical process and includes an example of a memo. The second step involved sorting the codes into categories using constant comparisons between categories, codes, and interview protocols. In the third step, identified categories were fitted together using the constant comparative method. The theoretical sampling was a process of taking information from the data collection and comparing it to emerging categories. The parallel process of data collection and data analysis allowed specification of relationships between categories and abstraction to theoretical concepts. The analysis resulted in a substantive theoretical model with 8 categories resting on 3 concepts and 1 core concept. The analysis process was discussed by 3 of the authors (U.L., K.A., and K.S.), who read and/or analyzed a sample of the transcripts. Emerging codes and categories were compared and collectively discussed with all the authors. Final concepts were then agreed. All the authors are experienced researchers, and 1 has long experience from working with GT (K.A.). The authors are either clinically experienced nurses (U.L., K.S., P.F., B.J., E.O.N., and K.A.) or clinically experienced physicians (T.B.E. and P.W.). During the whole analysis process, the researchers' preunderstanding was constantly discussed.

■ Results

The aim of this study was to explore the process of symptom management in patients with brain tumor receiving PBT. An overall model (Figure 1) describing symptom management as a process was developed. The analysis extracted "The art of living

with symptoms" as a core concept, which encompassed 3 interconnected symptom management concepts: "Adapting to limited ability," "Learning about oneself," and "Creating new routines." The symptoms that the participants experience ranged from severe symptoms (eg, consequences of epilepsy) to less severe symptoms (eg, low-intensity headaches). Participants' experiences of symptoms were not different in relation to whether it was a benignant or malignant tumor that was treated. Common for all participants were the increasing intensity of symptoms over time and the major impact on daily life. Despite the presence of symptoms and significant restrictions on everyday life, participants expressed living a satisfactory life as they handled the situation by different strategies based on their own action and personal resources.

Adapting to Limited Ability

The theoretical concept "Adapting to limited ability" described how the patients manage the challenges related to the symptoms and comprised 4 categories: "Lack of multitasking," "Priority of doing," "The body as a barrier," and "Limitations in daily life." "Lack of multitasking" reflected participants' diminished capacity to perform daily chores owing to limited multitasking capability. They expressed an ability to only perform 1 activity at a time. Several participants spoke of experiencing difficulties after completing treatment every day and returning home to their family and multiple obligations.

> Then it's not only to get back into the everyday routine. To get back when you have kids, take care of daycare and school and that is the home, which is a stress in itself. Right after the radiation. It's just a lot. (10)

"Priority of doing" included the ability to prioritize and opt out of certain actions, including social activities (eg, holidays) and domestic labor.

Partly I have to think first...before I head into things...almost every weekend we were on a summer holiday and other adventures. And all of those things we have to set aside because of my illness. (1)

"The body as a barrier" was a category that became obvious when participants described how they had to adapt their daily lives after being diagnosed and started treatment. They described how ordinary events, such as going to the toilet, now demanded rigorous planning, effort, and time. The same was reported for more extensive activities.

Because one is not fast. Just to go to the bathroom takes 3 times as long. I just sit down. I sit down like this. Then I sit. I almost have to count 'til 3 to get up and do something. I don't know what it is. (20)

The category "Limitations in daily life" reflected how participants became aware of possible obstacles because of symptoms

✳ **Table 2 •** The Analytical Process			
Quote	Category	Concept	Memo
"Because one is not fast. Just to go to the bathroom takes 3 times as long. I just sit down. I sit down like this. Then I sit. I almost have to count til 3 to get up and do something. I don't know what it is".	The body as a barrier	Adapting to limited ability	"The patient is very limited in everyday life. She feels a strong worry for the future and is significantly affected by her disease. She shares her emotions and trying to describe how the disease and treatment affects her."

The table gives an example in the analysis process through coding, category and concept, including a memo in the category "The body as a barrier."

Reprinted with permission from Langegard, U., et al. (2020). The art of living with symptoms: A qualitative study among patient with primary brain tumors receiving proton beam therapy. *Cancer Nursing, 43*(2), E79–E86.

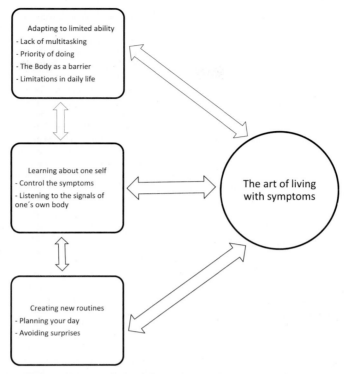

Figure 1. Process of symptoms management in patients with brain tumor receiving proton beam therapy.

experienced and how even simple chores (eg, emptying the dishwasher) became impossible tasks. Furthermore, participants reported having to give up beloved pastimes. Concurrent with existing obstacles, they were no longer allowed to perform activities such as driving a car, which placed major limitations on their everyday lives.

What are obvious are the epileptic cramps. And that I get tired in public but otherwise I am not in pain. There are some things I cannot do. I cannot drive a car. I shall not expose myself to some contexts. One shall not be intoxicated. One shall not be at high altitudes. One shall not swim in deep water. So one is a little limited. (13)

Learning About Oneself

The theoretical concept "Learning about oneself" was also a way to manage the symptoms and comprised 2 categories: "Controlling the symptoms" and "Listening to the signals of one's own body." In the "Controlling the symptoms category," participants described the importance of managing their daily lives by gaining control of the intensity and frequency of their symptoms. Participants reported experiencing several symptoms of varying intensity that had a major influence on their daily lives and led to considerable changes in most cases. Participants managed to control their symptoms by getting to know their own body. They expressed

developing increased awareness of how to lead their life to gain control over symptoms by prioritizing good sleep, obtaining a balance between rest and physical activity, and having regular meals; otherwise, an increased intensity and number of symptoms was expected.

But it's one of those things that the brain has taught itself. Furthermore, I know how to act to get more or less of the symptoms. Healthy living. Too little sleep, too little food, and too much work. Then the symptoms increase. (11)

The category "Listening to the signals of one's own body" reflected how participants learned to anticipate symptoms by listening to their own body's signals and taking them more seriously. Not listening to one's own body led to an increase in symptoms.

With the epileptic cramps it's the same. Too much stress and it says "bang." Stress is bad. It cannot be eliminated through medication. I have to live normally. If I live badly the cramps will come knocking at my door. (3)

Creating New Routines

"Creating new routines in daily life" was a distinguishing that reflected how participants found a new daily balance. This encompassed creating practical routines and new roles. Participants' life patterns underwent radical transformation as a result of their symptoms. The theoretical concept of creating new

Reprinted with permission from Langegard, U., et al. (2020). The art of living with symptoms: A qualitative study among patient with primary brain tumors receiving proton beam therapy. *Cancer Nursing, 43*(2), E79–E86.

routines comprised 2 categories: "Planning your day" and "Avoiding surprises." In the category "Planning your day," participants expressed the importance of planning or structuring their day in advance. This involved scheduling minor to major activities, from taking care of personal hygiene to performing work. All chores needed to be planned in detail. Before committing to different activities, participants reflected on what was required to ensure that they could manage those activities. Several participants mentioned the need to write notes about how their day would be structured. Fatigue that increased over time was considered an enemy; participants endeavored to create new routines to avoid fatigue. For example, resting at midday was a routine that was not included in earlier life patterns.

It has to do with my brain tiredness; I sort of want to plan everything ahead. (1)

The category "Avoiding surprises" reflected how participants experienced increased stress levels. This left no room for surprises, such as a friend or relative asking for help or making a spontaneous visit. Fatigue increased when habitual routines were disrupted, which in turn increased the risk of other symptoms such as epilepsy and headache. Most life events were undertaken in low gear.

I have to know in advance what the day will look like. Something unplanned cannot happen that I have to focus on. It will only mess up the head. (7)

■ Discussion

This is the first qualitative study worldwide to explore symptom management among patients who received PBT for primary benign or malignant brain tumors. "The art of living with symptoms" emerged as the core concept, illustrating an ongoing process of action and thoughts throughout the treatment period. Our findings showed that participants had to consider how to live their life in terms of the new conditions of illness and treatment. In the process of achieving symptom relief, participating patients used themselves as a resource through strategies such as adapting to their limited ability, learning about oneself, and creating new routines. The present results are discussed in relation to existing theories in the field.

Participants' comments indicated that they were important actors in the process of symptom management. The data showed that participants managed their symptoms in similar ways, regardless of whether they were treated for a malignant or benignant tumor. However, it is important to note that most participants stayed at the patient hotel during their 5-week PBT treatment. These circumstances might have influenced the experience of a better QoL and also increased capability for self-care compared with those who received conventional treatment at their local clinic. In addition, participating patients might have been selected for PBT because of their better health-status.

The number of symptoms that the participants described and the treatment period contributed to a perception of increased intensity of symptom experience. The present analysis highlighted the challenge of understanding how patients managed to live a satisfactory life despite the presence of symptoms and limited ability in their everyday lives. Similar findings have been described in other studies among patients with primary brain tumor.[22–24] Bitterlich and Vordermark[22] found no decrease in patients' QoL despite radiotherapy and associated side effects. Piil et al[24] reported that patients adjusted to symptom limitations through an ongoing process of becoming aware of, and adapting to, the loss of functioning. Bennett et al[23] explored the impact of symptoms on QoL and found that a consistent theme was an underlying determination to "get on with life" and not be bound by symptomatic implications. These studies showed how patients maintained their QoL by taking part in daily living and focusing on positive aspects in their lives. Therefore, how well an individual participant tolerated symptoms over time may reflect a higher tolerance for perceived symptoms in that person and indicate their symptom management strategies were effective.

Participants in this study perceived that it was important to establish a balance and create new everyday routines when their existence and fundamental security were threatened by illness. During the latter part of the treatment period, participants were affected by fatigue; despite this, they reported that it was important to continue with their everyday life routines. Participants planned their days carefully, which gave them control and reassurance. This is consistent with the response shift theory, which describes how a patient confronted with a life-threatening disease adapts to the disease and modifies his/her internal norms, values, and conceptualization of what he/she is experiencing. When health is no longer manageable and available energy does not allow work to be performed as before, attention may be refocused on developing resources and properties other than professional accomplishments, such as intimate relationships.[25]

Response shift processes have been documented in various cancer populations.[26–28] Sprangers and Schartz[25] discussed the integration of response shift in QoL. When participants in the present study were confronted with a life-threatening or chronic disease, they also faced the need to adapt to their illness and symptoms. Sprangers and Schwartz interpreted response shift as an important mediator in this adaptation process, involving changing internal standards, values, and the conceptualization of QoL. An explanation for why most participants in this study achieved a satisfactory life might be that they had the resources to change their internal standards.[25]

Most participating patients had no permanent symptoms before diagnosis with a brain tumor. A debut symptom of a tumor may be an acute epileptic seizure or slowly deteriorating eyesight. Therefore, a patient's adaptation to being diagnosed with a tumor and experiencing symptoms might have been abrupt. This transition represents dramatic changes in health status, relationships, and roles. It also involves a change in human needs, as an individual has to assimilate new knowledge and change their behavior accordingly. This transition includes meaning, expectations, knowledge, environment, planning, and well-being. Participants in the present study talked about their own essential personal development when transitioning from a state of good health to facing a potentially life-threatening primary brain tumor. An important factor indicating how well participants managed their symptoms was their reflection on how they perceived their surroundings, how their life should be lived, and what relationships were important to them, as well as learning how to accept their new situation.

Several previous studies have discussed posttraumatic growth as an outcome of highly stressful life events. Posttraumatic growth may result in greater appreciation for life, better relationships with others, and a commitment to live a healthier life.[29,30] Groarke et al[31] presented evidence to support a hypothesis that stress was related to higher posttraumatic growth; higher cancer-specific stress was found 6 months after diagnosis. The findings of the present study provide additional support for positive growth among those who struggle with a challenging illness.

The substantive theoretical model developed during the present analysis (Figure 1) described the process of how participants expressed their symptoms, and presents the abstracted core concept and an interpretation of how they managed their symptoms. The arrows illustrate the development of participants' personal resources and how they reached the core concept ("The art of living with symptoms").

Methodological Considerations

Data from 22 participants provided diverse views on patients' experiences, particularly regarding how participants managed their symptoms. A strength of the present study was the large number of interviews included in the analysis. In addition, the wide age range of participants, inclusion of both sexes, and participants remitted from all over Sweden increased the likelihood that our findings may be transferable to other patients in the studied diagnosis group. The present study focused on exploring symptom management in patients with primary brain tumors receiving PBT. We chose not to separate the analysis based on whether the patient had a benign or malignant tumor, as benign tumors may become life threatening if they are not treated.

Furthermore, when collecting and comparing data on patient reported symptom during the treatment for patients with benign or malignant brain tumor, we saw that reported symptoms seem to be as frequent among the 2 groups. However, further research is required to elucidate potential differences that might affect the patient with brain tumor during and after the process of treatment. Qualitative studies with focus on the disease experience as well as comparative studies of the 2 groups treated with PBT and with adequate follow-up are suggested.

The Skandion Clinic is a novel facility using a new care strategy and required most patients to stay at a hotel. These circumstances may limit the transferability of the findings to patients treated in ordinary Swedish cancer care facilities. To ensure credibility, 2 authors (U.L. and K.A.) started the analysis process and created the concepts together, using classic GT.[18] The first author (U.L.) has many years of experience in oncology nursing. During the inductive phase, memos and regular discussion were conducted among the research group. The memos provided a trustworthy data source for the analysis, as they were obtained by regular use of a reflective research diary. To gain a deeper understanding of symptom management, many participants completed 2 interviews. Interviews were conducted by telephone when face-to-face interviews were not possible, but we assessed these telephone interviews as being of value.

■ Implications for Nursing

It is important to increase knowledge about how patients manage the symptoms to effectively support patients with brain tumors receiving PBT. When nursing for these patients, it is essential to support their own personal resources and their strategies in symptom management and, thus, maintaining daily life. The substantive theoretical model developed in this study can be used to increase caregivers' understanding of a patient's individual resources in managing symptoms and can be used for initiating discussion about a patient's symptom experience and symptom management.

■ Conclusion

Grounded Theory was used to develop a substantive theoretical model to explain the symptom management process in patients with primary brain tumors receiving PBT. Most participants in the present study struggled with their symptoms (eg, fatigue, seizures, and sleep disorders). In finding new rhythms and routines, they reported that it was important to establish a balance to avoid symptoms becoming overwhelming. Increased fatigue was central to the development of other aggravating symptoms (eg, seizures). Although participants experienced symptoms differently, symptom management was described as a process of action, thoughts, and emotions. Increasing symptoms over time and the major impact of symptoms on daily life were factors common to all participants. Participants described how they used their own resources to manage their symptoms. "The art of living with symptoms" was the core concept that reflected how participants achieved a satisfactory life by "Adapting to limited ability," "Learning about oneself," and "Creating new routines" despite the number and intensity of symptoms experienced.

ACKNOWLEDGMENTS

The authors thank the study participants for sharing their experiences and thank all employees at Skandion Clinic for support with data collection, especially Caroline Wenngren, RN. We also thank Anette Löfgren, MSc, RN, University Hospital in Lund, for support with data collection.

References

1. The National Board of Health and Welfare. 2017. http://www.socialstyrelsen.se/statistics/statisticaldatabase/cancer. Accessed September 30, 2018.
2. Wen PY, Kesari S. Malignant gliomas in adults. *N Engl J Med*. 2008;359(5):492–507.
3. Ahlberg K, Ekman T, Gaston-Johansson F, Mock V. Assessment and management of cancer-related fatigue in adults. *Lancet (London, England)*. 2003;362(9384):640–650.
4. Scoccianti S, Detti B, Cipressi S, Iannalfi A, Franzese C, Biti G. Changes in neurocognitive functioning and quality of life in adult patients with brain tumors treated with radiotherapy. *J Neurooncol*. 2012;108(2):291–308.
5. Yuh GE, Loredo LN, Yonemoto LT, et al. Reducing toxicity from craniospinal irradiation: using proton beams to treat medulloblastoma in young children. *Cancer J*. 2004;10(6):386–390.
6. Schulz-Ertner D, Tsujii H. Particle radiation therapy using proton and heavier ion beams. *J Clin Oncol*. 2007;25(8):953–964.

7. Verma V, Simone CB2nd, Mishra MV. Quality of life and patient-reported outcomes following proton radiation therapy: a systematic review. *J Natl Cancer Inst.* 2018;110(4):341–353.

8. Maquilan G, Grover S, Alonso-Basanta M, Lustig RA. Acute toxicity profile of patients with low-grade gliomas and meningiomas receiving proton therapy. *Am J Clin Oncol.* 2014;37(5):438–443.

9. Taphoorn MJ, Sizoo EM, Bottomley A. Review on quality of life issues in patients with primary brain tumors. *Oncologist.* 2010;15(6):618–626.

10. Payne C, Wiffen PJ, Martin S. Interventions for fatigue and weight loss in adults with advanced progressive illness. *Cochrane Database Syst Rev (Online).* 2012;1(1): CD008427.

11. Combs SE, Adeberg S, Dittmar J-O, et al. Skull base meningiomas: long-term results and patient self-reported outcome in 507 patients treated with fractionated stereotactic radiotherapy (FSRT) or intensity modulated radiotherapy (IMRT). *Radiother Oncol.* 2013;106(2):186–191.

12. Molassiotis A, Wilson B, Brunton L, Chaudhary H, Gattamaneni R, McBain C. Symptom experience in patients with primary brain tumours: a longitudinal exploratory study. *Eur J Oncol Nurs.* 2010;14(5):410–416.

13. Osoba D, Brada M, Prados MD, Yung WK. Effect of disease burden on health-related quality of life in patients with malignant gliomas. *Neuro Oncol.* 2000;2(4):221–228.

14. Lenz ER, Suppe F, Gift AG, Pugh LC, Milligan RA. Collaborative development of middle-range nursing theories: toward a theory of unpleasant symptoms. *ANS Adv Nurs Sci.* 1995;17(3):1–13.

15. Rhodes VA, Watson PM. Symptom distress—the concept: past and present. *Semin Oncol Nurs.* 1987;3(4):242–247.

16. Dodd MJ, Miaskowski C, Paul SM. Symptom clusters and their effect on the functional status of patients with cancer. *Oncol Nurs Forum.* 2001;28(3):465–470.

17. Liu R, Page M, Solheim K, Fox S, Chang SM. Quality of life in adults with brain tumors: current knowledge and future directions. *Neuro Oncol.* 2009;11(3):330–339.

18. Glaser BG, Strauss AL, Strutzel E. The discovery of grounded theory; strategies for qualitative research. *Nursing Research.* 1968;17(4):364.

19. Glaser BG. *Getting Out of the Data: Grounded Theory Conceptualization.* Mill Valley: Sociology Press; 2011.

20. PRO-CNS. Proton radiotherapy for primary central nervous system tumours in adult. https://clinicaltrials.gov/ct2/show/NCT02797366. 2015. Accessed February 02, 2018.

21. Morse JM, Barrett M, Mayan M, Olson K, Spiers J. Verification strategies for establishing reliability and validity in qualitative research. *Int J Qual Methods.* 2002;1(2):13–22.

22. Bitterlich C, Vordermark D. Analysis of health-related quality of life in patients with brain tumors prior and subsequent to radiotherapy. *Oncol Lett.* 2017;14(2):1841–1846.

23. Bennett SR, Cruickshank G, Lindenmeyer A, Morris SR. Investigating the impact of headaches on the quality of life of patients with glioblastoma multiforme: a qualitative study. *BMJ Open.* 2016;6(11):e011616.

24. Piil K, Juhler M, Jakobsen J, Jarden M. Daily life experiences of patients with a high-grade glioma and their caregivers: a longitudinal exploration of rehabilitation and supportive care needs. *J Neurosci Nurs.* 2015;47(5):271–284.

25. Sprangers MA, Schwartz CE. Integrating response shift into health-related quality of life research: a theoretical model. *Soc Sci Med.* 1999;48(11):1507–1515.

26. Visser MR, Oort FJ, Sprangers MA. Methods to detect response shift in quality of life data: a convergent validity study. *Qual Life Res.* 2005;14(3):629–639.

27. Oort FJ, Visser MRM, Sprangers MAG. An application of structural equation modeling to detect response shifts and true change in quality of life data from cancer patients undergoing invasive surgery. *Qual Life Res.* 2005;14(3):599–609.

28. Sharpe L, Butow P, Smith C, McConnell D, Clarke S. Changes in quality of life in patients with advanced cancer: evidence of response shift and response restriction. *J Psychosom Res.* 2005;58(6):497–504.

29. Sears SR, Stanton AL, Danoff-Burg S. The yellow brick road and the emerald city: benefit finding, positive reappraisal coping and posttraumatic growth in women with early-stage breast cancer. *Health Psychol.* 2003;22(5):487–497.

30. Tedeschi RG, Calhoun LG. The Posttraumatic Growth Inventory: measuring the positive legacy of trauma. *J Trauma Stress.* 1996;9(3):455–471.

31. Groarke A, Curtis R, Groarke JM, Hogan MJ, Gibbons A, Kerin M. Posttraumatic growth in breast cancer: how and when do distress and stress contribute?. *Psychooncology.* 2016;967–974.

Reprinted with permission from Langegard, U., et al. (2020). The art of living with symptoms: A qualitative study among patient with primary brain tumors receiving proton beam therapy. *Cancer Nursing, 43*(2), E79–E86.

Increasing Colorectal Cancer Screening Using a Quality Improvement Approach in a Nurse-Managed Primary Care Clinic

Diane Hountz, Jennifer Coddington, Karen J. Foli, Janet Thorlton

Introduction

Colorectal cancer (CRC) is the third most common type of cancer in men and women in the United States and is the second leading cause of cancer-related deaths in the United States.[1] In 2016, more than 134,000 new cases of CRC will be diagnosed with more than 49,000 of these resulting in a patient death.[2] Individuals with Stage 1 CRC have a 92% 5-year survival rate when detected and treated; however, only 39% of these individuals are diagnosed at Stage 1.[2] With early detection through screening procedures, CRC can be prevented or treated sooner with increased potential for positive patient outcomes.

Colorectal cancer screening modalities are widely available throughout the United States and can detect early-stage cancer and adenomatous polyps.[3] For average risk individuals, the U.S. Preventive Services Task Force recommends CRC screening to begin at age 50 and continue until age 75 years, and to begin at age 40 for those adults with a high risk for CRC.[4] National benchmarks recommend that at least 70% of all adults aged 50 to 75 be screened for CRC.[5]

Recommendations are for CRC screening to be accomplished by either colonoscopy or fecal immunochemical tests (FITs).[3,4] Colonoscopy is the gold standard in CRC screening and can be performed every 10 years if the screening is negative. It is an invasive procedure that allows for direct visualization of the colon, and the physician is able to remove polyps if discovered during the procedure. The FIT is a noninvasive test that relies on the individual to collect a stool sample to send

Abstract: According to the American Cancer Society, 1 in 23 Americans will be diagnosed with colorectal cancer (CRC) in their lifetime. Screening for CRC is an effective, yet underused preventive approach. This is especially true in rural areas, where only 35% of patients were found to be up to date on their screenings in 2014. Increasing CRC screening can produce positive patient outcomes by early recognition and removal of precancerous polyps. The purpose of this project was to use quality improvement (QI) interventions to increase CRC screening rates at a nurse-managed clinic in rural Indiana. Using Deming's Plan-Do-Study-Act QI model, multiple interventions were implemented which resulted in a 37% increase in the number of screenings ordered on eligible patients and an overall increase of 28% in the completion of the screenings. This project contributes to healthcare quality knowledge by also suggesting that the fundamental principles of encouraging staff feedback to gain buy-in, improving processes informed by patient data, and valuing frequent performance feedback to staff, strengthened this QI project and ensured adoption and sustainability of these results.

in to the laboratory and is recommended annually if negative. If the FIT is positive, a colonoscopy is recommended to identify and remove any adenomatous polyps.[3,6]

Purpose

Although screening rates have increased overall in recent years, the rates for patients seen at Federally Qualified Health Clinics (FQHCs) remain around 35% (Figure 1).[7] The purpose of this project was to use a quality improvement (QI) approach to increase CRC screening rates in a rural FQHC nurse-managed health clinic (NMHC). The goals of this project were to

- Review the current CRC screening process used at the NMHC.

Keywords
colorectal cancer
screening
preventive care
quality improvement
nurse-managed health
clinics
nurse led

Journal for Healthcare Quality
Vol. 0, No. 0, pp. 1–12
© 2017 National Association for
Healthcare Quality

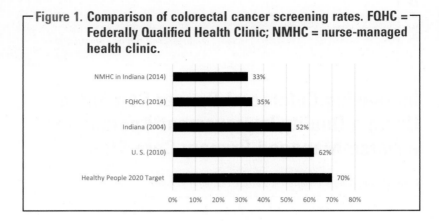

Figure 1. Comparison of colorectal cancer screening rates. FQHC = Federally Qualified Health Clinic; NMHC = nurse-managed health clinic.

- Develop interventions based on results.
- Implement QI interventions to improve the process.
- Evaluate the progress of the interventions implemented.
- Sustain process changes.

Background

In the United States, office-based primary care medicine is the foundation of the healthcare system. Nurse-managed health clinics are one of the venues that provide primary healthcare in medically underserved rural and urban areas.[8] Nurse-managed health clinics are clinics operated by nurses and use nurse practitioners (NPs) as primary care providers. These clinics face challenges to provide high-quality, patient-centered care with limited financial resources while trying to continuously improve preventive screening rates through QI initiatives, (e.g., CRC screening). Currently there are more than 250 NMHCs operating throughout the United States with 2.5 million patient visits per year.[9] Many NMHCs operate in geographic areas with health professional shortages and provide care to low-income and minority individuals, where the primary sources of payment are Medicaid, Medicare, private, and federal grants.[9]

Review of Literature

Barriers. Low rates of CRC screening are a complex problem involving patients, providers, and healthcare systems. Barriers reported for underserved or low-income patients include lack of knowledge on importance of screenings, language barriers, fear of the screening procedure, suffering as a result of the procedures, lack of insurance coverage, and low literacy levels.[10,11] Additional barriers, specific to colonoscopies, reported were the lack of time, scheduling issues, bowel preparation time and discomfort, and lack of transportation. Fecal immunochemical test–specific barriers included being too busy, problems keeping track of cards, and not remembering to mail cards back.[12]

Healthcare system barriers include the inability to provide colonoscopies for patients with a positive FIT due to lack of insurance, lack of time during patient visit, lack of transportation, lack of insurance coverage, and lack of an electronic health record (EHR) tracking system.[10,11,13] A lack of physician/provider recommendation for CRC screening was a common healthcare system barrier in FQHCs, resulting in low screening rates.[14,15]

Interventions to Increase Screening Rates. Numerous approaches to increase CRC screening rates have demonstrated small increases. Menon et al[16] used tailored telephone education and observed a 23% increase in colonoscopy and FIT rates among patients. Tailored navigations through a CRC screening booklet and materials, matched patient preferences for screening, increased screening rates by 6.5% over nontailored interventions.[17] Client reminder postcards yielded a 16% increase in CRC screenings.[18] Lasser et al[19] found patient navigators increased the CRC screening rates at clinics by 13.6%. Hendren et al[20] used a multifaceted approach through letters, automated phone calls, and mailed FIT kits, netting a 21% increase in screening rates. Provider recommendation was found to increase screening rates in one study by 34%.[14]

Methods

Increasing quality of care outcomes in settings involves a problem-solving and iterative approach. The Deming Plan-Do-Study-Act (PDSA) Framework, when applied to systems problems, is shown to improve morale, organizational effectiveness, and efficiency, whereas reducing costs.[21] Throughout this process, the PDSA model emphasized staff input as an integral process for ensuring buy-in and success of any QI project.[22] Therefore, this model was selected as a guiding framework for this project.

Setting

The setting used for this QI project is a NMHC that provides primary care to patients in medically underserved, rural areas of Indiana. A QI committee serves to assess, implement, and monitor all QI initiatives. In 2015, clinic NPs saw more than 3,212 patients, with more than 8,500 patient encounters. About 50% of patients seen are at 100% or above the poverty level. This NMHC received full recognition in 2014 as a Level Two Patient-Centered Medical Home provider. To ensure financial viability, ongoing reporting and improvement of quality of care measures had been in place for the past 15 years. One of these measures was CRC

screenings. A summary of the PDSA methods used to address each of the five main goals of the project are summarized in Table 1.

Institutional Review Board Approval

Our University's Institutional Review Board approved this study in April 2015 (IRB study number 1504015943).

Results

Goal 1: Review the Current CRC Screening Process

A comprehensive assessment of the current CRC screening process was completed. Input was given by all staff involved in the process (i.e., NPs, nurses, medical assistants, administration, QI committee). The QI committee previously established a CRC screening rate goal of 70% for patients aged 51–74. The NMHC is required by Health Resources and Services Administration to monitor, improve, and report different quality initiatives through Uniform Data Sets (UDS) measures. The UDS measurement for CRC screening is from age 51 to 74, so was decided to keep this consistent with monitoring and reporting for these requirements. During May–July 2015, a retrospective review of 200 medical records was conducted for this population. All patients between ages of 51 and 74 who were seen and treated for a medical condition by a NP at the NMHC were included. Patients who were less than 51 years or greater than 74 years and those patients who were not seen or treated by a NP were excluded from the record review.

Data points were then entered into the Research Electronic Data Capture (REDCap) database. Of the 200 charts reviewed, 76 (38%) had either screenings ordered by the provider or were up to date with screenings (see Table 2 for CRC screening definitions). In addition, 60 of the 200 charts (30%) had their screenings ordered by the provider and completed by the patient or were up to date with their screenings. Of those charts with no

Reprinted with permission from Hountz, D., et al. (2017). Increasing colorectal cancer screening using a quality improvement approach in a nurse-managed clinic. *Journal of Healthcare Quality*, *39*, 379–390.

Table 1. Quality Improvement Methods Overview

Goal	PDSA framework	Timeframe	Project tasks
1. Review the current CRC screening process.	Plan	May–July 2015	Determined current CRC screening process. Develop process flow map Retrospective chart review of 200 charts
	Plan		Obtained organizational goal from NMHC QI committee.
	Plan		Reviewed pertinent literature and current practice guidelines.
	Plan		
	Plan	August–September 2015	Informal interviews of NPs and registered nurse staff at NMHC.
	Plan		Analyzed preintervention data with identification of problems.
2. Develop QI interventions.	Plan	August–September 2015	Used problems from predata, staff interviews, review of literature, and clinical guidelines to shape intervention development.
3. Implement QI interventions to improve the process.	Do	October 2015	Educated staff at staff meeting on predata and proposed interventions.
	Do		Obtained staff feedback on proposed interventions and modified interventions.
	Do	Oct 2015–February 2016	Performed weekly chart audits and sent findings to individual providers for feedback.
	Do		Compiled data and sent to providers and posted at NMHC.
	Do		Answered questions and educated staff on new processes.
4. Evaluate the interventions implemented.	Study	Feb 2016–March 2016	Performed biweekly chart audit and sent findings to individual providers
	Study		Retrospective review of 200 charts 2 months postimplementation
	Study		Completed pre and postdata comparison and analysis.
5. Sustain process changes.	Act	April–May 2016	Continue to provide education to staff as needed.
	Act		Post data by provider monthly at NMHC.
	Act		Establish process owners.

CRC = colorectal cancer; NMHC = nurse-managed health clinic; NP = nurse practitioner; PDSA = Plan-Do-Study-Act; QI = quality improvement.

Reprinted with permission from Hountz, D., et al. (2017). Increasing colorectal cancer screening using a quality improvement approach in a nurse-managed clinic. *Journal of Healthcare Quality, 39,* 379–390.

Table 2. Colorectal Cancer Screening Process Definitions

Colorectal cancer screening process term	Definition
Screening ordered	Colonoscopy or FIT was ordered by the NP.
Screening up to date	Patient had colonoscopy within past 10 years or FIT within past 1 year
Screening completed	Patient completed screening procedure (colonoscopy or FIT)

FIT = fecal immunochemical test; NP = nurse practitioner.

screenings ordered, only 5 (4%) indicated a patient refusal.

Data were analyzed to illuminate problems with existing processes and guide semistructured staff interviews with the researcher. These interviews revealed process strengths and weaknesses, along with proposed interventions for overcoming the problems with the screening process (Table 3).

Goal 2: Develop Interventions Based on Findings

Six interventions were developed using an iterative, multifaceted approach,

Table 3. Problems Identified and Quality Improvement Interventions Completed

Problem	Intervention
1) Lack of defined CRC screening protocol	Protocol/algorithm for CRC screening posted at nursing stations and given to all providers.
2) Inefficient process for ordering FIT	Simplified FIT ordering process in EHR to allow NPs to order FIT at same time as other laboratories and support staff to split orders to print requisitions to be sent home with patient.
3) Low numbers of ordering CRC screenings on those who are eligible	Clinical decision support tools (pop-up reminders in EHR) to NPs on patients who are eligible but not up to date on screenings.
4) Lack of follow-up for outstanding FIT that were ordered	Outstanding FITs will be queried monthly and letters sent to all patients with outstanding FIT.
5) Lack of patient education information regarding CRC screening options	Educational brochure on colonoscopy and FIT explanations, preparations for tests, and frequency of tests placed in patient rooms.
6) Inadequate documentation of patient refusals of CRC screening tests	Utilization of comments box in EHR within screening window of colonoscopy and FIT

CRC = colorectal cancer; EHR = electronic health record; FIT = fecal immunochemical test; NP = nurse practitioner.

Reprinted with permission from Hountz, D., et al. (2017). Increasing colorectal cancer screening using a quality improvement approach in a nurse-managed clinic. *Journal of Healthcare Quality, 39*, 379–390.

considering stakeholder input, current practice guidelines, and pertinent literature.

Goal 3: Implement QI Interventions to Improve the Process

We began by educating the clinic staff in a meeting. An overview of the problem, project goals, and proposed interventions were presented. Interventions were modified based on staff feedback through informal discussions and email correspondence. To improve overall CRC screening rates, ongoing communication with the NMHC staff during the first few weeks of the implementation was critical to support successful interventions.

Data were compiled and provided to all NPs after weekly chart audits; NPs were given the number of patients eligible for CRC screening along with the actual number of screenings ordered. Data were also organized by NP name and posted on the clinic QI board weekly. Specific feedback was also given through individual flags in the EHR, which were sent to NPs requesting clarification of documentation.

Two weeks postimplementation, FIT follow-up letters were sent to all patients with uncompleted FITs. Letters were written in English and Spanish, and included in the EHR for tracking purposes. Monthly follow-up letters continued to be mailed to all patients with uncompleted FITs.

Goal 4: Evaluate the Progress of the Interventions Implemented

A retrospective review of 200 new charts began in March 2016. To ensure consistency in pre and postintervention data analysis of these two patient groups, identical data points were collected in the postintervention chart review (Table 4).

Postintervention results showed 150 charts of 200 (75%) had CRC screenings ordered by the NP or were up to date. We compared the proportions of CRC screening for the two independent samples by calculating z scores to test our hypothesis. The z statistic was determined to be -7.4635 (p value $<.0001$), which correlates with significant improvement from pre to postdata equating to a 74% increase in screenings ordered, and

Table 4. Sample Characteristics of Pre and Postintervention Data

Characteristic	Preintervention (02/2015), n = 200	Postintervention (01/2016), n = 200
Age group, n (%)		
51–59	120 (60)	116 (58)
60–69	75 (38)	73 (37)
70–75	5 (2)	11 (5)
Sex, n (%)		
Female	116 (58)	137 (68)
Male	84 (42)	63 (32)
Race/ethnicity, n (%)		
Caucasian	176 (88)	192 (96)
Hispanic	20 (10)	7 (4)
Other	4 (2)	1 (1)
Health insurance coverage type, n (%)		
Medicaid	59 (29.5)	86 (43)
Self-pay	53 (26.5)	27 (14)
Medicare	45 (22.5)	55 (28)
Private insurance	43 (21.5)	32 (16)

Reprinted with permission from Hountz, D., et al. (2017). Increasing colorectal cancer screening using a quality improvement approach in a nurse-managed clinic. *Journal of Healthcare Quality*, 39, 379–390.

a 56% increase in screenings completed (Figure 2).

Of the 200 charts, 116 (58%) had CRC screenings ordered and completed or were up to date. By almost doubling this measure, the NMCH is closer to their goal of 70%. The z statistic was determined to be -5.64 (p value $<.0001$), which also correlates with significant improvement from pre to postdata (Table 5). Post-intervention also revealed that 12 (24%) charts had a patient refusal documented compared with 4% in predata results. Seventy-eight letters were mailed one time to patients who had not completed their FIT. The mean rate of return was 42% for the FITs.

One month postimplementation, increases in the overall numbers for CRC screening were seen at the NMHC. Because of this increase, provider feedback was decreased to biweekly and included overall screening rates and NP documentation of patient refusals. Overall screening rates continued to be posted biweekly by provider on the QI bulletin board and were reported monthly at the QI meeting.

Because interventions were implemented, the impact on the overall screening completions has been positive. Since October 2015, 19 patients have had either a positive FIT or colonoscopies. Of

these, 11 patients had polyps removed, thus preventing the potential growth of these polyps into CRC.

Confounding factors could have also contributed to this increase in ordering and completion of screening. In 2015, the clinic hired a QI Coordinator to drive QI initiatives and also an additional patient navigator to patient enrollment for insurance through the Affordable Care Act.

Goal 5: Sustain Process Changes

Monthly feedback was given to individual providers and continues to be posted at the NMHC. Pre and postintervention data were presented to the QI committee, where ideas were discussed for ongoing sustainability. First, the committee wanted to educate the staff on project outcomes to encourage staff to help with sustainability. Next, it was determined to continue to post the monthly data on the number of CRC screenings ordered by provider at the NMHC. The QI committee also determined the positive value of the FIT follow-up letter and will continue this intervention.

Limitations

There are several limitations to this project. The Affordable Care Act was

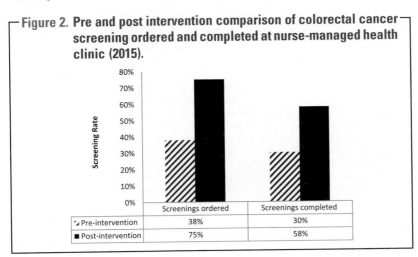

Figure 2. Pre and post intervention comparison of colorectal cancer screening ordered and completed at nurse-managed health clinic (2015).

	Screenings ordered	Screenings completed
Pre-intervention	38%	30%
Post-intervention	75%	58%

Reprinted with permission from Hountz, D., et al. (2017). Increasing colorectal cancer screening using a quality improvement approach in a nurse-managed clinic. *Journal of Healthcare Quality, 39*, 379–390.

Table 5. Pre and Postintervention Comparison of Colorectal Cancer Screenings for Those Patients Who Were Up to Date or Had Screenings Ordered and Those Patients Where Screening Was Completed

	Predata (n = 200), n (%)	Postdata (n = 200), n (%)	% Change (increase)	Z statistic	p value
Colorectal cancer screening up to date or ordered	76 (38)	150 (75)	74	−7.4635	<.001
Colorectal cancer screening completed	60 (30)	116 (58)	56	−5.64	<.001

changing the payer system structure in the United States, especially for the underserved population, during the project implementation. Those patients who had suboptimal or no health insurance were now able to afford preventive screenings. This influx of patients with health insurance could have influenced the results. This project was completed at one NMHC in a rural, underserved setting and, therefore, generalizability of the results may vary across geographic areas.

Discussion

The six goals outlined in this project were achieved and assisted in the improvement of CRC screening rates in this NMHC. Based on the positive results, the QI interventions that were developed and implemented had a significant impact not only on the numbers of CRC screenings ordered on patients but also on the numbers of patients who completed their CRC screenings.

Four main themes emerged that influenced the increase in the CRC screening rates. The first theme, using multiple interventions, summarizes the implementation of this QI project. Healthcare QI processes are multidimensional and complex. Assessing these processes brings about identification of multiple problems that require various interventions to positively bring about change. In this project, six different QI interventions were implemented concurrently to target the six problems identified. This multifaceted approach to

increase screening rates was also previously noted in the literature. Using an approach with multiple interventions helped to improve CRC screening rates in primary care settings by 13–23%.[16,20]

The utilization of staff input, theme two, helped to guide the project development and will strengthen sustainment. According to The Deming Institute,[23] utilization of staff input is crucial to the success of QI initiatives. Staff input was used from the inception to the end of this project. The NMHC staff were presented with the initial data and asked for their recommendations on how to improve the findings. Staff had many ideas for improvement and were then motivated to be a part of the solution. With this initial buy-in, additional feedback throughout the process was given freely, with minimal prompting, as providers were excited to see how their ideas positively affected CRC screening rates.

Within this feedback, NPs repeatedly discussed the difficulty remembering the numerous preventive screenings they needed to address with patients. Reminder systems, theme three, were incorporated into workflow to trigger NPs to order the CRC screenings. These findings verify that a lack of provider reminders is a barrier in ordering CRC screenings in the literature.[11,15] For this project, pop-up reminders in the EHR were initiated to serve as reminders for the NPs.

Strategic reminders applied to the patients who needed CRC screenings and the providers. Low-income patients often

Reprinted with permission from Hountz, D., et al. (2017). Increasing colorectal cancer screening using a quality improvement approach in a nurse-managed clinic. *Journal of Healthcare Quality*, 39, 379–390.

have competing health priorities and financial challenges that contribute to their complicated lives.[24] Within this project, a process was developed and implemented to provide patients with reminders to complete their CRC screenings. Reminder letters, which were sent to patients through postal mail 2–4 weeks after their visit to those who had not completed their FITs, were effective. Reminder systems, whether for NPs or for patients, are useful tools to provide and receive quality healthcare.

Theme four, the value of performance feedback, is an often underused and underestimated method for producing positive results in QI. The Deming PDSA model emphasizes the importance of data-driven continuous improvement that focuses on the needs of the staff and providing current performance feedback.[25] Healthcare personnel want to see the result of their nursing interventions to grasp whether these strategies were impactful, from both micro and macrosystem perspectives. After the implementation of the QI interventions, performance feedback was given to the individual NPs on a weekly basis through emails. These weekly numbers were also posted on the QI bulletin board for entire NMHC staff to view. This visualization created peer pressure to improve individual performances, and therefore, have an impact on the organization's overall goal.

Conclusion

Colorectal cancer is one of the most common cancers with high patient morbidity and mortality; the disease also provides a significant financial burden to the patient and healthcare system. However, positive outcomes can result for patients afflicted with CRC through the early detection and diagnosis through screening methods (i.e., colonoscopy and FIT). Through the Deming PDSA QI model, an assessment was completed and multiple interventions were developed and implemented that successfully increased CRC screening rates at a NMHC. These interventions incorporated the QI principles of using multiple interventions, using staff input to develop and sustain lasting change, implementing staff and patient reminders, and using data-driven information to provide performance feedback to staff. This project demonstrates that applying QI principles to the challenge of increasing CRC screening rates at a NMHC can result in positive patient and healthcare organization outcomes.

Implications for Practice

Using these QI interventions has had a substantial impact on the quality of care for patients in this NMHC at minimal organizational cost. This project used existing EHR technology to provide patient and staff reminders and to establish an easier workflow for ordering and following up of the FIT. In addition, a minimal time commitment was necessary to provide valuable performance feedback, which will be sustained through the QI committee.

The economic impact on the patients was also significant. The overall increase in the number of patients screened for CRC will ultimately lead to a decreased need for CRC treatment. Through CRC screening, polyps are discovered and removed at an earlier stage. Because these polyps were identified early, they are less likely to progress into more complicated CRC treatment regimens, thus decreasing the burden of cost to patients and third party payers.

Primary care providers and leaders in healthcare may find this project's design and findings useful and easily transferred to primary care organizations. The overall impact of this project resulted in the prevention of CRC in 11 patients; thus, decreasing the morbidity and mortality of this underserved patient population. These QI interventions could also be applied to additional preventive screening practices in primary care clinics. Adoption of reminders for NPs or patients could be easily transferred to screenings such as mammograms for the detection of breast cancer or cervical cancer screenings.

Reprinted with permission from Hountz, D., et al. (2017). Increasing colorectal cancer screening using a quality improvement approach in a nurse-managed clinic. *Journal of Healthcare Quality, 39*, 379–390.

References

1. Meester RG, Doubeni CA, Lansdorp-Vogelaar I, et al. Colorectal cancer deaths attributable to nonuse of screening in the United States. *Ann Epidemiol.* 2015;25:208-213.

2. Survival rates for colorectal cancer screening. American Cancer Society Website. http://www.cancer.org/cancer/colonandrectumcancer/detailedguide/colorectal-cancer-survival-rates. Updated January 20, 2016. Accessed June 22, 2016.

3. Smith RA, Manassaram-Baptiste D, Brooks D, et al. Cancer screening in the United States, 2015: A review of current American Cancer Society guidelines and current issues in cancer screening. *Cancer.* 2015;65:30-54.

4. United States Preventive Services Task Force (USPSTF). Screening for colorectal cancer: U.S. Preventive Services Task Force recommendation statement. *Ann Intern Med.* 2008;149:627-637.

5. Healthy people 2020 topics and objectives. Healthy People 2020 Website. https://www.healthypeople.gov/2020/leading-health-indicators/2020-lhi-topics/Clinical-Preventive-Services/data#c16. Accessed October 5, 2015.

6. Daly J. Fecal immunochemical tests for colorectal cancer screening. *Am J Nurs.* 2012;112:67-69.

7. Centers for Disease Control and Prevention (CDC). Vital signs: Colorectal cancer screening test use—United States. *MMWR Morb Mortal Wkly Rep.* 2013;62:881-888.

8. Policy brief: Nurse-managed health clinics: Increasing access to primary care and educating the healthcare workforce. American Association of Colleges of Nursing Website. http://www.aacn.nche.edu/government-affairs/FY13NMHCs.pdf. Published 2013. Accessed December 16, 2015.

9. Hansen-Turton T, Bailey DN, Torres N, Ritter A. Nurse-managed health centers: Key to a healthy future. *Am J Nurs.* 2010;110:23-26.

10. Daly JM, Levy BT, Moss CA, Bay CP. System strategies for colorectal cancer screening at federally qualified health centers. *Am J Public Health.* 2015;105(1):212-219.

11. Garcia-Dominic O, Lengerich EJ, Wray LA, et al. Barriers to colorectal cancer screening among latino adults in Pennsylvania: ACCN results. *Am J Health Behav.* 2012;36(2):153-167.

12. Quick B, Hester C, Young K, Greiner K. Self-reported barriers to colorectal cancer screening in a racially diverse, low-income study population. *J Community Health.* 2013;38(2):285-292.

13. Guessous I, Dash C, Lapin P, Doroshenk M, Smith RA, Klabunde CN. Colorectal cancer screening barriers and facilitators in older persons. *Prev Med.* 2010;50(1-2):3-10.

14. Davis TC, Arnold CL, Rademaker AW, et al. FOBT completion in FQHCs: Impact of physician recommendation, FOBT information, or receipt of the FOBT Kit. *J Rural Health.* 2012;28(3):306-311.

15. Lopez-Class M, Luta G, Noone AM, et al. Patient and provider factors associated with colorectal cancer screening in safety net clinics serving low-income, urban immigrant Latinos. *J Health Care Poor Underserved.* 2012;23(3):1011-1019.

16. Menon U, Belue R, Wahab S, et al. A randomized trial comparing the effect of two phone-based interventions on colorectal cancer screening adherence. *Ann Behav Med.* 2011;42(3):294-303.

17. Lairson DR, Dicarlo M, Deshmuk AA, et al. Cost-effectiveness of a standard intervention versus a navigated intervention on colorectal cancer screening use in primary care. *Cancer.* 2014;120(7):1042-1049.

18. McFall AM, Ryan JE, Hager P. Implementing a client reminder intervention for colorectal cancer screening at a health insurance worksite. *Prev Chronic Dis.* 2014;11:E20.

19. Lasser KE, Murillo J, Lisboa S, et al. Colorectal cancer screening among ethnically diverse, low-income patients: A randomized controlled trial. *Arch Intern Med.* 2011;171(10):906-912.

20. Hendren S, Winters P, Humiston S. Randomized, controlled trial of a multimodal intervention to improve cancer screening rates in a safety-net primary care practice. *J Gen Intern Med.* 2014;29(1):41-49.

21. Elmulti D, Kathawala Y. A preliminary analysis of Deming's quality improvement program: Some insights. *Prod Inventory Manage J.* 1994;1994(35):52-56.

22. Science of improvement: How to improve. Institute for Healthcare Improvement (IHI) Website. http://www.ihi.org/resources/Pages/HowtoImprove/ScienceofImprovementHowtoImprove.aspx. Accessed March 21, 2016.

23. The PDSA cycle. The Deming Institute Website. https://www.deming.org/theman/theories/pdsacycle. Accessed April 13, 2016.

24. Khankari K, Eder M, Osborn C, et al. Improving colorectal cancer screening among the medically underserved: A Pilot study within a federally qualified health center. *J Gen Intern Med.* 2007;22(10):410-1414.

25. Clark D, Silvester K, Knowles S. Lean management systems: Creating a culture

of continuous quality improvement. *J Clin Pathol.* 2013;66:638-643.

Authors' Biographies

Diane Hountz, DNP, MS, ANP, RN is a Clinical Assistant Professor, School of Nursing, Purdue University, West Lafayette, IN. She holds a Yellow Belt Certification and currently teaches quality improvement to undergraduate nursing students. She has acted as the Quality Improvement Coordinator for the North Central Nursing Clinics.

Jennifer Coddington, DNP, MSN, RN, CPNP is a Clinical Associate Professor, School of Nursing, Purdue University, West Lafayette, IN. She is also the Director of the Primary Care Pediatric Nurse Practitioner Master's Program, Director of Practice and Outreach and the Medical Director of North Central Nursing Clinics.

Karen J. Foli, PhD, RN is an Associate Professor, School of Nursing, Purdue University, West Lafayette, IN. She is also the director of the PhD program in Nursing at Purdue and holds Yellow Belt Certification in Lean Healthcare Six Sigma.

Janet Thorlton, PhD, RN is a Clinical Associate Professor, School of Nursing, Purdue University, West Lafayette, IN. She is also a member of the Center for Health Outcomes & Policy Safety Net Research team at the Purdue Regenstrief Center for Healthcare Engineering. Across the curriculum, she teaches Evidence Based Practice and Health Policy.

For more information on this article, contact Jennifer Coddington at jsundell@purdue.edu.

The authors declare no conflicts of interest.

Journal for Healthcare Quality is pleased to offer the opportunity to earn continuing education (CE) credit to those who read this article and take the online posttest at www.nahq.org/journal/ce. This continuing education offering, JHQ [269] (39.6), will provide 1 hour to those who complete it appropriately.

Core CPHQ Examination Content Area
IV. [**Domain** #3 Performance Measurement and Improvement]

Continuing Education (CE) Objectives and Questions: Increasing Colorectal Cancer Screening Utilizing a Quality Improvement Approach in a Nurse-Managed Primary Care Clinic

Learning Objectives
After reading this article and taking this test, the learner should be able to:

1. Define the importance of colorectal cancer screening and the modalities used.
2. Describe the goals of this project to increase the CRC screening rates in a rural FQHC NMHC.
3. Describe the 4 major themes that were determined to influence CRC screening rates.

Questions
1. Approximately how many people in the United States will be diagnosed with colorectal cancer in their lifetime?
   a. 1 in 15
   b. 1 in 23
   c. 1 in 54
   d. 1 in 100

2. What quality improvement conceptual framework was utilized for this project?
   a. Define, Measure, Analyze, Improve, Control (DMAIC)
   b. Plan, Do, Study, Act (PDSA)
   c. Model for Improvement (MFI)
   d. Continuous Quality Improvement (CQI)

3. What is the recommended screening modality for colorectal cancer?
   a. Fecal Immunochemical Tests (FIT)
   b. Colonoscopy
   c. CT Abdomen
   d. Either Fecal Immunochemical Tests (FIT) or Colonoscopy

4. Nurse-managed health clinics utilize which healthcare professional as primary care providers?
   a. Physicians

b. Physician Assistants (PA)
c. Nurse Practitioners (NP)
d. Registered Nurses (RN)

5. All of the following were goals of this Quality Improvement project except:
   a. Convince patients to receive colorectal cancer screenings
   b. Review the current colorectal cancer screening process utilized at this nurse-managed health clinic
   c. Develop and implement quality improvement interventions based upon results
   d. Sustain process changes

6. In order to increase the completion of Fecal Immunochemical Tests (FIT), which of the following interventions was implemented?
   a. Tailored telephone education by patient navigators
   b. Follow-up phone calls by RNs
   c. Follow-up letters mailed
   d. Counseling by RNs during discharge from primary care visit

7. Low numbers of screening for colorectal cancer for those who were eligible was identified as one of the problems during this project. What intervention was developed in order to help with this problem?
   a. Clinical decision support tool in Electronic Health Record (EHR)
   b. Educational brochure on colorectal cancer screens given to patients
   c. Revised colorectal cancer screening protocol
   d. Simplification of the ordering process for screenings

8. As a result of the interventions, what percentage increase in the number of eligible patients being screened for colorectal cancer was seen in the nurse-managed health clinic?
   a. 11%
   b. 25%
   c. 37%
   d. 53%

9. This project's positive results indicate that utilizing staff input throughout the entire quality improvement process was important. At what point during the project was staff input utilized?
   a. Initially during a staff meeting, prior to implementation
   b. During implementation and for 1 month after implementation
   c. During the sustainability phase of the project
   d. Prior to implementation and during implementation

10. All of the following were themes identified from this project except:
    a. Patient and family centered care
    b. The value of data-driven performance feedback
    c. Utilizing multiple interventions simultaneously
    d. Importance of reminder systems to providers and patients

The Effectiveness of Medication Adherence Interventions Among Patients With Coronary Artery Disease
A Meta-analysis

Jo-Ana D. Chase, PhD, APRN-BC; Jennifer L. Bogener, BSN; Todd M. Ruppar, PhD, RN; Vicki S. Conn, PhD, RN, FAAN

Background: Despite the known benefits of medication therapy for secondary prevention of coronary artery disease (CAD), many patients do not adhere to prescribed medication regimens. Medication nonadherence is associated with poor health outcomes and higher healthcare cost. **Objective:** The purpose of this meta-analysis was to determine the overall effectiveness of interventions designed to improve medication adherence (MA) among adults with CAD. In addition, sample, study design, and intervention characteristics were explored as potential moderators to intervention effectiveness. **Methods:** Comprehensive search strategies helped in facilitating the identification of 2-group, treatment-versus-control–design studies testing MA interventions among patients with CAD. Data were independently extracted by 2 trained research specialists. Standardized mean difference effect sizes were calculated for eligible primary studies, adjusted for bias, and then synthesized under a random-effects model. Homogeneity of variance was explored using a conventional heterogeneity statistic. Exploratory moderator analyses were conducted using meta-analytic analogs for analysis of variance and regression for dichotomous and continuous moderators, respectively. **Results:** Twenty-four primary studies were included in this meta-analysis. The overall effect size of MA interventions, calculated from 18,839 participants, was 0.229 ($P < .001$). The most effective interventions used nurses as interventionists, initiated interventions in the inpatient setting, and informed providers of patients' MA behaviors. Medication adherence interventions tested among older patients were more effective than those among younger patients. The interventions were equally effective regardless of number of intervention sessions, targeting MA behavior alone or with other behaviors, and the use of written instructions only. **Conclusions:** Interventions to increase MA among patients with CAD were modestly effective. Nurses can be instrumental in improving MA among these patients. Future research is needed to investigate nurse-delivered MA interventions across varied clinical settings. In addition, more research testing MA interventions among younger populations and more racially diverse groups is needed.

KEY WORDS: coronary artery disease, medication adherence, meta-analysis, patient compliance

Jo-Ana D. Chase, PhD, APRN-BC
Assistant Professor, S343 School of Nursing, University of Missouri, Columbia.

Jennifer L. Bogener, BSN
Nursing Student, School of Nursing School of Health Professions, University of Missouri, Columbia.

Todd M. Ruppar, PhD, RN
Assistant Professor, S423 School of Nursing, University of Missouri, Columbia.

Vicki S. Conn, PhD, RN, FAAN
Potter-Brinton Professor and Associate Dean for Research, S317 School of Nursing University of Missouri Columbia.

Supported by Award Number R01NR011990 (Conn-PI) from the National Institute of Nursing Research. The content is solely the responsibility of the authors and does not necessarily represent the official views of the National Institute of Nursing Research or the National Institutes of Health.

The authors have no conflicts of interest to disclose.

Correspondence
Jo-Ana D. Chase, PhD, APRN-BC, S343 School of Nursing, University of Missouri, Columbia, MO 65211 (chasej@missouri.edu).

DOI: 10.1097/JCN.0000000000000259

Introduction

Heart disease is the leading cause of death among adults in the United States.[1,2] Coronary artery disease (CAD), the most common form of heart disease, is responsible for 385,000 deaths and $108.9 billion in healthcare expenditures annually.[1,2] Secondary prevention for CAD is a multi-intervention approach involving therapeutic lifestyle changes and evidence-based medical therapies, such as prescribed medications. Between 1980 and 2000, these therapies have contributed to a 50% reduction in CAD-related deaths.[3] Research suggests that the greatest contributor to this reduction is medications for secondary prevention of CAD.[3]

Unfortunately, medication nonadherence is highly prevalent.[4] Approximately one-third of patients who have had a myocardial infarction do not adhere to prescribed

175

medication regimens.[5] Nonadherence is associated with increased risk for all-cause and cardiovascular mortality, revascularization procedures, hospitalization, and higher healthcare cost.[6–8] Effective interventions to improve medication adherence (MA) in this population are critically needed.

Efficacy of MA interventions varies.[9–14] Few systematic reviews have focused on MA interventions among patients with CAD.[15–18] Prior reviews have been limited by narrow search strategies, unclear inclusion criteria, lack of a quantitative synthesis, or absent exploration of potential moderating variables.[16] To date, no current meta-analyses addressing MA intervention effectiveness among patients with CAD exist. Thus, the overall effectiveness of MA interventions in this population is unclear; furthermore, the most effective types of interventions are yet unknown.

A meta-analysis and moderator analysis of MA interventions among patients with CAD could promote efficiency in developing future interventions and provide clinicians with guidance to promote MA in clinical practice. The purposes of this systematic review and meta-analysis were to describe and quantify the overall effectiveness of the body of MA intervention research among patients with CAD and to explore potential moderators of intervention effectiveness. In addition, we identified limitations in the extant research and suggested areas for future study.

The following research questions guided this study:

1) What is the overall effectiveness of MA interventions on MA outcomes among patients with CAD?
2) Does intervention effectiveness vary based on intervention, sample, or design characteristics?

Methods

The systematic review and meta-analysis were performed using standard meta-analysis techniques and PRISMA guidelines.[19,20] This project was part of a larger parent study examining MA outcomes of MA interventions across multiple chronic and acute illnesses.

Search Strategies

We consulted an expert health sciences reference librarian to ensure comprehensive search strategies.[21] Databases that were searched included the following: MEDLINE, PubMED, PsychINFO, CINAHL, EBSCO, PQDT, Cochrane Central Trials Register, Cochrane Database of Systematic Reviews, IndMed, ERIC, International Pharmaceutical Abstracts, EBM Reviews-Database of Abstracts of Reviews of Effects, as well as Communication and Mass Media. Broad MeSH terms were used, which included the following: *patient compliance, medication adherence, drugs, prescription drugs, pharmaceutical preparations, generic, dosage, compliant, compliance, adherent, adherence, noncompliant, noncompliance, nonadherent,* *nonadherence, medication(s), regimen(s), prescription(s), prescribed, drug(s), pill(s), tablet(s), agent(s), improve, promote, enhance, encourage, foster, advocate, influence, incentive, ensure, remind, optimize, increase, impact, prevent, address, decrease.* Fifty-seven relevant journals were hand-searched, and author searches and ancestry searches of prior reviews' bibliographies were conducted to identify additional potentially eligible studies.

Inclusion Criteria

We included 2-group, treatment-versus-control comparison studies testing interventions to increase MA in patients 18 years or older with a diagnosis of CAD, defined by the primary studies. Medication adherence interventions are deliberate actions performed or directed by investigators to increase adherence to specified medication regimens. Examples include education, reminders, and special packaging. Studies with varied types of MA measurement (eg, electronic monitoring devices, pharmacy refills, self-report) were included, given the diversity of MA measures in this research area. Eligible studies needed to contain enough data to calculate an effect size (ES). The research team attempted to contact corresponding authors to obtain missing outcome data.

Data Extraction

To extract relevant data from primary studies, a coding strategy was developed from prior research and expert consultations. The codebook was developed through an iterative process and pilot tested. Data extracted included the primary study source, publication date, dissemination type (eg, journal article, dissertation), presence of funding, participant demographics (eg, age, gender, ethnicity, comorbidities), research methods, intervention details, and MA outcomes. Multiple descriptors of primary study research methods were coded, such as sample size, randomization, and intention-to-treat analyses. Method of MA measurement and follow-up interval were recorded. Varied intervention characteristics were coded, including content (eg, problem solving, self-monitoring, goal setting), delivery (eg, face-to-face, telephone), dose (eg, length/number of sessions), and setting (eg, clinic, home).

Included studies were independently coded by 2 extensively trained research specialists, then compared and discussed until consensus was reached. A doctorally prepared senior research specialist supervised the coding process to ensure coding integrity and reviewed all ES data. Questionable items were resolved in team meetings with the study principal investigator.

Data Analysis

All data were analyzed using Comprehensive Meta-Analysis Software.[22] Standardized mean difference effect sizes (d, ES) were calculated for each 2-group treatment-versus-control posttest comparison. The

Reprinted with permission from Chase, J., et al. (2016). The effectiveness of medication adherence interventions among patients with coronary artery disease. *Journal of Cardiovascular Nursing, 31,* 357–366.

standardized mean difference ES between the groups was calculated by dividing the difference between treatment and control group postintervention means by the pooled standard deviation. Additional ES analyses were conducted within the groups by subtracting the outcome scores from the baseline scores and dividing by the baseline standard deviation. Effect sizes were weighted by the inverse of variance to account for sample size and adjust for bias, then synthesized using a random-effects model.[23] A random-effects model was chosen a priori, given the expected within- and between-study variance across primary studies. Data were examined for possible outliers on the basis of standardized residuals of each primary study's ES. Publication bias was examined by assessing the symmetry of a funnel plot constructed by plotting each primary study's standard error against its ES.[23]

Homogeneity of variance was tested using a conventional heterogeneity statistic (Q), to quantify observed heterogeneity across studies, and I^2 to determine the proportion of observed heterogeneity due to true differences in effects across studies.[23] Exploratory moderator analyses were used to examine possible associations between study characteristics and intervention effectiveness. Dichotomous variables were evaluated using subgroup analysis, and continuous variables were evaluated using meta-regression.[23]

Results

Twenty-four primary reports were eligible for analysis.[9–14,24–41] Additional coding information was found in 4 companion reports about the same primary studies.[42–45] Three primary study reports contained multiple comparison groups.[33,36,37] There were 28 treatment-versus-control-group posttest comparisons, 9 treatment group pretest-posttest comparisons, and 6 control group pretest-posttest comparisons. Few smaller studies with negative findings were included, indicating evidence of publication bias.

Primary Study Characteristics

The primary studies that were included in this meta-analysis included 24 journal articles, 3 dissertations, and 1 presentation. Six studies were disseminated before 2000. Seventeen studies were supported by funding.

Primary study characteristics are presented in Table 1. Majority of the samples were males. The median of the mean age for participants was 62.9 years. Only 7 studies reported data on ethnicity. Of those, most subjects were white. Some studies reported additional chronic diseases among their subjects including the following: hypertension ($k = 17$), undifferentiated diabetes ($k = 16$), hyperlipidemia ($k = 12$), heart failure ($k = 4$), stroke ($k = 3$), lung disease ($k = 3$), renal disease ($k = 2$), osteoarthritis ($k = 1$), asthma ($k = 1$), atrial fibrillation ($k = 1$), nephritic syndrome ($k = 1$), thyroid disorder ($k = 1$), and cerebral vascular disease ($k = 1$).

Primary studies reported diverse methods. The median number of intervention sessions was 2 ($k = 17$). The median number of days for MA intervention duration was 35 ($k = 23$). Only 1 study reported intervention session duration. Outcome data of MA were collected with a median of 124.5 days after intervention ($k = 14$). Studies reported diverse methods of collecting MA outcomes including pharmacy refill ($k = 7$), self-report ($k = 18$), biological measures ($k = 2$), and pill counts ($k = 1$).

Overall Effects of Medication Adherence Interventions of Medication Adherence Outcomes

Overall MA ESs are presented in Table 2. The ESs were calculated for 28 treatment-versus-control-group comparisons containing 18,839 subjects. The overall ES for these comparisons was 0.229 ($P < .001$), indicating significant improvements in MA outcomes in the treatment over the control group (Figure). When the 3 largest sample studies were excluded, the ES for these comparisons demonstrated minimal change ($d = 0.269$, $P < .001$). The ESs were significantly heterogeneous.

We also calculated overall ESs for the 9 treatment group pretest-posttest comparisons and for the 6 control group pretest-posttest comparisons. Although the former ES was positive (0.183) and the latter negative (-0.014), neither were statistically significant. Lack of

TABLE 1. Characteristics of Primary Studies Included in Medication Adherence Meta-analyses						
Characteristic	k	Min	Q_1	Median	Q_3	Max
Treatment group sample size	28	4	18.75	86.5	246.5	3635
Control group sample size	24	5	21	82	562	3010
Percentage attrition	23	0	0	4.545	14.646	65.282
Percentage of females	23	0	25	40	51.05	67.4
Percentage underrepresented group subjects	7	7	24.1	48	90.4	92.9
Mean age, y	21	53.7	58.4	62.9	64	72.22
Median number of intervention sessions	17	1	1	2	5	12
Median duration of interventions, d	23	1	1	35	126	365
Median duration postintervention for MA outcome data collection, d	14	12	40.25	124.5	175.5	700

k, number of comparisons in which characteristic was reported; Min, minimum; Max, maximum; Q_1, first quartile; Q_3, third quartile.

Reprinted with permission from Chase, J., et al. (2016). The effectiveness of medication adherence interventions among patients with coronary artery disease. *Journal of Cardiovascular Nursing, 31*, 357–366.

TABLE 2 Overall Effects of Medication Adherence Interventions Among Patients With Coronary Artery Disease

Comparison	k	d	P (d)	95% Confidence Interval	SE	Q	I^2	P (Q)
Treatment vs control groups at posttest[a]	28	0.229	<.001	0.138–0.321	0.047	78.201	65.474	<.001
Treatment vs control groups at posttest[b]	25	0.269	<.001	0.135–0.403	0.068	65.384	63.294	<.001
Treatment group pretest vs posttest	9	0.183	.106	−0.039 to 0.405	0.113	69.462	88.483	<.001
Control group pretest vs posttest	6	−0.014	.887	−0.208 to 0.180	0.099	11.124	55.052	.049

d, standardized mean difference effect size; I^2, proportion of observed variance across effect size due to true differences in effects; k, number of comparisons; Q, conventional homogeneity statistic; SE, standard error.
[a]All studies included.
[b]Three larger sample studies excluded.

statistical significance may reflect low power from the small number of comparisons.

Moderator Analyses

Continuous and dichotomous moderator analyses are displayed in Tables 3 and 4, respectively. Although all studies from the main analysis were examined for moderating variables, only those moderators reported for a

sufficient number of comparisons were included in the analyses.

Intervention Moderators
Studies in which health care providers were given information about subjects' MA revealed a significantly greater ES (0.387) than when the providers were not given information on MA (0.151). An example of this type of intervention component could involve using a

FIGURE. *Forest plot of main effects. Forest plot of meta-analysis of two-group posttest comparisons of medication adherence outcomes listed by year of publication. Effect sizes calculated using a random effects model. Study weight is proportional to the area of each square.*

Reprinted with permission from Chase, J., et al. (2016). The effectiveness of medication adherence interventions among patients with coronary artery disease. *Journal of Cardiovascular Nursing, 31*, 357–366.

Continuous Moderator Results				
Moderator	k	B	SE	P
Report and methods moderators				
Year of publication	28	−0.005	0.004	.205
Sample size	28	−0.000	0.000	.004
Sample attribute moderators				
Age	21	0.014	0.004	.001
Percentage of women	23	−0.000	0.002	.968
Underrepresented groups	7	0.000	0.001	.810
Intervention feature moderator				
No. sessions	17	−0.013	0.013	.304
Duration of intervention	23	−0.000	0.000	.972
Time point for MA outcome data collection	14	−0.000	0.000	.213

B, meta-regression coefficient (unstandardized); k, number of comparisons; p, value for B; SE, standard error.

questionnaire on participants' baseline MA and barriers to MA.[24] Studies with nurse interventionists (0.428) reported significantly higher MA than studies without nurse interventionists (0.127). Studies with and without physician and pharmacist interventionists had similar ESs. Interventions started when participants were inpatients had significantly larger effects (0.590) than interventions that did not start with inpatients (0.141); however, there was little difference when the intervention was delivered at home versus in the clinic. With regards to the mode of intervention delivery, we saw no significant differences among telephone, written materials only, or face-to-face delivery. Interventions using mail delivery were less effective (0.060) than interventions without mail delivery interventions (0.292). There were several nonsignificant variables, including: utilization of theory, number of sessions, duration of intervention, time point for measuring outcome MA, goal setting, interventions delivered at home, interventions delivered in clinic, problem solving, succinct written instructions, any written instructions, behavior target (MA or multiple behaviors), physician or pharmacist interventionists, telephone and face-to-face delivery, and written instructions only.

Report and Sample Moderators

The age of subjects had a significant positive slope (0.014), revealing that MA interventions led to greater adherence improvement in samples of older patients. Interventions were equally effective regardless of publication status, funding, and location. Other nonsignificant moderators included year of publication, percentage of women and underrepresented groups, and socioeconomic status.

Design and Methods Moderators

Although sample size had a statistically significant negative slope, this finding is not clinically substantive. Other potential moderators related to design, such as blinding, allocation concealment, random assignment, and intention-to-treat analyses, were not associated with MA effectiveness.

Discussion

Findings from this meta-analysis, which is the first of its kind, that suggest interventions to increase MA among participants with CAD were significantly effective. These positive findings are similar to prior meta-analyses examining MA outcomes from MA interventions among underrepresented groups and from packaging intervention effects.[46,47] Although poor MA has been linked to negative health outcomes in patients with CAD,[4,6,7] consensus on how much MA is needed to improve varied CAD-related outcomes is not yet clear. Prior research exploring MA and blood pressure outcomes[48,49] as well as cardiovascular disease risk exists.[49] However, further research is needed to quantify the amount of MA needed to mitigate additional CAD-related outcomes. Moreover, the dose of MA intervention needed to change MA behavior among patients with CAD is yet to be determined. Due to the small number of comparisons using similar measures of MA, we were unable to convert the ES to a clinical metric of adherence. Future MA intervention research among patients with CAD should include explicit information regarding intervention dose.

Moderator Findings

We found several interesting moderators. Interventions in which healthcare providers were given information regarding participants' MA were more effective than interventions without this component. Awareness of patients' MA behavior can motivate and guide providers to address issues related to MA. Clinicians working with patients with CAD should assess issues with or barriers to MA to identify the possible need to intervene. Future research might directly compare an intervention that provides patient MA status to healthcare providers to a similar intervention without this provision.

Medication adherence interventions delivered by nurses were especially effective. Nurses have considerable access to patients with CAD in outpatient settings, such as cardiac rehabilitation and clinics. In addition, nurses working in the inpatient setting spend approximately 25% to 37% of their time providing direct patient care and 11% to 21% of their time in medication-related tasks.[50,51] In addition to substantial access to this patient population, nurses also have clinical skills to promote MA. For example, nurses have delivered efficacious MA interventions through counseling,[52] follow-up communication,[27,53,54] and case management.[55,56] Nurses should play an active role in developing and implementing MA interventions among patients with CAD. Research exploring nursing interventions to increase MA among patients with CAD could focus on testing or comparing specific intervention strategies such as education, counseling, and managing barriers. Specific nurse type and training were not clearly reported among the studies, hindering the comparison of

Reprinted with permission from Chase, J., et al. (2016). The effectiveness of medication adherence interventions among patients with coronary artery disease. *Journal of Cardiovascular Nursing, 31,* 357–366.

Dichotomous Moderator Results

Moderator	k	d	SE	Q_B	P
Report moderators					
Publication status				1.267	.260
Unpublished (eg, dissertation, presentation)	4	0.724	0.474		
Published article	24	0.189	0.037		
Presence of funding for research				1.911	.167
Unfunded	11	0.452	0.192		
Funded (any funding reported or acknowledged)	17	0.182	0.040		
Socioeconomic status				0.194	.660
Not reported as low income	24	0.237	0.046		
Reported as low income	4	0.352	0.259		
Location				0.531	.466
Not North America	7	0.380	0.125		
North America	21	0.182	0.045		
Research methods moderators					
Allocation to treatment and control groups				0.200	.655
Not random assignment	8	0.199	0.068		
Random assignment	20	0.244	0.072		
Allocation concealment				1.222	.269
Allocation not concealed	15	0.188	0.050		
Allocation concealed	13	0.319	0.108		
Theory				0.167	.683
No theory	23	0.239	0.050		
Any theory	5	0.184	0.124		
Data collectors blinded				0.481	.488
Data collectors not blinded	18	0.207	0.052		
Data collectors blinded	10	0.293	0.112		
Intention-to-treat				0.000	.997
No intention-to-treat	23	0.236	0.063		
Intention-to-treat	5	0.237	0.097		
Intervention feature moderators					
Goal setting				0.095	.758
No goal setting	23	0.227	0.050		
Goal setting	5	0.183	0.135		
Healthcare provider given information about MA				3.899	.048
Healthcare provider NOT given information about MA	20	0.151	0.042		
Healthcare provider given information about MA	8	0.387	0.112		
Intervention delivered at home				0.676	.411
Not at home	23	0.254	0.053		
At home	5	0.129	0.143		
Intervention delivered at clinic				0.705	.401
Not at clinic	23	0.213	0.049		
At clinic	5	0.320	0.118		
Intervention started while subjects were inpatients				8.448	.004
Not inpatients	19	0.141	0.037		
Inpatients	9	0.590	0.150		
Problem solving				0.307	.580
No problem solving	22	0.245	0.054		
Problem solving	6	0.188	0.088		
Self-monitoring of medications				1.198	.274
No self-monitoring	25	0.195	0.045		
Self-monitoring	3	0.492	0.267		
Succinct written instructions				1.820	.177
No succinct written instructions	22	0.255	0.054		
Succinct written instructions	6	0.124	0.080		
Any written instructions				2.868	.090
No written instructions	19	0.287	0.065		
Any written instructions	9	0.149	0.049		
Behavior target				1.212	.271
Multiple behaviors	11	0.306	0.109		
MA only	17	0.179	0.038		

(continues)

Reprinted with permission from Chase, J., et al. (2016). The effectiveness of medication adherence interventions among patients with coronary artery disease. *Journal of Cardiovascular Nursing, 31*, 357–366.

Moderator	k	d	SE	Q_B	P
Part of intervention delivered to providers				0.476	.490
Not delivered to providers	24	0.213	0.053		
Delivered to providers	4	0.311	0.131		
Nurse interventionist				6.502	.011
No nurse	18	0.127	0.020		
Any nurse	10	0.428	0.116		
Physician interventionist				0.397	.529
No physician	21	0.223	0.050		
Physician	7	0.322	0.148		
Pharmacist interventionist				0.310	.578
No pharmacist	21	0.240	0.056		
Pharmacist	7	0.193	0.062		
Mail delivery				10.845	.001
No mail delivery	23	0.292	0.059		
Mail delivery	5	0.060	0.038		
Telephone delivery				0.701	.403
No telephone delivery	14	0.192	0.065		
Telephone delivery	14	0.280	0.082		
Written materials ONLY				2.985	.084
No written intervention	26	0.248	0.049		
Written intervention	2	0.008	0.130		
Face-to-face delivery				2.604	.107
No face-to-face	7	0.143	0.048		
Face-to-face	21	0.288	0.076		

Table G. Dichotomous Moderator Results, Continued

k, number of comparisons; d, standardized mean difference effect size; SE, standard error; Q_B, sum of weighted sum of squares of subgroup means about overall mean; p, value for Q_B.

MA intervention effectiveness across different types of nurses. Investigators of future studies should explicitly identify types of nurses delivering MA interventions among patients with CAD.

Medication adherence interventions initiated in the inpatient setting were more effective. The inpatient setting may provide an opportunity for clinicians to inform patients and families about the importance of medications for secondary prevention of CAD as well as strategies for MA. Moreover, the dire nature of hospitalization may influence patient and family receptivity to MA interventions. Most MA interventions initiated in the inpatient setting included follow-up intervention content after discharge. Continued reinforcement of MA after discharge may positively affect MA outcomes. For those patients who may start medications outside the hospital, interventions delivered at home or in the clinic were equally effective. Future research might directly compare MA interventions initiated in the inpatient setting to MA interventions initiated after hospitalization.

Regarding sample characteristics, only age appeared to impact intervention effectiveness. As the age of the sample increased, so did the intervention effectiveness. These findings support prior research related to statin MA and low-density lipoprotein goal attainment.[57,58] Chi and colleagues[57] postulated that older individuals are more likely to have multiple comorbidities and may be more attentive to prescribed medication regimens. Additional primary research is needed to identify effective MA interventions among younger populations with

CAD. Furthermore, more primary research involving more diverse samples is needed. Deaths related to CAD are higher among African Americans than whites and other groups.[2,59] Rates of MA for various chronic diseases also differ across race and ethnicity, with minority groups being less adherent to prescribed medications.[60,61] However, few primary studies included in this meta-analysis reported racially or ethnically diverse groups. Thus, future primary research testing MA interventions among patients with CAD must strive to include minority groups to reduce this disparity.

We found some interesting nonsignificant moderators. Interventions focusing solely on MA were as effective as interventions that had multiple behavioral foci. Thus, clinicians may take the opportunity to introduce strategies for MA while discussing other health behaviors with CAD patients. The use of only written material did not impact intervention effectiveness, suggesting that providers should consider using more than this type of delivery when promoting MA among patients with CAD. Future MA intervention research among patients with CAD should incorporate additional forms of intervention delivery beyond written materials. Number of intervention sessions did not appear to be a significant moderator. It is possible that even 1 or 2 intervention sessions may be effective in changing MA behavior among patients with CAD. However, additional research testing or comparing various aspects of intervention dose could help identify the most effective dose needed to change MA behavior. We did not identify any specific

Reprinted with permission from Chase, J., et al. (2016). The effectiveness of medication adherence interventions among patients with coronary artery disease. *Journal of Cardiovascular Nursing, 31*, 357–366.

What's New and Important

- Interventions designed to increase MA among patients with CAD are modestly effective.
- In this patient population, nurse-delivered MA interventions were more effective than interventions not delivered by nurses.
- Among patients with CAD, MA interventions initiated in the inpatient setting can be more effective than interventions initiated in the outpatient setting.

should consider using objective measures of MA to reduce bias.

Meta-analyses are observational studies. The moderator findings of this study are intended to promote additional exploration in this area of study. The scope of this meta-analysis is limited to MA among patients with CAD. Therefore, interpretation of these findings may not be possible among patients with other chronic illnesses or other forms of heart disease.

Conclusion

Medication management is an important aspect of secondary prevention for CAD. Nonadherence to prescribed medications for CAD has been linked with multiple poor outcomes. Findings from this meta-analysis suggest that MA interventions among patients with CAD are effective, especially among older patients. Clinicians working with patients with CAD evaluate patients' MA behavior before initiating interventions to improve MA. Nurses are on the front lines of health behavior promotion among these patients and can be effective MA interventionists. Future research is needed to explore MA interventions among younger populations and more racially diverse groups.

intervention strategy that increased MA intervention effectiveness; however, lack of statistical significance of these moderators may be related to the small number of comparisons.

Medication adherence interventions delivered by physicians or pharmacists were equally effective as interventions not delivered by these providers. Although these findings suggest that involving these providers may not increase MA intervention effectiveness, the number of studies incorporating these types of interventionists was small. Future research could directly compare similar MA interventions among patients with CAD delivered by different clinicians. Additional research may also explore variations in MA intervention delivery across diverse healthcare providers.

This meta-analysis was limited by some primary study characteristics. Although efforts were made to contact corresponding authors, some studies were excluded because critical data were missing from primary study reports. Primary study reporting limits the generalizability of this study's findings to more diverse populations. Primary study quality is an important issue in meta-analysis work. Multiple strategies are recommended to manage primary study quality.[62,63] We used specific inclusion criteria to capture reports with more rigorous study designs, employed analysis techniques accounting for study heterogeneity, and explored study quality empirically through moderator analyses. Some publication biases were present. Smaller, negative studies are less likely to be published; therefore, access to these studies is limited. Despite extensive search strategies, capturing these relevant studies was a challenge.

Primary study reporting affected the ability to identify effective combinations of MA components. Several studies used multiple intervention strategies; however, combinations of strategies were inconsistent. Thus, determining the most effective combination of MA intervention strategies was not possible.

Measurement error within the primary studies could have introduced bias toward overestimation of MA intervention effects. Objective measures are the most sensitive and specific means of measuring MA[64,65]; however, most included studies used self-reported MA, which is known to overestimate patients' MA.[66] Future MA intervention research conducted among patients with CAD

REFERENCES

1. Centers for Disease Control and Prevention. *Heart Disease Facts*. 2014. http://www.cdc.gov/heartdisease/facts.htm. Accessed July 16, 2014.
2. National Heart, Lung, and Blood Institute. *Morbidity and Mortality: 2012 Chart Book on Cardiovascular, Lung, and Blood Diseases*. Washington, DC: National Institutes of Health; 2012.
3. Ford ES, Ajani UA, Croft JB, et al. Explaining the decrease in U.S. deaths from coronary disease, 1980–2000. *N Engl J Med.* 2007;356(23):2388–2398.
4. Ho PM, Bryson CL, Rumsfeld JS. Medication adherence its importance in cardiovascular outcomes. *Circulation.* 2009; 119(23):3028–3035.
5. Naderi SH, Bestwick JP, Wald DS. Adherence to drugs that prevent cardiovascular disease: meta-analysis on 376,162 patients. *Am J Med.* 2012;125(9):882–887.
6. Chowdhury R, Khan H, Heydon E, et al. Adherence to cardiovascular therapy: a meta-analysis of prevalence and clinical consequences. *Eur Heart J.* 2013;34(38):2940–2948.
7. Sokol MC, McGuigan KA, Verbrugge RR, Epstein RS. Impact of medication adherence on hospitalization risk and healthcare cost. *Med Care.* 2005;43(6):521–530.
8. Ho PM, Magid DJ, Shetterly SM, et al. Medication nonadherence is associated with a broad range of adverse outcomes in patients with coronary artery disease. *Am Heart J.* 2008; 155(4):772–779.
9. Kelly JM. Sublingual nitroglycerin: improving patient compliance with a demonstration dose. *J Am Board Fam Pract.* 1988;1(4):251–254.
10. Nicoleau, CM. *Evaluation of a comprehensive cardiac rehabilitation program* [dissertation]. New York, NY: Yeshiva University; 1985.
11. Zhao Y. Effects of a discharge planning intervention for elderly patients with coronary heart disease in Tianjin, China:

Reprinted with permission from Chase, J., et al. (2016). The effectiveness of medication adherence interventions among patients with coronary artery disease. *Journal of Cardiovascular Nursing, 31,* 357–366.

a randomized controlled trial. 2004. http://search.proquest.com.proxy.mul.missouri.edu/pqdt/docview/305041963/abstract/CE2FD56D4F7B49F2PQ/1?accountid=14576. Accessed June 11, 2014.

12. Costa e Silva R, Pellanda L, Portal V, Maciel P, Furquim A, Schaan B. Transdisciplinary approach to the follow-up of patients after myocardial infarction. *Clin Sao Paulo Braz.* 2008;63(4):489–496.

13. Lourenco L, Rodrigues RCM, Gallani CB, Spana TM. Effectiveness of the combination of planning strategies in adhering to the drug therapy and health related quality of life among coronary heart disease outpatients. Paper presented at: International Nursing Intervention Conference; 2011; Montreal, Canada.

14. Miller P, Wikoff R, Garrett MJ, McMahon M, Smith T. Regimen compliance two years after myocardial infarction. *Nurs Res.* 1990;39(6):333–336.

15. Ara S. A literature review of cardiovascular disease management programs in managed care populations. *J Manag Care Pharm.* 2004;10(4):326–344.

16. Cutrona SL, Choudhry NK, Fischer MA, et al. Targeting cardiovascular medication adherence interventions. *J Am Pharm Assoc (2003).* 2012;52(3):381–397.

17. Maddox TM, Ho PM. Medication adherence and the patient with coronary artery disease: challenges for the practitioner. *Curr Opin Cardiol.* 2009;24(5):468–472.

18. Schadewaldt V, Schultz T. Nurse-led clinics as an effective service for cardiac patients: results from a systematic review. *Int J Evid Based Healthc.* 2011;9(3):199–214.

19. Cooper H, Hedges LV, Valentine JC, eds. *The Handbook of Research Synthesis and Meta-Analysis.* 2nd ed. New York, NY: Russell Sage Foundation; 2009.

20. Moher D, Liberati A, Tetzlaff J, Altman DG. Preferred reporting items for systematic reviews and meta-analyses: the PRISMA statement. *BMJ.* 2009;339:b2535.

21. Reed JG, Baxter PM. Using reference databases. In: *The Handbook of Research Synthesis and Meta-Analysis.* 2nd ed. New York, NY: Russell Sage Foundation; 2009:73–101.

22. Borenstein M, Hedges LV, Higgins JPT, Rothstein HR. *Comprehensive Meta-Analysis.* Englewood, NJ: Biostat; 2005.

23. Borenstein M, Hedges LV, Higgins JPT, Rothstein HR. *Introduction to Meta-Analysis.* 1st ed. West Sussex, UK: Wiley; 2009.

24. Calvert SB, Kramer JM, Anstrom KJ, Kaltenbach LA, Stafford JA, Allen LaPointe NM. Patient-focused intervention to improve long-term adherence to evidence-based medications: a randomized trial. *Am Heart J.* 2012;163(4):657–665.

25. Campbell N, Ritchie L, Thain J, Deans H, Rawles J, Squair J. Secondary prevention in coronary heart disease: a randomised trial of nurse led clinics in primary care. *Heart.* 1998;80(5):447–452.

26. Choudhry NK, Avorn J, Glynn RJ, et al. Full coverage for preventive medications after myocardial infarction. *N Engl J Med.* 2011;365(22):2088–2097.

27. Edworthy SM, Baptie B, Galvin D, et al. Effects of an enhanced secondary prevention program for patients with heart disease: a prospective randomized trial. *Can J Cardiol.* 2007; 23(13):1066–1072.

28. Faulkner MA, Wadibia EC, Lucas BD, Hilleman DE. Impact of pharmacy counseling on compliance and effectiveness of combination lipid-lowering therapy in patients undergoing coronary artery revascularization: a randomized, controlled trial. *Pharmacotherapy.* 2000;20:410–416.

29. Gould KA. A randomized controlled trial of a discharge nursing intervention to promote self-regulation of care for early discharge interventional cardiology patients. *Dimens Crit Care Nurs.* 2011;30(2):117–125.

30. Guthrie RM. The effects of postal and telephone reminders on compliance with pravastatin therapy in a national reg- istry: Results of the first myocardial infarction risk reduction program. *Clin Ther.* 2001;23(6):970–980.

31. Jiang X, Sit JW, Wong TK. A nurse-led cardiac rehabilitation programme improves health behaviours and cardiac physiological risk parameters: Evidence from Chengdu, China. *J Clin Nurs.* 2007;16(10):1886–1897.

32. Kotowycz MA, Cosman TL, Tartaglia C, Afzal R, Natarajan MK, et al. Safety and feasibility of early hospital discharge in ST-segment elevation myocardial infarction—a prospective and randomized trial in low-risk primary percutaneous coronary intervention patients (the Safe-Depart Trial). *Am Heart J.* 2010;159(1):117.

33. Kripalani S, Schmotzer B, Jacobson TA. Improving medication adherence through graphically enhanced interventions in coronary heart disease (IMAGE-CHD): A randomized controlled trial. *J Gen Intern Med.* 2012;27(12):1609–1617.

34. Lehr BK. *A comparative study of self-management and cognitive behavioral therapies in the treatment of cardiac rehabilitation patients* [dissertation]. Milwaukee, WI: University of Wisconsin; 1986.

35. Muñiz J, Gómez-Doblas JJ, Santiago-Pérez MI, et al. The effect of post-discharge educational intervention on patients in achieving objectives in modifiable risk factors six months after discharge following an episode of acute coronary syndrome, (CAM-2 Project): A randomized controlled trial. *Health Qual Life Outcomes.* 2010;8:137.

36. Polack J, Jorgenson D, Robertson P. Evaluation of different methods of providing medication-related education to patients following myocardial infarction. *Can Pharm J.* 2008;141(4):241–247.

37. Shemesh E, Koren-Michowitz M, Yehuda R, et al. Symptoms of posttraumatic stress disorder in patients who have had a myocardial infarction. *J Consult Liaison Psychiatry.* 2006; 47(3):231–239.

38. Sherrard H, Struthers C, Kearns SA, Wells G, Mesana T. Using technology to create a medication safety net for cardiac surgery patients: a nurse-led randomized control trial. *Can J Cardiovasc Nurs.* 2009;19(3):9–15.

39. Smith DH, Kramer JM, Perrin N, et al. A randomized trial of direct-to-patient communication to enhance adherence to beta-blocker therapy following myocardial infarction. *Arch Intern Med.* 2008;168(5):477–483.

40. Yilmaz MB, Pinar M, Naharci I, et al. Being well-informed about statin is associated with continuous adherence and reaching targets. *Cardiovasc Drugs Ther.* 2005;19(6):437–440.

41. Zuckerman IH, Weiss SR, McNally D, Layne B, Mullins CD, Wang J. Impact of an educational intervention for secondary prevention of myocardial infarction on Medicaid drug use and cost. *Am J Manag Care.* 2004;10(7 part 2):493–500.

42. Miller P, Wikoff R, McMahon M, Garrett MJ, Ringel K. Influence of a nursing intervention on regimen adherence and societal adjustments postmyocardial infarction. *Nurs Res.* 1988;37(5):297–302.

43. Miller P, Wikoff R, McMahon M, et al. Personal adjustments and regimen compliance 1 year after myocardial infarction. *Heart Lung.* 1989;18(4):339–346.

44. Choudhry NK, Brennan T, Toscano M, et al. Rationale and design of the Post-MI FREEE trial: a randomized evaluation of first-dollar drug coverage for post-myocardial infarction secondary preventive therapies. *Am Heart J.* 2008;156(1):31–36.

45. Gould KA. A randomized controlled trial of a discharge nursing intervention to promote self-regulation of care for early discharge interventional cardiology patients. *Dimens Crit Care Nurs.* 2009;30(2):117–125.

46. Conn VS, Enriquez M, Ruppar TM, Chan KC. Cultural relevance in medication adherence interventions with underrepresented adults: systematic review and meta-analysis of outcomes. *Prev Med.* 2014;69:239–247.

47. Conn V. Packaging interventions to increase medication adherence: systematic review and meta-analysis. *Curr Med Res Opin.* 2015;31(1):145–160.

48. Burnier M, Schneider MP, Chioléro A, Stubi CL, Brunner HR. Electronic compliance monitoring in resistant hypertension: the basis for rational therapeutic decisions. *J Hypertens.* 2001; 19(2):335–341.

49. Lowy A, Munk VC, Ong SH, et al. Effects on blood pressure and cardiovascular risk of variations in patients' adherence to prescribed antihypertensive drugs: role of duration of drug action. *Int J Clin Pract.* 2011;65(1):41–53.

50. Westbrook JI, Duffield C, LiL, Creswick NJ. How much time do nurses have for patients? A longitudinal study quantifying hospital nurses' patterns of task time distribution and interactions with health professionals. *BMC Health Serv Res.* 2011;11:319.

51. Jones M, Johnston D. Understanding phenomena in the real world: the case for real time data collection in health services research. *J Health Serv Res Policy.* 2011;16(3):172–176.

52. Krantz MJ, Havranek EP, Haynes DK, Smith I, Bucher-Bartelson B, Long CS. Inpatient initiation of beta-blockade plus nurse management in vulnerable heart failure patients: a randomized study. *J Card Fail.* 2008;14(4):303–309.

53. Kirscht JP, Kirscht JL, Rosenstock IM. A test of interventions to increase adherence to hypertensive medical regimens. *Health Educ Q.* 1981;8(3):261–272.

54. Piette JD, Weinberger M, McPhee SJ, Mah CA, Kraemer FB, Crapo LM. Do automated calls with nurse follow-up improve self-care and glycemic control among vulnerable patients with diabetes? *Am J Med.* 2000;108(1):20–27.

55. Logan AG, Milne BJ, Achber C, Campbell WP, Haynes RB. Work-site treatment of hypertension by specially trained nurses. A controlled trial. *Lancet.* 1979;2(8153):1175–1178.

56. Rudd P, Miller NH, Kaufman J, et al. Nurse management for hypertension. A systems approach. *Am J Hypertens.* 2004; 17(10):921–927.

57. Chi MD, Vansomphone SS, Liu I-LA, et al. Adherence to statins and LDL-cholesterol goal attainment. *Am J Manag Care.* 2014;20(4):e105–e112.

58. Nag SS, Daniel GW, Bullano MF, et al. LDL-C goal attainment among patients newly diagnosed with coronary heart disease or diabetes in a commercial HMO. *J Manag Care Pharm.* 2007;13(8):652–663.

59. Coronary Heart Disease and Stroke Deaths—United States, 2006. http://www.cdc.gov/mmwr/preview/mmwrhtml/su6001a13.htm. Accessed June 6, 2014.

60. Gerber BS, Cho YI, Arozullah AM, Lee S-YD. Racial differences in medication adherence: A cross-sectional study of Medicare enrollees. *Am J Geriatr Pharmacother.* 2010;8(2): 136–145.

61. Rolnick SJ, Pawloski PA, Hedblom BD, Asche SE, Bruzek RJ. Patient characteristics associated with medication adherence. *Clin Med Res.* 2013;11(2):54–65.

62. Valentine JC. Judging the quality of primary research. In: Cooper HM, Hedges LV, Valentine JC, eds. *The Handbook of Research Synthesis and Meta-Analysis.* 2nd ed. Russell Sage Foundation; 2009:122–146.

63. Conn VS, Rantz MJ. Research methods: managing primary study quality in meta-analyses. *Res Nurs Health.* 2003;26(4): 322–333.

64. Dunbar-Jacob J, Sereika SM, Houze M, Luyster FS, Callan JA. Accuracy of measures of medication adherence in a cholesterol-lowering regimen. *West J Nurs Res.* 2012; 34(5):578–597.

65. Hansen RA, Kim MM, Song L, Tu W, Wu J, Murray MD. Comparison of methods to assess medication adherence and classify nonadherence. *Ann Pharmacother.* 2009;43(3): 413–422.

66. Zeller A, Ramseier E, Teagtmeyer A, Battegay E. Patients' self-reported adherence to cardiovascular medication using electronic monitors as comparators. *Hypertens Res.* 2008; 31(11):2037–2043.

Reprinted with permission from Chase, J., et al. (2016). The effectiveness of medication adherence interventions among patients with coronary artery disease. *Journal of Cardiovascular Nursing, 31,* 357–366.

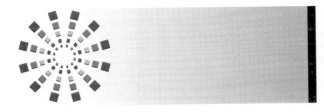

Tracey L. Carr, PhD

Gary Groot, MD, PhD

David Cochran, BSc

Lorraine Holtslander, PhD, RN

Patient Information Needs and Breast Reconstruction After Mastectomy

A Qualitative Meta-Synthesis

KEY WORDS

Breast cancer

Delayed breast reconstruction

Immediate breast reconstruction

Information needs

Meta-synthesis

Qualitative

Background: Although many women benefit from breast reconstruction after mastectomy, several studies report women's dissatisfaction with the level of information they were provided with before reconstruction. **Objective:** The present meta-synthesis examines the qualitative literature that explores women's experiences of breast reconstruction after mastectomy and highlights women's healthcare information needs. **Methods:** After a comprehensive search of 6 electronic databases (CINAHL, Cochrane Library, EMBASE, MEDLINE, PsycINFO, and Scopus), we followed the methodology for synthesizing qualitative research. The search produced 423 studies, which were assessed against 5 inclusion criteria. A meta-synthesis methodology was used to analyze the data through taxonomic classification and constant targeted comparison. **Results:** Some 17 studies met the inclusion criteria, and findings from 16 studies were synthesized. The role of the healthcare practitioner is noted as a major influence on women's expectations, and in some instances, women did not feel adequately informed about the outcomes of surgery and the recovery process. In general, women's desire for normality and effective emotional coping shapes their information needs. **Conclusion:** The information needs of women are better understood after considering women's actual experiences with breast reconstruction. It is important to inform women of the immediate outcomes of reconstruction surgery and the recovery process. **Implications for Practice:** In an attempt to better address women's information needs, healthcare

Author Affiliations: Department of Community Health and Epidemiology (Drs Carr and Groot and Mr Cochran) and College of Nursing (Dr Holtslander), University of Saskatchewan, Saskatoon, Canada.

This work was supported by the University of Saskatchewan College of Medicine Research Award (grant number: N/A).

The authors have no conflicts of interest to disclose.

This is an open-access article distributed under the terms of the Creative Commons Attribution-Non Commercial-No Derivatives License 4.0 (CCBY-NC-

Correspondence: Tracey L. Carr, PhD, Department of Community Health and Epidemiology, University of Saskatchewan, 107 Wiggins Rd, Saskatoon, SK, Canada S7N 5E5 (tracey.carr@usask.ca).

DOI: 10.1097/NCC.0000000000000599

185

Reprinted with permission from Carr, T., et al. (2019). Patient information needs and breast reconstruction after mastectomy: A qualitative meta-synthesis. *Cancer Nursing*, 42, 229–241.

> practitioners should discover women's initial expectations of reconstruction as a starting point in the consultation. In addition, the research revealed the importance of the nurse navigator in terms of assisting women through the recovery process.

Mastectomy after breast cancer can negatively affect physical and psychosocial functioning.[1,2] In response, some women elect to have breast reconstruction (BR). Breast reconstruction surgery takes the form of either immediate BR (IBR), which is initiated at the same time as the mastectomy, or delayed BR (DBR), which is performed at some point after mastectomy.[3] Women's motives for either form of reconstruction are similar and include a desire to return to (or maintain) normality,[4] to restore a sense of wholeness,[5] and to avoid wearing a prosthesis.[6,7] Furthermore, the return of the breast may mark a symbolic end of cancer treatment in the case of IBR or a literal end of treatment for those pursuing DBR. Ultimately, BR may allow women to move past the cancer experience and restore their physical and psychological selves.[5,8,9]

The decision to opt for reconstruction and the timing of reconstruction are influenced by several factors. Women's decisions are influenced by general body image and sexual functioning concerns, in addition to a need to feel whole and restore femininity.[6,10] The choice of IBR is often motivated by consideration of the impact a prosthesis would have on daily functioning. Some women are concerned about their ability to obtain a surgical appointment if they waited until after recovering from mastectomy and cancer.[11] Moreover, women who chose IBR rated interactions with their doctor more favorably than those who chose DBR.[10] Many women who delayed reconstruction wanted to ensure that they had recovered from cancer before seeking reconstruction.[11] In addition, for some who did not initially consider reconstruction, their prosthesis struggle and body image concerns motivated an acceptance of reconstruction.[6]

Although women are generally satisfied with the outcome of BR,[12–16] many encounter unanticipated struggles during the recovery period.[17] Patients have expressed dissatisfaction with the physical result of surgery.[17] Beyond this dissatisfaction, women struggle with adjusting to a new reality within their intimate relationships, revising a new conception of their femininity, and modifying their daily routine. These challenges are present whether the reconstruction is immediate or delayed.[18–20]

The unexpected struggles of recovery from BR have caused women to question the accuracy of information provided by their plastic surgeon.[15] Women felt ill-informed about their BR options, expressed regret about not knowing more about the recovery process,[17,21] and felt that surgeons did not adequately inform them of postoperative realities.[21–23] Some women felt deceived by healthcare professionals who emphasized the potential psychological benefits of reconstruction without acknowledging the difficulty of the recovery.[19,22,23]

Informing women about BR options while acknowledging both the risks and benefits is a complex process. The initial BR consultation typically occurs around the time of cancer diagnosis. Researchers have documented the negative impact a cancer diagnosis can have on a woman's ability to retain information.[24]

Description of the complexities of BR treatment, combined with the fear experienced in the context of a diagnosis, can impair patient recall.[25] Accordingly, some researchers have suggested using audio recordings, written summaries, and one-to-one conversations to improve information exchange.[26–28] If patients' information needs are better understood, the quality of provider-patient communication may also improve.[22]

To better understand women's information needs, we performed a qualitative meta-synthesis on the relevant literature. A qualitative meta-synthesis involves integrating findings from several qualitative studies. This methodology seeks to clarify differences and highlight overlapping concepts and themes from multiple studies.[29] By using this approach, we can encompass the disparate experiences of women who have undergone BR. This approach is particularly useful when considering the differences between various women's access to information about BR, and it can provide insight into women's information needs.

To date, no meta-synthesis exists that explores women's experiences with BR. The primary objectives of this study were to explore the qualitative research regarding women's experiences with BR and to synthesize the findings in relation to women's information needs. A better understanding of women's information needs can translate into improved patient-centered care. A secondary objective was to determine whether women's information needs differ for those who choose IBR or DBR.

■ Methods

We used the methodology for qualitative meta-synthesis outlined by Sandelowski and Barroso.[29] This process was guided by a multidisciplinary clinical research team in consultation with a health sciences librarian. After a comprehensive search of the literature on women's experiences of BR surgery, the results were synthesized using a 3-stage process: (1) study appraisal, (2) study classification, and (3) synthesis of findings.

Search Method

For this review, we searched the following electronic databases and filtered results by the corresponding date ranges: CINAHL (1982 to May 2016), Cochrane Library (2008–2016), EMBASE (1980 to May 2016), MEDLINE (1950 to May 2016), PsycINFO (1985 to May 2016), and Scopus (2003 to May 2016). For the search, we generated key search terms and subject headings that encompassed breast cancer surgery, patient experience, and qualitative research. The specific search terms were "breast cancer," "breast reconstruction," "breast tumor," "mammoplasty," and "support groups," in addition to the MESH search terms of "breast neoplasms," "mastectomy," "breast implantation," and "psychology." The pilot search in MEDLINE rendered 28 titles.

The research team established the following inclusion and exclusion criteria to screen the results. Titles were included when (a) the focus was on women's experiences with the process and outcomes of breast cancer surgery, (b) 1 aspect of cancer treatment was BR surgery, (c) the impact of BR surgery was on different psychosocial aspects (body image, sexuality, relationships, satisfaction, etc), and (d) the study identified qualitative methods. Titles were excluded when (a) the focus was exclusively on other forms of breast cancer treatment (eg, mastectomy or radiography), (b) only the decision-making process leading to BR surgery (ie, preoperative experience) was considered, or (c) sources were non-English.

SEARCH OUTCOME

The online search of the 6 databases yielded 423 titles. After the duplicates were removed, 364 titles remained. The inclusion and exclusion criteria were applied by 2 independent reviewers. Agreement on the selection process was greater than 95%. The remaining titles underwent further review until a consensus was reached. For this review, we considered only those studies that examined patients' experiences with BR using qualitative methodology. When the screening criteria were applied to the abstracts, 348 titles were excluded and the remaining 17 were retrieved in full text (see PRISMA diagram in the Figure). Although no specific quality appraisal tool was applied to each article, we ensured that each study had a clear statement of aims, used a qualitative methodology appropriately, used a method of data collection that appropriately addressed the research question, and had a clear statement of findings.[30]

Most studies were conducted in the United Kingdom (n = 8). The other studies were conducted in the United States (n = 3), Canada (n = 2), Australia (n = 2), Sweden (n = 1), and Taiwan (n = 1). A total of 258 female participants were included across the 17 studies. A total of 201 female participants from the studies underwent BR. Two studies included interviews with women's partners. A total of 16 partners were interviewed across two of the studies. In the process of data collection, we only included statements or researcher inferences from the women undergoing BR and not their partners. Furthermore, the women were interviewed separately from their partners. Considering the studies as a whole, 193 of the participants were interviewed one-on-one, whereas a single study[31] used a focus group with 8 participants. For the synthesis, we focused on the women's experiences rather than their partners' perspectives. In Table 1, we outline the study method and objectives and the finding classification and rigor analysis of each study.

APPRAISING THE FINDINGS

We examined each study's methods and findings and evaluated the degree of analytical rigor. The evaluation was based on team discussions[32,33] and an existing meta-synthesis study that used Sandelowski and Barroso's[29] meta-summary technique.[34] When considering a particular analysis, we noted the interview structure and whether an interview guide was used.[32,33] We also noted whether the researchers verified their analysis with an outside source.[34] In addition, we assessed the studies to determine

whether the ratio of researcher interpretation to presented data was reasonable and well presented.[32,33] This criterion evaluated whether the quantity of interview data presented was sufficient to support the authors' inferences. It also evaluated whether the inferences seemed reasonable in relation to the data presented.[33] We also used another set of criteria to ensure that the data were neither too specific nor too general.[32] The summary of our observations is recorded in the Analysis Rigor column of Table 1.

CLASSIFYING THE FINDINGS

We used the criteria from Sandelowski and Barroso[29] to categorize each study's findings. Four categories of findings, ranging from least to most elaboration, are distinguished: topical survey, thematic survey, conceptual/thematic description, and interpretative explanation.[29] Topical surveys are removed from the meta-synthesis because of the survey's low level of elaboration.[29] One member of the research team categorized each study based on the degree to which the authors elaborated on the participant interviews. One study met this classification for low-level elaboration and was removed.[35] Of the remaining 16 studies, 12 were thematic surveys and four were classified as conceptual/thematic description. The classification process was verified by a second member of the research team.

The methodologies reported by the studies' authors were diverse: five were thematic analysis, and two were modified thematic analysis (thematic narrative analysis and phenomenological thematic analysis). In addition, there were 2 grounded theory studies, a qualitative feminist analysis, a hermeneutic phenomenology study, an interpretive phenomenological analysis, a framework analysis, an iterative coding study, and a study that used a heuristic approach. A description of the studies and their classifications is reported in Table 1.

SYNTHESIS OF FINDINGS

Following Sandelowski and Barroso's[29] methodological approach to synthesizing qualitative research findings, we performed a taxonomic analysis of the findings, which involved organizing individual concepts from the findings into a hierarchy. Following the authors'[29] methodology, when performing the taxonomic analysis, we focused on broadening the conceptual range over simply noting prevalent themes. After the taxonomic analysis, a constant targeted comparison was performed. Such a comparison contrasts different conceptual groups found during the taxonomic analysis. Contrasting the different conceptual groups reveals similarities and differences that clarify conceptual boundaries. Specifically, we contrasted the experiences of women who had undergone IBR with those who had undergone DBR.

COMPARING STUDY DEMOGRAPHICS AND METHODOLOGY

Reported participant demographic information varied from study to study. Table 2 details the demographic data extracted from each study. Although the precise form of demographic reporting varied, participant age, marital status, and type of surgical procedure are most frequently reported. Comparing the data presented in Tables 1 and 2, the studies differ noticeably in

Reprinted with permission from Carr, T., et al. (2019). Patient information needs and breast reconstruction after mastectomy: A qualitative meta-synthesis. *Cancer Nursing, 42,* 229–241.

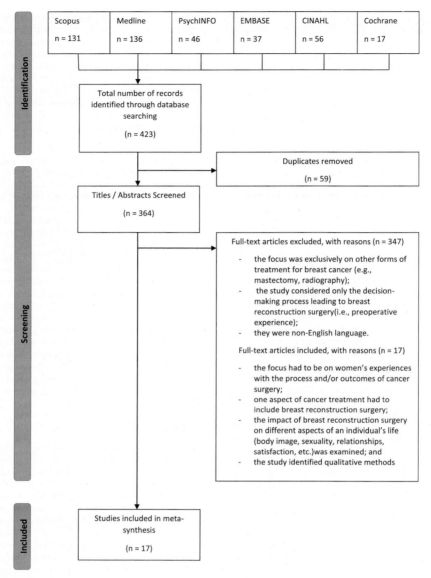

Figure ■ PRISMA diagram.

terms of both methodology and participants. Thus, performing a direct one-to-one association between studies may not produce meaningful comparisons.

Lack of methodological and demographic resemblance could be a concern in a meta-analytic study; however, Sandelowski and Barroso's meta-synthesis technique accommodates the varying individual study methodologies and demographics. The emphasis in a meta-synthesis is on the integration of results instead of comparison alone. Subsequently, the present analysis notes the similarities in women's information needs despite the diversity

or unknown demographics of participants. Although, by using Sandelowski and Barroso's methodology, we explored the similarities of women's experiences, we were also able to reveal the contrasting experiences of those who chose IBR over DBR.

■ Results

Our synthesis revealed the importance of the role played by the information provided by healthcare providers to patients

Reprinted with permission from Carr, T., et al. (2019). Patient information needs and breast reconstruction after mastectomy: A qualitative meta-synthesis. *Cancer Nursing, 42*, 229–241.

✳ Table 1 • Study Attributes

Authors	Objective	Methodology	Data Collection Method[a]	Analysis Rigor	Finding Classification
Abu-Nab and Grunfeld[39] (2007) (England)	Investigate patient's perception of scaring as a result of breast reconstruction	Thematic analysis	Semistructured interviews; interviewed individually (N = 15)	The interview schedule was described by its general themes. Sample transcripts were verified by an independent researcher. The data were well presented.	Thematic survey
Crompvoets[19] (2006) (Australia)	Examine women's efforts to accept their changed body	Qualitative, feminist analysis	Interviews; interviewed individually (N = 4)	No interview guide and method of analysis verification was described. The data were presented well.	Conceptual/ thematic description
Denford et al[41] (2011) (United States)	Aim of study was to investigate women's conceptualization of normality	Thematic analysis	Semistructured interviews; interviewed individually (N = 35)	An interview schedule was described by its general themes. The initial themes were verified by a second researcher. The data were reasonably well presented.	Thematic survey
Fallbjörk et al[36] (2012) (Sweden)	Examine women's breast reconstruction experiences	Thematic narrative analysis	Interviews; interviewed individually (N = 6)	An initial question was used to guide discussion. Consensus between the authors was reached regarding the products of analysis. Data were reasonably well presented.	Thematic survey
Fang et al[15] (2010) (Taiwan)	Examine women's breast reconstruction experiences	Hermeneutic phenomenology	Open-ended interviews; interviewed individually (N = 7)	The interview was guided by 5 prompt questions. Two participants reviewed the findings and provided feedback. Findings were well presented.	Thematic survey
Hill and White[14] (2008) (Australia)	Examine women's transverse rectus abdominis musculocutaneous flap breast reconstruction experiences	Thematic analysis	Semistructured interviews; interviewed individually (N = 10)	Researchers described the list of topics discussed in the interview. Participants verified the findings in a focus group setting. The findings were reasonably well presented.	Thematic survey
Kasper[12] (1995) (United States)	Investigate how women manage social and psychological threats to themselves and how do they maintain or modify their female identity	Thematic analysis	Unstructured interview; interviewed individually (N = 16)	No interview guide was used; the researcher only had the participant freely express their experience. No method of verification was stated. Findings were reasonably well presented.	Conceptual/ thematic description
Loaring et al[40] (2015) (United Kingdom)	Study examines couple's experience of breast reconstruction and how it affects body image and sexuality	Interpretative phenomenological analysis	Semistructured interviews; interviewed individually (N = 4)[b]	Interview schedule was used, and the broad themes were described. The third and fourth authors reviewed the late-stage analysis.	Conceptual/ thematic description
Marshall and Kiemle[13] (2005) (England)	Explore how breast reconstruction affects sexual intimacy and what coping strategies are used and identify what healthy support is needed	Grounded theory	Semistructured interviews; interviewed individually (N = 12)[c]	The topic areas were described, and the researchers provided some sample questions. The key themes uncovered were reviewed by participants. The presentation of results was acceptable.	Thematic survey

(continues)

Reprinted with permission from Carr, T., et al. (2019). Patient information needs and breast reconstruction after mastectomy: A qualitative meta-synthesis. *Cancer Nursing, 42,* 229–241.

✳ Table 1 • Study Attributes, Continued

Authors	Objective	Methodology	Data Collection Method[a]	Analysis Rigor	Finding Classification
McKean et al[16] (2013) (Scotland)	Using grounded theory, examine how breast reconstruction restores a perception of normality in terms of body image and a sense of self	Grounded theory	Semistructured interviews; interviewed individually (N = 10)	Example questions from the interview were provided. The participants verified the findings. The presentation of results was acceptable.	Thematic survey
Murray et al[38] (2015) (England)	Explored women's immediate breast reconstruction experiences to understand what affects patient satisfaction	Thematic analysis, phenomenological approach	Semistructured interviews; interviewed individually (N = 9)	The topics of the interview questions were described. Participants provided feedback on the themes uncovered. The presentation of results was acceptable.	Thematic survey
Snell et al[37] (2010) (England)	Explore women's preoperative experiences of breast reconstruction	Iterative coding	Open-ended interviews; interviewed individually (N = 28)	A copy of the interview guide was provided in the article. The method of analysis was somewhat vague. No method of verification was specified. The findings were well presented.	Thematic survey
Spector et al[20] (2011) (Canada)	Explore women's expectations and information needs in relation to breast reconstruction	Thematic analysis	Semistructured interviews; interviewed individually (N = 21)	An interview guide was used, and some sample questions were provided. The results were verified by a qualitative research expert. The results were well presented.	Thematic survey
Spector et al[22] (2010) (Canada)	Explore women's experience of breast reconstruction recovery	Thematic analysis	Semistructured interviews and survey; interviewed individually (N = 20)	An interview guide was used, and some sample questions were provided. The results were verified by a qualitative research expert. The results were reasonably well presented.	Thematic survey
Truelsen[18] (2003) (Scotland)	Explore how mastectomy affected the decision to pursue breast reconstruction	Heuristic approach	Open-ended interviews; interviewed individually (N = 6)	Prompt questions were used to guide the interview. The analysis was verified by a counseling supervisor. The results were well presented.	Conceptual/ thematic description
Wolf[31] (2004) (England)	Examines women's information needs as it relates to breast reconstruction	Framework analysis	Focus group interviews (N = 8)	The interview guide was described as having prompts and memory aids to guide discussion. The analysis was verified by a breast care nurse. The results were reasonably well presented.	Thematic survey

[a]The N value refers to the number of women in the study who underwent breast reconstruction.
[b]Study also interviewed women's partners (N = 4); partner data were not included in the analysis.
[c]Study also interviewed women's partners (N = 12); partner data were not included in the analysis.

considering BR. The focus of this synthesis is on women's information needs as they relate to the most challenging aspect of BR: recovery from surgery. Although many women's experiences with the initial result of surgery and recovery were negative, many other women were very happy with their decision to have BR postrecovery.[14–16,36] We grouped our findings regarding information needs into 2 main categories: expectations do not match

BR experience and assessing patient information needs. A summary of our key findings is provided in Table 3.

Expectations Do Not Match BR Experience

Women's information needs came from several sources. Although the specific route of referral varies by jurisdiction,

Reprinted with permission from Carr, T., et al. (2019). Patient information needs and breast reconstruction after mastectomy: A qualitative meta-synthesis. *Cancer Nursing, 42,* 229–241.

Table 2 • Study Participant Demographic Information

Authors	IBR/DBR	Age, y	Marital Status	Surgery type	Employment	Socioeconomic Status/Education/Misc	Ethnicity	Time between surgery and interview
Abu-Nab and Grunfeld[39] (2007) (England)	IBR, 8; DBR, 7	Mean, 50 (38–59)	73% Married	TRAM flap: all participants			14 white, 1 Afro-Caribbean	Mean, 13.6 mo (5–30 mo)
Crompvoets[19] (2006) (Australia)	IBR, 0; DBR, 3; Mastr, 1; IBR/DBR, 1	(33–53)		TRAM flap, 2; saline implant, 2				
Denford et al[41] (2011) (United States)	IBR, 32; DBR, 3	30–39 = 6; 40–49 = 16; 50+ = 13		TRAM flap, 12; tissue expander, 20; LD and tissue expander, 2; none, 1	Working, 23; homemaker, 5; unemployed, 2; retired, 3; no answer, 2		Black, 8; white Hispanic, 2; white/European American, 23; Asian, 2	
Fallbjörk et al[36] (2012) (Sweden)	DBR, 6	Mean, 49 (39–61)	Married, 3; divorced, 1; common law, 1; widow, 1		75%–100% of full time	Healthcare publicly financed; all had 10+ y of education	All Swedish	
Fang et al[15] (2010) (Taiwan)	IBR, 7	(36–52)	Married, 6; not married, 1;	Autologous BR, 5; saline Implant, 2				
Hill and White[14] (2008) (Australia)	IBR, 5; DBR, 5	Mean, 48.5 (39–59)	Married, 9; widowed, 1;	TRAM flap, 10				Mean, 18.5 mo (10–31 mo)
Kasper[12] (1995) (United States)	BR, 16; mastectomy, 4; lumpectomy, 9	Mean, 47 (29–74)	Married, 15; divorced, 6; single, 3; widowed, 2; living with partner, 2			Middle class; heterosexual, 25; lesbian, 4	White	
Loaring et al[40] (2015) (United Kingdom)	IBR, 4	(37–55) Women and spouses	All married	TRAM flap, 2; DIEP, 1; LD, 1			White British, 2; Asian British, 1; African British, 1	(7 mo to 3 y)
Marshall and Kiemle[13] (2005) (England)	IBR, 11; DBR, 1	(38–58)	Married, 8; partnered, 2; unknown, 2	LD, 5; implant, 2; LD/implant, 2; rectus abdominis, 3			All white British	
McKean et al[16] (2013) (Scotland)	IBR, 6; DBR, 4	(31–60)	Married, 7; divorced, 1; partner, 1; single, 1	LD flap, 5; implant, 3; TRAM flap, 1; unknown, 1	Employed, 8; unemployed, 2			(<1 to 9 y)
Murray et al[38] (2015) (England)	IBR, 9	30–35 = 1; 40–45 = 3; 45–50 = 2; 50–55 = 1; 60–65 = 1; 65–70 = 1	Married, 6; single, 2; partnered, 1	Implant, 5; LD, 4				3.5–9 mo
Snell et al[37] (2010) (England)	IBR, 28	Average, 49	~50% Married	All implant				
Spector et al[20] (2011) (Canada)	Unknown whether immediate or delayed BR	Mean, 52.9 (20–65)		Either implant or TRAM flap		Living in Canada with Canadian health insurance	85% white	
Spector et al[22] (2010) (Canada)	Unknown whether immediate or delayed BR	(20–65)	~50% Married			Living in Canada with Canadian health insurance	85% white	
Truelsen[18] (2003) (Scotland)	IBR, 4; DBR, 2; mastectomy, 2	(40–58)	Married, 7; divorced, 1		Work at shop, 2; shop manager, 1; factory worker, 1; office worker, 1; help at dance school, 1; community health worker, 1; sewing machinist, 1		Scottish, 7; Irish, 1	

(continues)

Reprinted with permission from Carr, T., et al. (2019). Patient information needs and breast reconstruction after mastectomy: A qualitative meta-synthesis. *Cancer Nursing*, *42*, 229–241.

Table 2 • Study Participant Demographic Information, Continued								
Authors	IBR/DBR	Age, y	Marital Status	Surgery type	Employment	Socioeconomic Status/Education/Misc	Ethnicity	Time between surgery and Interview
Wolf[31] (2004) (England)	Unknown whether immediate or delayed BR	Mean, 51.5 (41–61)		Pedicled latissimus dorsi musculocutaneous flap, 5; tissue expansion, 2; free TRAM muscle flap, 1	Professional, 6; housewife, 2	Private healthcare, 3; NHS, 5; social class A: professional people, senior managers, 4; social class B: middle management executives, principal officers in local government, civil service, 4	All white	8.6 mo (4–14 mo)

Abbreviations: BR, breast reconstruction; DBR, delayed breast reconstruction; DIEP, deep inferior epigastric perforators; IBR, immediate breast reconstruction; LD, latissimus dorsi; NHS, National Health Service; TRAM, transverse rectus abdominis musculocutaneous.

the most significant information exchange occurs between the surgeon (plastic or breast) and the patient.[15,19,37,38] When this information is lacking, women's expectations are inaccurate and they react with disappointment to the outcome of surgery and the reality of recovery. Women also relied on information from a surgical consultation and from the Internet, friends, and relatives.[19,22] Yet, consultation with a plastic surgeon initiated the BR process. The surgeon discussed surgery options, informed the patient of the anticipated surgery outcome, and outlined any potential complications.[15,19,22,31,37] Women were often presented with pictures of a reconstructed breast. The quality of the interaction with the surgeon varies from woman to woman. In some instances, the prospective patients were led to "[imagine] a 'wonderful future' in which their bodies would not be greatly altered after mastectomy."[15] In addition to receiving a surgical consultation, many women used the Internet to find other pictures and written descriptions of surgical outcomes.[22,36–38] Such information played a role in shaping women's expectations of what their new breast would look and feel like. Women expected, based on their surgical consultation, to have their body return to normal or even improve.[15,19,38] Unfortunately, when the information did not match the outcome of surgery and the process of recovery, women experienced disappointment.

INFORMATION CONFLICTS WITH OUTCOME

Despite women's expectations, in some cases, the surgery produced unanticipated outcomes. The unmet expectations could be grouped into 1 of 2 categories: the unexpected appearance of the breast or the unexpected feel of the breast.[12,15,22,37–40] In the case of the aesthetic breast, some women expected their breast to more closely resemble photos they had seen during their surgical consultation, and others felt the breast looked unnatural.[37–40] Referring to photos provided by a surgeon, a participant remarked: "There are photographs in the booklets they give you, but mine bears no resemblance to that at all."[38] In a different study, a participant expressed similar dissatisfaction with photos: "I expected to look like that, like the photos of everyone else."[39]

Other women, in contrast, expressed dissatisfaction with the lack of a "natural" look for the breasts, and one woman exclaimed that "they really they look nothing like what I wanted and was used to looking like. So it was, it was very, very distressing."[40] One research team noted the dissatisfaction of patients for whom the outcome failed to meet expectations.[37] Excessive scarring was described by researchers as a major component of dissatisfaction.[22,36,37,39] One participant described her experience with scarring: "I expected to have one scar and I accepted that. I can't accept the other ones because they shouldn't be there."[39]

Other unexpected outcomes included the unnatural feeling of the breast and the limited movement of the breast.[12,15,20,37,39] As 1 research team described, "Photographs conveyed little information about the sensation and texture of the reconstructed breast."[39] One patient in a separate study expressed dissatisfaction with the "foreign" feeling of the breast: "I don't like

Reprinted with permission from Carr, T., et al. (2019). Patient information needs and breast reconstruction after mastectomy: A qualitative meta-synthesis. *Cancer Nursing, 42,* 229–241.

✳ Table 3 • Key Findings

Key Findings	Source Article
Theme 1: Expectations do not match BR experience	
Primary information exchange between doctor and patient	15, 19, 37, 38
Internet, friends, and relatives as other sources of information	19, 22
Topics discussed in consultation	15, 19, 22, 31, 37
Information about surgical outcomes from the Internet	22
Expectation of normality or improvement after surgery	15, 19, 38
Subtheme: Information conflicts with outcome	
Unmet expectations: appearance and sensation	12, 15, 22, 37, 38, 39, 40
Perception that breast looked unnatural	37, 38, 39, 40
Unnatural feel and limited movement of the breast	12, 15, 20, 37, 39
Unexpected degree or location of pain	15, 22
Regret having surgery due to excessive pain or bodily changes	37, 39
Subtheme: Information inaccurately reflects process	
Unanticipated recovery period and difficulty adapting to changes	20, 31
Subtheme: Overwhelmed by information	
Struggle to retain information	31
Theme 2: Assessing patient information needs	
Concerns that motivate breast reconstruction	12, 15, 41
Desire to achieve the same look as before surgery	12, 41
Consideration of emotional outcome of surgery	15, 38
Experience of mastectomy and motives for reconstructive surgery	12, 18, 19, 41
Emotional struggle of mastectomy	14, 16, 19
Subtheme: Need for greater patient-centered care	
Sense of being objectified by surgeon	40

the way it feels. It still feels like something that's been grafted onto my body. I wasn't prepared for it being quite so fake."[12] Participants described the breast as feeling "hard as a snow-ball."[36] Regarding the struggle of dealing with skin toughened by radiation treatments after surgery, 1 participant explained, "My radiated skin was too tough so it curved inwards into the ribs instead of outwards."[36] In a different study, a participant described her breast in the following way: "I just felt it was artificial."[15]

The lack of preoperative discussion about breast movement was discussed. One participant expressed, "I did expect them to be more—they do not move…so I guess I wouldn't have expected them to move more."[37] Other women described the discomfort associated with the foreign body sensation of the breast: "There is a constant feeling that there is something there that should not be there."[36] The foreign body sensation proved to be a reminder of the surgery: "I didn't expect to always think of it, to always be reminded of it and always have it in my mind. I thought it would just eventually feel like part of me. And it doesn't."[34]

Participants were also surprised by the location and degree of pain. Some experienced unexpected pain under their arms and in their upper back. A participant described the aspects of recovery that interfered with day-to-day exercises: "…I felt it was tight and limited my stretches."[15] In 1 instance, the pain was so excessive that the woman believed it to be a sign of an infection.[22] One woman directly admonished her surgeon for failing to inform her of the potential extent of the pain.[15]

For some women, the outcome of surgery was so severe and unexpected that they regretted having the surgery. Such regrets were often the result of the perception of excessive damage to the body and/or surgical complications.[12,37,39] Some women felt that scarring was excessive. One woman described, "I've got a scar from hip to hip and a 6 inch scar down my back…. I've got scars everywhere…they are hideous."[37] The excessive scarring was perceived as permanent damage to the body: "When you're in the shower, you sort of think oh my god is this my body now? And you feel less than you were before because you are not perfect anymore—and you never will be…. I feel less confident and less attractive."[39] The damage to a woman's self-confidence proved to be an especially pernicious outcome.

INFORMATION INACCURATELY REFLECTS PROCESS

In addition to being surprised by the surgery outcomes, many patients were surprised by the process of recovery. Several women did not expect the length of recovery time, which in some cases included additional procedures and significant adjustment to their changed bodies.[20,31] One patient described the recovery process as "not a quick fix but like doing a marathon."[31] Different researchers emphasized that the process could take more than a year in some cases.[14,16,20,31,39,40] Participants expressed frustration at the time required to return to normal. One patient explained, "It was months before I felt, you know, anywhere near normal and even then, you know, it still took a while for my body, for my skin to stretch too, because I was hunched over for a while."[20]

OVERWHELMED BY INFORMATION

The success of informing BR patients about the process and outcome of surgery was affected by the patients' ability to

Reprinted with permission from Carr, T., et al. (2019). Patient information needs and breast reconstruction after mastectomy: A qualitative meta-synthesis. *Cancer Nursing, 42,* 229–241.

engage with the physicians and to retain information.[31] One researcher explored patients' struggle to retain information about BR options during the surgical consult. A participant stated: "You see I must have read it at least twice at the time but I can't remember it at all."[31] The researcher suggested that the inability to process information had nothing to do with the complexity of the information itself; instead, the emotional stress of the cancer diagnosis made it difficult for the patient to focus on the discussion.[31]

Assessing Patient Information Needs

The findings reveal that a patient's information needs are influenced by the individual woman's concerns and circumstances. These circumstances include whether a woman has IBR or DBR. For example, women who chose IBR might do so because they fear the outcome of mastectomy alone. Women were concerned about their ability to wear clothes properly, to maintain their self-confidence and femininity, and to avoid the burdens of prosthesis.[12,15,38,41] In 1 study, women expressed concern about their ability to wear clothes in an orderly manner.[15] One participant explained, "If you wear a bra, you may appear to be more tidy and demure, as though your clothes are more perfectly fitted."[15]

In other studies, participants were concerned about looking the same as they did before the surgery or like those in the pictures they were shown.[12,37,39,41] One patient hoped to have "virtually the same look as I had before."[41] A participant in a different study stated: "When I went in for the mastectomy, I knew I was definitely losing something, and when I went in for the reconstruction I was getting something back."[12] Although the concerns outlined here refer to having a mastectomy, they show that women have information needs that involve understanding how their clothes will fit postsurgery and they feel a need to look the same.

When they considered IBR, women contemplated the emotional ramifications of mastectomy in addition to the physical ones.[15,38] One woman explained, "I just wondered whether I would lose my self-confidence if I lost my breast and will end up having problems in coping."[15] Researchers found that women's motivations for undergoing IBR included the desire to feel "normal," "to maintain femininity," and to "feel attractive."[38] They suggested that the perception of feeling normal was tied to feeling comfortable in an intimate relationship.[38] Awareness of women's emotional concerns is an important feature of women's information needs in the context of BR.

The experiences of women who delayed their BR reveal some informational needs that differ from those of women who underwent IBR. For women who delayed BR, their motivations to undergo the surgery were colored by their experiences living with a mastectomy and struggling with a prosthesis. The decision was mainly driven by a desire to return to "normality" in looks, sexuality, and routines.[12,18,19,41] One participant described wearing a prosthesis once and hating it; she also described her frustration over not being able to "just pull on clothes and just go."[19] She described her postsurgery daily dressing routine as "[getting] back to normal again, you know, just put on a bra without having to fiddle around with anything."[19] Another participant in Crompvoets's[19] study described wanting to return to normality in the context of her sexuality; she described "losing" her sexuality and "[wanting] to make it whole again."[19] A different study emphasized women's desire to return to their body's premastectomy state; 1 woman explained, "All I want is to look like I looked. I don't want to go bigger or smaller, I just want to look like me."[41] There are some similarities between the experiences of women recovering from IBR and those recovering from DBR. However, women who underwent DBR have experienced the reality of the struggle with the mastectomy and prosthesis. Firsthand knowledge of such experiences may be valuable to women considering BR.

These findings suggest that women are not fully informed about the emotional struggles that accompany mastectomy. Many participants described how living without a breast brought emotional turmoil.[12,14,16,18,19,41] One woman described her struggle with her self-image before having surgery: "I've never had a very good, my self-image isn't very good, but then after this happened [the mastectomy] I thought, 'well, you didn't have anything to complain about before.'"[19] Other women expressed revulsion at the sight of their body: "I couldn't look at myself, I was absolutely disgusted, my body image was…Just disgust, absolute disgust in my whole body…. I couldn't look, it was just…horrible, and I never did look, except for that once, I stood and looked in the mirror and I could feel my stomach churning."[16] One woman emphasized that her motivation for the surgery was based on being relatively young and wanting to live her life to the greatest extent possible.[14]

NEED FOR GREATER PATIENT-CENTERED CARE

Ultimately, paying closer attention to a patient's specific needs will yield better patient-centered care. When such care is neglected, the patient can feel alienated.[15,19,40] In some instances, women pursuing BR felt as though the surgeon was treating them as a "canvas" on which to produce his/her "art."[19,40] Researchers emphasized "the perceived artistry of the surgeons"[39] and suggested that "at times the doctor-patient relationship could almost be compared with that of artist and muse."[40] Greater focus on the needs of the individual patient would likely address these feelings of alienation.

▪ Discussion

This meta-synthesis explored qualitative research on women's information needs in relation to BR. Our findings suggest that women undergoing BR surgery need clear and comprehensive information. Satisfying women's specific information needs may lead to improved patient outcomes. Some women were dissatisfied with the initial outcome of BR and distressed by the process of recovery. These negative experiences with initial outcomes and recovery seem to be, to some degree, the

Reprinted with permission from Carr, T., et al. (2019). Patient information needs and breast reconstruction after mastectomy: A qualitative meta-synthesis. *Cancer Nursing, 42,* 229–241.

result of insufficient information from healthcare professionals during consultation. In terms of outcome, some women were disappointed by the look or feel of their reconstructed breast. Several women were not prepared for how much pain they would experience because of the surgery, and others were shocked by the degree of scarring. Women were also surprised by the tissue's lack of flexibility and tendency to restrict movement and routine tasks. Some women perceive the new breast as a foreign object and a reminder of the disease. In some instances, an undesirable physical outcome had a negative impact on the woman's self-confidence.

Other women were alarmed by the difficult realities of the recovery process. Some did not anticipate the length of time the recovery process required, whereas others were surprised by the need for additional surgical procedures. The excessive length of the surgery ultimately delayed women's ability to return to a normal routine and to overcome the entire cancer experience. These findings are consistent with other research that notes that women feel unprepared to deal with the changes in their body and the emotional challenges of the recovery process.[21] Furthermore, some women have expressed that they were dissatisfied with their surgeons for not providing more information about the recovery process before surgery.[21]

Despite methodological and population differences between the 16 studies, women's experience of BR, especially as it relates to their information needs, is quite similar. Although the studies took place in different countries, with participant samples who varied in terms of demographics, women experienced the pain of reconstruction and the struggle with recovery in similar ways. At the same time, understanding women's BR experience would be improved with research that explores women's experiences using comparable methodologies and investigates the influence of different demographic features.

The secondary purpose of this study was to determine whether women's information needs differed between those who had DBR and those who had IBR. This study's findings demonstrate that women have unique information needs in regard to their expectations of the surgery and preparation for recovery. Although women's experience of IBR and DBR is similar, the findings suggest that there are some unique features of each experience that reflect different information needs depending on the timing of the procedure. Specifically, women worried that, if they did not undergo immediate reconstruction, they would have difficulty wearing clothes properly, feel loss, struggle to cope with the loss, and face the challenge to maintain self-confidence.[12,18,36]

In contrast to the anticipatory concerns of those who elected to have IBR, women whose reconstruction was delayed were motivated to have BR by their experiences living with a mastectomy and a prosthesis.[42] The surgery signaled an opportunity to return to normality, both physically and in their daily routines. These women sought to regain their femininity and sexuality and to overcome depression. Other research has found that younger women elect to have BR more often than older women.[6]

In addition to revealing women's reactions to surgical outcomes, 1 study considered the influence of a woman's emotional state as the result of a cancer diagnosis on the consultation process.[31] The researchers of the study suggested that the shock of the cancer diagnosis caused women to be overwhelmed by the BR consultation process.[31] This finding is likely relevant to understanding women's information needs but requires further investigation to distinguish the precise nature of how the cancer diagnosis affects the BR consultation. Presumably, if the surgical consultation takes place much later, as in the case of DBR, the emotional weight of the cancer diagnosis would have less of an impact on the patient's information needs.

When considering the contrast in experiences of women who had IBR compared with those who had DBR, many women's experiences of pain and adjustment were similar. However, the 2 groups of women generally differed in terms of their motivations for choosing reconstruction in 1 general respect. Women who chose IBR are, to some degree, anticipating what life would be like without a breast and attempt to avoid that hypothetical reality. Women who chose reconstruction after experiencing living with mastectomy are motivated by their day-to-day experiences. Furthermore, for some women who had DBR, IBR may not have been an option for economic reasons such as women whose healthcare system or insurance plan does not provide coverage for BR. However, women whose reconstruction decision was not impinged by economic factors could benefit from knowledge of another's experience of life without reconstruction when deciding between IBR and DBR.

Despite the need for further investigation, it is worth noting that the use of audio recordings during consultation was helpful in terms of increasing patient recall and allowed patients to review information at their own convenience. There also was evidence that audio recordings enhanced patient participation in future decision-making.[28,36] Some participants also suggested that having a support person at the consultation to assist with the interaction helped ease the feeling of being overwhelmed.[31]

This study demonstrated that women's information needs are defined by women's dissatisfactory BR experiences. Many women experienced unexpected physical outcomes, a body image threat, in addition to a recovery period of unanticipated duration. The unexpected nature of these experiences points to a need for greater information from healthcare providers. These women felt they not properly informed about the typical realities of BR. Consideration of each individual patient in terms of their disease, life circumstances, and values is necessary when delineating their information needs.

To improve patient care at the time of consultation, these findings emphasize the importance of the surgeon's understanding of the patient's unique situation and motives. Loaring et al[40] commented on the feelings of objectification women experienced during the process. Specifically, women felt as though they were being treated as a living work of art who became a muse and canvas for the surgeon.[40] Other research has demonstrated that the surgeon's perception of the patient's needs can differ from the patient's perception of those same needs.[43,44] Such disconnection from the patient's information needs is a significant barrier to effective patient care. If information needs are better assessed, women can be more engaged in

Reprinted with permission from Carr, T., et al. (2019). Patient information needs and breast reconstruction after mastectomy: A qualitative meta-synthesis. *Cancer Nursing, 42,* 229–241.

the process and develop realistic expectations; patient-centered care can be achieved, and the BR recovery process may be improved.

Limitations

This study is subject to some limitations. Because the meta-synthesis process integrates the interpretation of findings of different researchers, it relies heavily on the quality of the researchers' interpretations. Thus, the limitations of the meta-synthesis are affected by the characteristics of the original studies. Similarly, common speech is used to describe women's experience of BR. Without a standardized language to articulate women's experiences, contrast between similar experiences within and across studies lacks some precision. Many of the studies used a retrospective design. It is difficult to know to what degree the women's recollections of their past experiences reflected their status at that time. Finally, this meta-synthesis is affected by the realities of differing healthcare systems, which make it such that women's experiences of BR are based on unique procedural aspects.

Future Research

There are questions raised by the findings that require further elucidation, namely, whether the experience of the surgical consultation is different for those pursuing IBR compared with those pursuing DBR. It seems likely that the consultation for IBR would be affected to some degree by the recent cancer diagnosis, but this was not explicitly stated in the studies examined in this meta-synthesis. Further investigation into women's information needs as they relate to IBR versus DBR is required to address these distinctions.

■ Conclusion

When women's information needs are not met, their experience of BR does not match their expectations. The shock of the cancer diagnosis has the potential to impinge on the exchange of information during the BR consultation. Nevertheless, when properly informed, women are able to better navigate recovery from BR and to ultimately move on from their breast cancer experience. If women are made aware of other women's experiences with BR, both the challenges and the benefits, their own experience can be improved. Ultimately, a successful recovery from BR can mark the end of recovery from the cancer itself.

■ Practice Implications

The results of this study suggest that more needs to be done by healthcare providers to address women's information needs in the case of BR. The relationship between the patient and the nurse navigator is an important service in healthcare. Nurse navigators are often in contact with the patients

throughout the recovery process and can help women with the different challenges they face. Two studies in the meta-synthesis commented on the role of the nurse navigator. Wolf[31] emphasized the importance of the nurse navigator in helping the patients through the psychological aspects of recovery. Furthermore, Murray et al[38] noted that women who had a supportive relationship with their nurse navigator tended to report a more positive perception of the recovery process than women who had a poor relationship. We suspect that greater awareness of patients' concerns and information needs has the potential to translate into better patient care.

Beyond the individual nurse providing care, the findings of this study suggest the need for system-wide modifications toward improving the quality and access to information for patients considering BR. Women recovering from BR have found support groups for emotional support and information resources, which are unique to women who have experienced BR.[38,44] If the healthcare institution provided women with access to such resources during the decision-making stage, women would likely benefit from speaking directly with those who had been through the process. When able to make a more informed choice, women can have more realistic expectations and a more favorable experience of BR overall. Because BR can lead to positive patient outcomes, providing the best patient-centered information to women considering and undergoing this procedure is imperative.

ACKNOWLEDGMENTS

The authors thank Health Science Librarian, Vicky Duncan, and Mikaela Vancoughnett for their research assistance. In addition, they are thankful for the financial support from the College of Medicine Research Award.

References

1. Ray C. Psychological implications of mastectomy. *Br J Soc Clin Psychol.* 1977;16(4):373–377.
2. Weitzner MA, Meyers CA, Stuebing KK, Saleeba AK. Relationship between quality of life and mood in long-term survivors of breast cancer treated with mastectomy. *Support Care Cancer.* 1997;5(3):241–248.
3. Canadian Institute for Health Information and the Canadian Partnership Against Cancer. Breast cancer surgery in Canada, 2007–2008 to 2009–2010. https://secure.cihi.ca/free_products/BreastCancer_7-8_9-10_EN.pdf. Accessed March 28, 2017.
4. Neill KM, Armstrong N, Burnett CB. Choosing reconstruction after mastectomy: a qualitative analysis. *Oncol Nurs Forum.* 1998;25(4):743–750.
5. Berger K, Bostwick JA. *Woman's Decision: Breast Care, Treatment & Reconstruction.* 3rd ed. Ann Arbor, MI: Quality Medical Publishing; 1998.
6. Reaby LL. Reasons why women who have mastectomy decide to have or not to have breast reconstruction. *Plast Reconstr Surg.* 1998;101(7):1810–1818.
7. Querci della Rovere G. Breast reconstruction following mastectomy: patients' expectations. In: Querci della Rovere G, Benson DJR, eds. *Oncoplastic and Reconstructive Surgery of the Breast.* London, UK: Taylor and Francis; 2004:187–190.
8. Matheson G, Drever JM. Psychological preparation of the patient for breast reconstruction. *Ann Plast Surg.* 1990;24(3):238–247.
9. Langellier KM, Sullivan CF. Breast talk in breast cancer narratives. *Qual Health Res.* 1998;8(1):76–94.
10. Ananian P, Houvenaeghel G, Protiere C, et al. Determinants of patients' choice of reconstruction with mastectomy for primary breast cancer. *Ann Surg Oncol.* 2004;11(8):762–771.

11. Harcourt D, Rumsey N. Mastectomy patients' decision-making for or against immediate breast reconstruction. *Psychooncol.* 2004;13(2):106–115.

12. Kasper AS. The social construction of breast loss and reconstruction. *Womens Health.* 1995;1(3):197–219.

13. Marshall C, Kiemle G. Breast reconstruction following cancer: its impact on patients' and partners' sexual functioning. *Sex Relatsh Ther.* 2005;20(2):155–179.

14. Hill O, White K. Exploring women's experiences of TRAM flap breast reconstruction after mastectomy for breast cancer. *Oncol Nurs Forum.* 2008;35(1):81–88.

15. Fang SY, Balneaves LG, Shu BC. "A struggle between vanity and life": the experience of receiving breast reconstruction in women of Taiwan. *Cancer Nurs.* 2010;33(5):E1–E4.

16. McKean LN, Newman EF, Adair P. Feeling like me again: a grounded theory of the role of breast reconstruction surgery in self-image. *Eur J Cancer Care.* 2013;22(4):493–502.

17. Lee CN, Hultman CS, Sepucha K. What are patients' goals and concerns about breast reconstruction after mastectomy? *Ann Plast Surg.* 2010;64(5):567–569.

18. Truelsen M. The meaning of 'reconstruction' within the lived experience of mastectomy for breast cancer. *Couns Psychother Res.* 2003;3(4):307–314.

19. Crompvoets S. Comfort, control, or conformity: women who choose breast reconstruction following mastectomy. *Health Care Women Int.* 2006;27(1):75–93.

20. Spector DJ, Mayer DK, Knafl K, Pusic A. Women's recovery experiences after breast cancer reconstruction surgery. *J Psychosoc Oncol.* 2011;29(6):664–676.

21. Rolnick SJ, Altschuler A, Nekhlyudov L, et al. What women wish they knew before prophylactic mastectomy. *Cancer Nurs.* 2007;30(4):285–291.

22. Spector D, Mayer DK, Knafl K, Pusic A. Not what I expected: Informational needs of women undergoing breast surgery. *Plast Surg Nurs.* 2010;30(2):70–74.

23. Wilkins EG, Cederna PS, Lowery JC, et al. Prospective analysis of psychosocial outcomes in breast reconstruction: one-year postoperative results from the Michigan Breast Reconstruction Outcome Study. *Plast Reconstr Surg.* 2000;106(5):1014–1025.

24. Fallowfield LJ, Hall A, Maguire GP, Baum M. Psychological outcomes of different treatment policies in women with early breast cancer outside a clinical trial. *BMJ.* 1990;301(6752):575–580.

25. Luker KA, Beaver K, Leinster SJ, Owens RG, Degner LF, Sloan JA. The information needs of women newly diagnosed with breast cancer. *J Adv Nurs.* 1995;22(1):134–141.

26. Griffiths M, Leek C. Patient education needs: opinions of oncology nurses and their patients. *Oncol Nurs Forum.* 1994;22(1):139–144.

27. Butow P, Brindle E, McConnell D, Boakes R, Tattersall M. Information booklets about cancer: factors influencing patient satisfaction and utilisation. *Patient Educ Couns.* 1998;33(2):129–141.

28. Scott JT, Entwistle VA, Sowden AJ, Watt I. Giving tape recordings or written summaries of consultations to people with cancer: a systematic review. *Health Expect.* 2001;4(3):162–169.

29. Sandelowski M, Barroso J. *Handbook for Synthesizing Qualitative Research.* New York, NY: Springer; 2007.

30. Critical Appraisal Skills Checklist. CASP Qualitative research checklist. http://docs.wixstatic.com/ugd/dded87_25658615020e427da194a325e7773d42.pdf. Accessed: February 18, 2017.

31. Wolf L. The information needs of women who have undergone breast reconstruction. Part II: information giving and content of information. *Eur J Oncol Nurs.* 2004;8(4):315–324.

32. Finset A. Qualitative methods in communication and patient education research. *Patient Educ Couns.* 2008;73(1):1–2.

33. Salmon P. Assessing the quality of qualitative research. *Patient Educ Couns.* 2013;90(1):1–3.

34. Lin WC, Gau ML, Lin HC, Lin HR. Spiritual well-being in patients with rheumatoid arthritis. *J Nurs Res.* 2011;19(1):1–12.

35. Goin MK, Goin JM. Growing pains: the psychological experience of breast reconstruction with tissue expansion. *Ann Plast Surg.* 1988;21(3):217–222.

36. Fallbjörk U, Frejeu E, Rasmussen BH. A preliminary study into women's experiences of undergoing reconstructive surgery after breast cancer. *Eur J Oncol Nurs.* 2012;16(3):220–226.

37. Snell L, McCarthy C, Klassen A, et al. Clarifying the expectations of patients undergoing implant breast reconstruction: a qualitative study. *Plast Reconstr Surg.* 2010;126(6):1825–1830.

38. Murray CD, Turner A, Rehan C, Kovacs T. Satisfaction following immediate breast reconstruction: experiences in the early post-operative stage. *Br J Health Psych.* 2015;20(3):579–593.

39. Abu-Nab Z, Grunfeld EA. Satisfaction with outcome and attitudes towards scarring among women undergoing breast reconstructive surgery. *Patient Educ Couns.* 2007;66(2):243–249.

40. Loaring JM, Larkin M, Shaw R, Flowers P. Renegotiating sexual intimacy in the context of altered embodiment: the experiences of women with breast cancer and their male partners following mastectomy and reconstruction. *Health Psychol.* 2015;34(4):426–436.

41. Denford S, Harcourt D, Rubin L, Pusic A. Understanding normality: a qualitative analysis of breast cancer patient's concepts of normality after mastectomy and reconstructive surgery. *Psycho-Oncol.* 2011;20(5):553–558.

42. Rowland JH, Holland JC, Chaglassian T, Kinne D. Psychological response to breast reconstruction: expectations for and impact on post mastectomy functioning. *Psychosomatics.* 1993;34(3):241–250.

43. Darisi T, Thorne S, Iacobelli C. Influences on decision-making for undergoing plastic surgery: a mental models and quantitative assessment. *Plast Reconstr Surg.* 2005;116(3):907–916.

44. Carr T, Groot G, Cochran D, Vancoughnett M, Holtslander L. Exploring women's support needs after breast reconstruction surgery: a qualitative study. *Cancer Nurs.* In press.

Answers to Selected Study Guide Exercises

CHAPTER 1

A. FILL IN THE BLANKS

1. clinical
2. club
3. paradigm
4. assumption
5. methods
6. Positivism
7. determinism
8. Quantitative
9. objectivity
10. Empirical
11. generalizability
12. constructivism
13. qualitative
14. cause
15. Therapy
16. Prognosis
17. Meaning
18. patient preferences and values
19. systematic review
20. meta-analysis
21. hierarchies
22. outcome
23. population
24. intervention (or influence)
25. comparison

B. MATCHING EXERCISES

1. a	2. b	3. d	4. b	5. a
6. b	7. d	8. b	9. c	10. a

C. STUDY QUESTIONS

C.3
a. Qualitative
b. Quantitative
c. Qualitative
d. Quantitative
e. Qualitative
f. Qualitative
g. Quantitative

C.4 P (Population) = middle-aged men
I (Intervention) = formal exercise program
C (Comparison) = the absence of a formal exercise program (or an alternative intervention)
O (Outcome) = blood pressure, cholesterol levels

D. APPLICATION EXERCISES

Exercise D.1: Questions of Fact (Appendix A)

a. Yes, this was a systematic study that tested the efficacy of a behaviorally based smartphone intervention designed to promote weight loss in young adults aged 18 to 25 years.
b. It was a quantitative study. The researchers systematically measured several outcomes (e.g., weight, body mass index, waist circumference, self-efficacy for healthy eating) using measures that yielded quantitative information.
c. The underlying paradigm was positivism/postpositivism.
d. Yes, the study involved the collection of information through the senses (i.e., through scrutiny of study participants' responses to series of questions and the observation of physical attributes).
e. Yes, this study was concerned with evaluating whether the intervention *caused* weight loss among the study participants exposed to the intervention. In this and most studies, there is an underlying assumption that phenomena are multiply

199

determined. Thus, the participants' weight and weight loss are *caused* by a number of factors, and this study tested whether one of the causes was participation in a special intervention.

f. This study directly addressed a question relevant to the *treatment* of young adults—a Therapy question. The results of this study, together with those from other similar studies, could provide guidance about evidence-based ways to help young adults manage their weight.

g. Here is a clinical question for this study in the PICO format: Among young adults aged 18 to 25 years (P), does participation in a special smartphone intervention (I), compared to nonparticipation in the intervention (C), result in reduced body mass index (O)?

Exercise D.2: Questions of Fact (Appendix B)

a. Yes, this was a systematic study of parents' perceptions of patient safety in a neonatal intensive care unit (NICU).

b. It was a qualitative study. Ottosen and colleagues used loosely structured methods (conversational interviewing and observations of parents' interactions within the NICU) to capture in an in-depth fashion parents' experiences of safe care.

c. The underlying paradigm for this study is constructivism (naturalism).

d. Yes, the study involved the collection of information through the senses (e.g., through conversations with and observations of parents and clinicians in the NICU).

e. No, this study is not cause probing per se. Qualitative studies seldom focus on causes and effects, although in-depth scrutiny of phenomena can sometimes suggest causal linkages.

f. This study addresses the evidence-based practice purpose described in the textbook as "Meaning/process," i.e., developing an in-depth understanding of parents' perceptions of safety in the NICU environment.

Exercise D.3: Questions of Fact (Appendix C)

a. The article does not describe an actual study. Rather, it describes the efforts of a team to undertake an evidence-based practice project designed to potentially result in improvements to patient care. Nevertheless, many aspects of the project included features of a study—that is, the team developed an intervention (various practice changes), gathered data on important outcomes before and after implementing the changes, and used statistical analyses to assess whether changes occurred.

b. No, the report did not articulate a clinical question stated in the PICO format. The team looked at evidence about various types of interventions that could improve the thermoregulation of trauma patients. As an example of a specific question that was considered in this project is the following: Does training a formal checklist and specific recommendations about temperature assessments (I), compared to the absence of any practice changes (C), for trauma patients being seen in the emergency department (P) result in a higher number of patients being assessed for core temperature (O)?

c. No, the report did not specifically state that the team looked at systematic reviews, but it did indicate that the clinical nurse specialist undertook a "systematic search" for relevant literature relating to thermoregulation. The search may have led to one or more systematic reviews.

d. No, the report did not mention evidence hierarchies or level-of-evidence scales. However, the authors did state that "evidence-based practice interventions were derived from the *best available clinical evidence*." This might mean that they derived some guidance from systematic reviews (Level I) or high-quality randomized controlled trials (Level II).

CHAPTER 2

A. FILL IN THE BLANKS

1. subject (study participant)
2. construct
3. theory
4. variable

5. dependent
6. independent
7. operational
8. data
9. relationship
10. causal (cause-and-effect)
11. experimental
12. observational
13. trial
14. grounded
15. phenomenology
16. ethnography
17. literature
18. design
19. population
20. sample
21. statistical
22. entrée
23. emergent
24. Saturation
25. themes; categories

B. MATCHING EXERCISES

B.1 1. a   2. c   3. b   4. a
        5. b   6. b   7. c   8. c
        9. b   10. c

B.2 1. b   2. c   3. a   4. c
        5. c   6. b   7. d   8. d

B.3 1. a   2. b   3. a   4. c
        5. b   6. c   7. d   8. c
        9. b   10. a

C. STUDY QUESTIONS

C.2

a. Independent variable (IV) = receipt versus nonreceipt of assertiveness training; dependent or outcome variable (DV) = psychiatric nurses' effectiveness
b. IV = patients' postural positioning; DV = respiratory function
c. IV = amount of touch by nursing staff; DV = patients' psychological well-being
d. IV = frequency of turning patients; DV = incidence of decubitus
e. IV = history of parental abuse during their childhood; DV = abuse of their own children
f. IV = patients' age; DV = tolerance for pain

g. IV = pregnant women's number of prenatal visits; DV = labor and delivery outcomes
h. IV = children's experience (vs. nonexperience) of a sibling death; DV = levels of depression
i. IV = gender; DV = compliance with a medical regimen
j. IV = participation versus nonparticipation in a support group among family caregivers of patients with AIDS; DV = coping
k. IV = time of day; DV = elders' hearing acuity
l. IV = location of giving birth—home versus other; DV = parents' satisfaction with the childbirth experience
m. IV = type of diet in the outpatient setting among patients undergoing chemotherapy; DV = incidence of positive blood cultures

C.5

a. An ethnographic study would not be experimental—no intervention would be introduced.
b. The independent variable is relaxation therapy (the intervention), and the dependent or outcome variable is pain.
c. Grounded theory studies are not clinical trials, which involve an intervention.
d. Study participants would not be exposed to an intervention in phenomenological studies (and they would not be called *subjects*).
e. In experimental studies, decisions about data collection would be made well before implementing the intervention.

C.6
a. Ethnographic
b. Phenomenological
c. Grounded theory

D. APPLICATION EXERCISES

Exercise D.1: Questions of Fact (Appendix D)

a. All five researchers were doctorally prepared nurses.
b. The study participants were patients diagnosed with heart disease.
c. Participants were recruited from one of two cardiology clinics. One clinic

served primarily urban minority patients, and the other served primarily Caucasian patients from a small city in a rural setting. The clinics were presumably located in the state of Illinois in the United States because all researchers were affiliated with institutions in that state. The data were collected during routine clinic appointments.

d. The central variable in this study is patients' level of *fatigue*. The authors did not specifically label any variables as *dependent* or *independent*, but the research questions indicate that fatigue was both an independent and dependent variable in the researchers' analyses. As stated in the abstract, one study objective was to assess whether demographic (age, education, income), physiological (hypertension, hyperlipidemia), or psychological (depressive symptoms) variables were correlated with fatigue. For this objective, fatigue is the outcome—the researchers considered the other factors as independent variables that were potentially associated with or that influenced levels of fatigue. A third objective was to examine whether fatigue was associated with the patients' quality of life. For this objective, it can be inferred that the researchers conceptualized levels of fatigue (the independent variable) as potentially influencing patients' quality of life (the outcome variable).

e. Fatigue was conceptually defined in the very first sentence of the report. Fatigue was operationally defined by participants' scores on a scale called the Fatigue Symptom Inventory or FSI. The FSI consists of 14 questions that ask about fatigue intensity, duration, and interference with activities of daily living. Each question is answered on an 11-point scale, from 0 (not at all fatigued/no interference) to 10 (as fatigued as I could be/extreme interference). The report also provided information on how responses to the 14 questions are scored to produce an overall fatigue score.

f. The researchers collected both quantitative and qualitative data in this study. The researchers not only administered a number of scales that yielded numeric information about participants' attributes (e.g., fatigue, quality of life)

but also asked in-depth questions, such as "Describe your fatigue." Responses to these questions were in narrative form and were analyzed qualitatively.

g. For the second study objective, the researchers investigated the relationship between the various demographic, physiological, and psychological factors on the one hand and fatigue on the other. In the context of this study, it is best to consider the relationships associative rather than causal, although it is certainly plausible that certain factors *caused* fatigue. The authors' conceptual model suggests the possibility of causal pathways, but the researchers judiciously noted (in the Discussion section) that "it remains to be determined if depression is the cause or consequence of fatigue." For their third objective, the researchers studied the relationship between fatigue and quality of life. Again, the model shown in their Figure 1 suggests the possibility that fatigue levels could affect patients' quality of life, but the authors did not explicitly infer a causal connection between fatigue and quality of life.

h. nonexperimental study

i. There was no intervention in this study. The researchers captured characteristics of the study participants at one point in time without intervening in any way.

j. The study involved the statistical analysis of the quantitative data as well as the qualitative analysis of the narrative data.

Exercise D.2: Questions of Fact (Appendix E)

a. This study was undertaken by a team of eight Swedish researchers, all of whom were health care professionals. Six of the authors were nurses and two were physicians. All of the nurses (except the first author) had PhDs. In a section of the report labeled "Data Analysis," it states that the authors were experienced researchers and either clinically experienced nurses or clinically experienced physicians. The authors had diverse institutional affiliations.

b. The study participants were 22 patients with primary brain tumor who were receiving proton beam therapy (PBT).

c. The researchers conducted interviews with the study participants in three health care settings in Sweden—the Skandion clinic (the first Nordic clinic to offer PBT) and two other university hospitals.

d. The key concept in this study was the management of symptoms among patients with primary brain tumors receiving PBT.

e. No, there were no *independent variables* or *dependent variables* in this qualitative study.

f. The data for this study were qualitative—rich narratives from interviews with study participants.

g. This study did not explicitly focus on relationships. However, the authors did look at whether there were differences in the pattern of symptom management between participants with a malignant or benign tumor.

h. This study was described as a grounded theory study.

i. This study was nonexperimental.

j. There was no intervention in this study.

k. The study did not report statistical "analyses" per se, but demographic characteristics were described in Table 1. For example, 10 of the 22 participants were women. The study data were analyzed qualitatively.

CHAPTER 3

A. FILL IN THE BLANKS

1. bias
2. title
3. reflexivity
4. trustworthy
5. significant
6. IMRAD
7. blinding (or masking)
8. abstract
9. confounding
10. journal
11. valid
12. inference
13. Reliability
14. control
15. Randomness
16. Transferability

B. MATCHING EXERCISES

1. c	2. d	3. b	4. a	5. c
6. e	7. d	8. b	9. c	10. e
11. b	12. d			

D. APPLICATION EXERCISES

Exercise D.1: Questions of Fact (Appendix A)

a. Yes, the structure of the Stephens and colleagues' article follows the IMRAD format. There is an Introduction that begins with the first words ("Overweight and obesity are major public health concerns"). Then, there are Methods, Results, and Discussion sections. The Methods and Results sections have several subsections. For example, the Methods section has subsections labeled "Setting and participants," "Outcome measures," "Interventions," and "Statistical analysis."

b. Yes, the abstract to this article includes all this information, organized into sections called Background, Objective, Methods, Results, and Conclusions.

c. The study methods were described mainly using the passive voice. For example, the first paragraph indicates that "participants were randomly assigned to intervention or control." In the active voice, this could have been "We randomly assigned participants to intervention or control."

d. This study is experimental. The researchers intervened by offering a smartphone intervention to some young adults but not to others.

e. Yes, the abstract stated that 62 young adults were *randomized* to receive either the smartphone application and health coach intervention and counseling or to a control group (right after the bolded Methods heading).

Exercise D.2: Questions of Fact (Appendix E)

a. Yes, the report by Langegård and colleagues followed the IMRAD format. The first part of the article is the Introduction, with a subsection labeled "Symptom experience and management." The next three major sections are called Methods, Results, and Discussion.

b. The abstract indicated the study purpose, using the bolded term **Objective** ("The aim of this study was to explore the process of symptom management in patients with brain tumor receiving PBT"). Then, there were three sentences that described the **Methods** (a grounded theory approach was used, and data were collected in interviews with 22 patients). Key **Results** were then highlighted. In the **Conclusion** section of the abstract, the authors offered brief interpretations, and this was followed by a sentence on the **Implications for Practice**.

c. The presentation was mostly written in the passive voice. As an example of the passive voice, the first sentence of the "Setting" subsection stated that "interviews *were conducted* at the Skandion Clinic and 2 university hospitals in Sweden."

d. Yes, this study was a grounded theory study, which is appropriate for understanding processes relating to a phenomenon. Here, the researchers were interested in understanding the processes by which the patients with a brain tumor who received proton beam therapy managed their symptoms.

CHAPTER 4

A. FILL IN THE BLANKS

1. codes
2. Anonymity
3. risk
4. Beneficence
5. Process consent
6. stipend
7. *Belmont*
8. implied
9. assent
10. confidentiality
11. disclosure
12. Institutional Review Board (IRB)
13. dilemma
14. vulnerable groups
15. Informed consent
16. Debriefing
17. minimal

B. MATCHING EXERCISES

1. d	2. b	3. c	4. b	5. a
6. d	7. b	8. a	9. c	10. a
11. b	12. d			

D. APPLICATION EXERCISES

Exercise D.1: Questions of Fact (Appendix D)

a. Yes, in the last paragraph of the "Sample and Setting" subsection under Methods, the researchers indicated that the study protocol was reviewed and approved by the IRBs of both cardiology clinics from which participants were recruited for the study.

b. No, the study participants were adults with a chronic illness (coronary heart disease); they would not be considered "vulnerable."

c. There is no reason to suspect that participants were subjected to any physical harm or discomfort or psychological distress. Only people who were medically stable were eligible to participate in the study. The content of the questionnaire and interview does not appear likely to induce stress or anxiety.

d. It does not appear that participants were deceived in any way.

e. There is no reason to suspect any coercion was used to force unwilling people to participate in the study. There is no information in the report concerning the number of prospective participants who declined to participate, but presumably some people who were recruited did not agree to take part in the study.

f. The report indicated that written informed consent was obtained from all participants. It is not possible to determine the extent to which disclosure was "full," but there does not appear to be any reason to conceal information in this study.

g. The report did not provide information about where data collection took place nor how the privacy and confidentiality of participants were protected. Adequate protections were likely in place, however, given that approval for the study protocols was given by two IRBs.

Presumably, statements regarding privacy and confidentiality were made in the informed consent form.

Exercise D.2: Questions of Fact (Appendix B)

a. Yes, the report indicated that this study was approved by the University of Texas Health Science Center at Houston Committee for the Protection of Human Subjects. This information was provided in the first sentence of the "Procedures" section.

b. The focus of the study was parents whose infants were in the neonatal intensive care unit (NICU)—not the infants themselves. The parents would not be considered "vulnerable" according to standard criteria. In the research team's fieldwork, observations were made of parents' interactions with clinicians, and the clinicians would also not be considered vulnerable.

c. Participants were not subjected to any physical harm or discomfort. Parents were observed during interactions with care providers, other parents, and their infants in the NICU. Parents were interviewed in a location of their own choosing. It is possible that there was a certain degree of self-consciousness when the study started, but it is likely that the parents and the clinicians became accustomed to the presence of the researcher.

d. There is no reason to suspect that participants were deceived. The article states that "parents were invited to participate . . . by the lead author who described the purpose, procedures, risks and benefits, and voluntary nature of study participation."

e. It does not appear that any coercion was involved.

f. The report stated that the researchers obtained written informed consent from the parents who participated in the study and that they were given a copy of the signed consent document.

g. The article stated that the parents were invited to select the location for the interviews. Parents were also asked whether they wanted to be interviewed individually, with their partner, or with other parents. Most of the parents opted to be interviewed with their partner in a conference room adjacent to the NICU.

h. Yes, the parents who participated in the study were offered a $50 gift card, which is a fairly generous stipend.

CHAPTER 5

A. FILL IN THE BLANKS

1. problem
2. statement of purpose
3. question
4. hypothesis
5. relationship
6. test
7. independent
8. nondirectional
9. proof
10. two
11. research
12. null

B. MATCHING EXERCISES

B.1

1. b	2. c	3. a	4. b
5. a	6. c	7. b	8. a

B.2

1. a	2. c	3. d	4. a
5. b	6. d	7. a	8. c
9. b	10. d	11. b	12. c
13. b	14. a	15. c	

C. STUDY QUESTIONS

C.4 Independent variable = IV, dependent/outcome variable = DV

2a. IV = type of stimulation (tactile vs. verbal); DV = physiological arousal

2b. IV = infants' birth weight; DV = hypoglycemia (or not) in term newborns

2c. IV = use versus nonuse of isotonic sodium chloride solution; DV = oxygen saturation

2d. IV = patients' fluid balance; DV = success/nonsuccess in weaning patients from mechanical ventilation

2e. IV = patients' sex; DV = amount of narcotic analgesics administered by nurses

3a. IV = prior blood donation versus no prior donation; DV = amount of anxiety

3b. IV = amount of conversation initiated by nurses; DV = patients' ratings of nursing effectiveness

3c. IV = ratings of nurses' informativeness; DV = amount of preoperative stress

3d. IV = pregnancy status (pregnant vs. not pregnant); DV = incidence of peritoneal infection

3e. IV = type of delivery (vaginal vs. cesarean) DV = incidence of postpartum depression

D. APPLICATION EXERCISES

Exercise D.1: Questions of Fact (Appendix D)

a. The first four paragraphs of this report stated the essence of the problem that the researchers addressed. In brief, the problem may be summarized as follows: Fatigue has been found to be a frequent symptom in patients with chronic health problems, including acute myocardial infarction and chronic heart failure. However, the severity and characteristics of fatigue in patients with stable coronary heart disease (CHD) has not been explored. It is important to better understand fatigue in this population because fatigue may be an indicator of a new onset or of progressive CHD.

b. The authors stated three objectives in the study abstract as well as in the introduction to the report. The purposes were to: "1. Describe fatigue (intensity, distress, timing, and quality) in patients with stable CHD; 2. determine if specific demographic (gender, age, education, income), physiological (hypertension, hyperlipidemia), or psychological (depressive symptoms) variables were correlated with fatigue; and 3. determine if fatigue was associated with health-related quality of life (HRQoL)." The authors used the verb "describe" for the first purpose, indicating that the study had a descriptive intent. The verb "describe" is appropriate in both quantitative

and qualitative studies—and in this study, both types of data were collected. The researchers used the verb "determine" for the next two purposes, which suggest a quantitative approach. However, given the limitations of any single study—particularly the reliance on relatively small samples from local populations—a verb such as "examine" or "assess" would have been preferable to "determine," which suggests a degree of conclusiveness that is not attainable.

c. The report did not explicitly state research questions, although they could be inferred from the purpose statement. For example, the question corresponding to the first descriptive aim might be What are the characteristics of fatigue—in terms of intensity, distress level, timing and quality—among patients with stable CHD? A question corresponding to the second purpose might be What factors, including demographic, physiological, and psychological factors, are associated with fatigue in patients with stable CHD? And a question corresponding to the third purpose would be Is fatigue associated with health-related quality of life in patients with stable CHD?

d. No hypotheses were formally stated in the body of the article. However, there are footnotes at the bottom of Tables 3 and 4 that indicate that the researchers *did* have hypotheses about factors that were related to fatigue intensity and fatigue interference, respectively. Based on the information in these tables, one research hypothesis could be stated as follows: We predict that a patient's age will be correlated with the level of pain intensity and pain interference. This is stated as a nondirectional hypothesis. A directional hypothesis might be the following: We predict that older patients will have higher levels of pain intensity and pain interference than younger patients.

e. Yes, the researchers used hypothesis-testing statistical tests. These are described in the Results section, under the subheading "Fatigue Intensity/Severity" and "HRQoL and Fatigue". For example, the researchers tested the hypothesis that fatigue intensity was related to a patient's gender. They found that fatigue intensity was significantly higher in women than in men ($p = .003$). The probability is less than 3 in 1,000 that this result is spurious.

Exercise D.2: Questions of Fact (Appendix B)

a. The research problem is articulated in the first few paragraphs of the report. The first paragraph indicates that the neonatal intensive care unit (NICU) environment is complex and can pose threats to patient safety and that building a culture of patient safety calls for input from parents—and yet their views are often not considered. The next paragraph notes the importance of understanding how parents of neonates perceive patient safety and how they perceive their roles in supporting patient safety in the NICU.

b. Ottosen and colleagues stated the purpose of their study in the abstract: "To determine how parents of neonates conceptualize patient safety in the NICU." They further stated the purpose of the article in the last sentence of the introduction: "The purpose of this article is to describe a conceptual model derived from the findings that depict how parents conceptualize patient safety and how they see their role as safety advocates in the NICU setting." These researchers used the verb "determine" in stating their study purpose in the abstract. Given the limitations of any single study, a verb such as "explore" or "understand" would have been preferable.

c. Specific research questions were not articulated. We could state a question as follows, which is simply the purpose rephrased interrogatively: How do parents of neonates conceptualize patient safety in the NICU?

d. No hypotheses were stated—nor would one have been appropriate in this qualitative study.

e. No, no hypotheses were tested. Qualitative studies do not use statistical methods to test hypotheses.

CHAPTER 6

A. FILL IN THE BLANKS

1. primary
2. secondary
3. ancestry
4. descendancy
5. bibliographic
6. mapping
7. keywords
8. CINAHL
9. Boolean
10. MeSH
11. PubMed
12. author

B. MATCHING EXERCISES

1. d	2. b	3. c	4. b	5. a
6. c	7. b	8. d		

D. APPLICATION EXERCISES

Exercise D.1: Questions of Fact (Appendix G)

a. This review was a systematic review that involved a meta-analysis.

b. Yes, the introduction described a research problem that the researchers addressed in the review. The problem might be stated as followed: Medication therapy provides known benefits for the secondary prevention of coronary artery disease (CAD). Yet, many patients do not adhere to prescribed medication regimens, and such nonadherence has been linked to poor health outcomes. Interventions to improve adherence in CAD patients have been developed and tested, but findings about their effectiveness have not been systematically integrated.

c. Yes, Chase and colleagues provided a statement of purpose in the abstract: "The purpose of this meta-analysis was to determine the overall effectiveness of interventions designed to improve medication adherence (MA) among adults with CAD. In addition, sample, study design, and intervention characteristics were explored as potential moderators to intervention effectiveness." Two research questions also were stated at the end of the Introduction: (1) What is the overall effectiveness of MA interventions on MA outcomes among patients with CAD? (2) Does intervention effectiveness vary based on intervention, sample, or design characteristics?" For students who not yet understand what the researchers meant by "moderators" in the purpose statement, the questions may be easier to understand. The researchers were interested in exploring whether beneficial effects on interventions was different for different types of people, for different types of interventions, or when different research designs were used in the primary studies.

d. The researchers used 13 different electronic databases in their literature search, including ones we discussed in Chapter 6 (PubMed, CINAHL) as well as others we did not.

e. The authors used many keywords (and MeSH terms) that included the following: *patient compliance, medication adherence, drugs, prescription drugs, pharmaceutical preparations, generic dosage, compliant, compliance, adherent, adherence, noncompliant, noncompliance, nonadherent, nonadherence, medication(s), regimen(s), prescription(s), prescribed, drug(s), pill(s), tablet(s), agent(s), improve, promote, enhance, encourage, foster, advocate, influence, incentive, ensure, remind, optimize, increase, impact, prevent, address, decrease.*

f. Yes, the report indicated that "ancestry searches of prior reviews' bibliographies were conducted."

g. The report did not state that the reviewers' search was restricted to English-language publications. It is unclear if there were any language restrictions—although it seems unlikely that studies reported in *all* languages would have been included.

h. This meta-analysis included 24 studies.

i. All studies included in the review were quantitative; meta-analyses integrate quantitative findings.

Exercise D.2: Questions of Fact (Appendix H)

a. Carr and colleagues undertook a systematic review of qualitative studies relating to women's experiences with breast reconstruction after mastectomy—a type of review called a metasynthesis, which will be explained in more detail in Chapter 17.

b. The abstract of this report described the purpose of this metasynthesis as an examination of "the qualitative literature that explores women's experiences of breast reconstruction after mastectomy and highlights women's healthcare information needs."

c. For this metasynthesis, Carr and colleagues searched six bibliographic databases: CINAHL, MEDLINE, the Cochrane library, EMBASE, PsycINFO, and Scopus.

d. The metasynthesis involved integrating results from 16 studies.

e. The 16 studies in the review included studies using several qualitative approaches, including grounded theory, phenomenology, and descriptive qualitative research, as shown in Table 1.

CHAPTER 7

A. FILL IN THE BLANKS

1. framework
2. conceptual
3. descriptive
4. middle
5. model; map
6. humans; environment; health; nursing
7. Pender
8. Parse
9. Adaptation
10. self-efficacy
11. stages; change
12. Planned Behavior

B. MATCHING EXERCISES

B.1 1. c   2. e   3. c   4. e
         5. d   6. a   7. b   8. d

B.2 1. c   2. d   3. e   4. a
         5. b   6. f

D. APPLICATION EXERCISES

Exercise D.1: Questions of Fact (Appendix D)

a. Eckhardt and colleagues stated that they used the Theory of Unpleasant Symptoms as the organizing framework for their study.

b. The Theory of Unpleasant Symptoms was not described in the textbook, but it is a theory that has been used by other nurse researchers.

c. The theory was not described in detail, but this likely reflects space constraints in the journal rather than the authors' negligence.

d. Yes, the article stated that the Theory of Unpleasant Symptoms was the basis for the researchers' framework, but that they adapted it for this study. The report did not specify what specific adaptations were made.

e. Yes, a schematic model of the organizing framework used in this research was presented in Figure 1.

f. The key concepts in the model are (1) physiological factors (e.g., hypertension, comorbid conditions), (2) psychological factors (e.g., depressed mood), (3) situational factors (e.g., age, sex, education), (4) symptom experiences (fatigue severity, fatigue interference), and performance (quality of life and functional status).

g. The schematic model did not show connections among concepts in a traditional manner; namely, with arrows between boxes. However, it seems reasonable to conclude that the model is intended to be read from the top down. That is, the physiological, psychological, and situational factors are presumed to affect patients' symptom experiences, which in turn influence performance concepts.

h. The report did not articulate formal conceptual definitions of each construct in the model. For example, there is no conceptual definition of "quality of life." However, operational definitions of all concepts were provided.

i. No, the researchers did not state formal hypotheses deduced from the conceptual framework—although they tested some, and these are consistent with our reading of the model, as explained in question G. For example, one hypothesis they tested was as follows: Situational factors (age, income), psychological factors (depression), and physiological factors (e.g., hypertension) are related to patients' fatigue intensity.

Exercise D.2: Questions of Fact (Appendix E)

a. The authors did not describe an a priori framework or theory that guided this research. For example, there was no mention of symbolic interactionism. The researchers were focused on developing a theory.

b. Yes, the purpose of the study was to generate a substantive theory that was grounded in the experiences of the study participants. The authors referred to their grounded theory as *The art of living with symptoms*.

c. Yes, Figure 1 of the report was a schematic model depicting the researchers' grounded theory. The figure was a good way to illustrate three processes contributing to the core concept: *Adapting to limited ability*, *Learning about one's self*, and *Creating new routines*.

d. Inasmuch as this was a grounded theory study, no hypotheses were tested. A grounded theory study sometimes results in the identification of hypotheses that can be tested in a future quantitative study. Indeed, the authors themselves stated that "increased understanding in this area will inform new hypotheses for future research . . . ."

CHAPTER 8

A. FILL IN THE BLANKS

1. validity
2. crossover
3. attrition
4. selection
5. random
6. blinding
7. control
8. Mortality
9. prospective (or cohort)
10. statistical
11. internal

12. external
13. cross-sectional
14. counterfactual
15. case-control
16. longitudinal
17. Matching
18. power
19. history
20. wait
21. baseline (or pretest)
22. quasi-experiments
23. relationships (or associations)
24. retrospective

B. MATCHING EXERCISES

1. b	2. b	3. a	4. c	5. b
6. a	7. c	8. a	9. b	10. c

C. STUDY QUESTIONS

C.2   2a. Both/either
2b. Nonexperimental
2c. Both/either
2d. Nonexperimental
2e. Nonexperimental
3a. Nonexperimental
3b. Both/either
3c. Nonexperimental
3d. Nonexperimental
3e. Nonexperimental

D. APPLICATION EXERCISES

Exercise D.1: Questions of Fact (Appendix A)

a. Yes, the researchers were evaluating the effectiveness of a weight loss intervention that used smartphone technology plus text messaging from a health coach.
b. The independent variable was participation versus nonparticipation in the special intervention. The dependent variables included body weight, body mass index, waist circumference, physical activity, and self-efficacy for healthy eating and exercise.
c. The design for this study was experimental.
d. Yes, randomization was used. Eligible participants were enrolled and then randomly assigned to either the intervention group or a control group, in blocks of four. Sixty-two participants were enrolled in the study—31 in each group.
e. The control group strategy in this study was the absence of a special intervention. The control group completed questionnaires but did not receive any special services. Control group members were asked not to use any smartphone applications focused on weight loss during the study. They were given the smartphone application used in the intervention (Lose It!), but not the text messages from a health coach, after the follow-up data were collected—this is a partial wait-list approach.
f. In this study, data were collected from experimental and control group members both before and after the intervention. Thus, we could call the design a pretest–posttest experimental design.
g. The article did not say anything about blinding, which usually means that no blinding was used.
h. The data were collected twice: before the intervention and 3 months later. This study could, therefore, be described as longitudinal.
i. Stephens and colleagues used randomization to groups to control confounding characteristics, which is the most effective strategy possible. It could also be said that they used another method; namely, homogeneity—although this method was not explicitly used as a control method. All of the study participants were between the ages of 18 and 25 years, were not diabetic, were not taking weight loss medications, and were not pregnant.
j. Through randomization, virtually all participant characteristics (e.g., sex, physical attractiveness, socioeconomic background, grade point average, weight) would have been controlled. Additionally, through homogeneity, age, pregnancy status, and so on were controlled (i.e., held constant).
k. Yes, there was modest attrition. As shown in Figure 1, 2 people out of 31 in the intervention group and 1 person out of 31 in the control group were not included in the final analyses. Thus, the overall rate of attrition was

4.8% (3 / 62). This is a modest rate of attrition for a 3-month study.

l. Selection was not a threat in this study because random assignment was used to equalize the groups. Table 2 shows that the two groups were not significantly different at baseline in terms of age, race, sex, and—most importantly—weight-related outcomes. That is, in the far right-hand column, the probability values (P) are all greater than .05, which means that the small group differences on these baseline variables were a function of chance.

m. No, the rate of attrition in this study was low and so the mortality threat likely did not undermine the study's internal validity.

Exercise D.2: Questions of Fact (Appendix D)

a. No, there was no intervention in this study.

b. The study design was nonexperimental. It had both descriptive components (e.g., What was fatigue like in patients with coronary heart disease?), and correlational components (What factors—demographic, physiological, psychological—were associated with fatigue? Is fatigue correlated with health-related quality of life?)

c. The article did not articulate a cause-probing intent. The stated purpose was to *describe* fatigue in patients with stable coronary heart disease and to examine factors *correlated with* fatigue. The authors were careful to avoid causal language. Indeed, they specifically noted that, with regard to the observed relationship between fatigue and depression, it could not be ascertained whether fatigue caused depression, or depression caused fatigue. They also specifically noted in their conclusion that it would be desirable to undertake longitudinal studies that might shed more light on the nature of the relationship between these variables.

d. The main dependent variable (the O) in this study was level of fatigue; the independent variables were demographic variables (gender, age, education, income), physiological variables (hypertension, hyperlipidemia), and

psychological (depression). However, the authors looked at level of fatigue (I and C) as an independent variable potentially affecting quality of life (O).

e. None of the variables in the study could be experimentally manipulated.

f. No, randomization was not used. This was a nonexperimental study.

g. This is a descriptive correlational study. It could also be described as retrospective: Eckhardt and colleagues were interested in identifying predisposing factors that could predict levels of fatigue.

h. No, blinding was not used in this study.

i. No, this study was cross-sectional, and it was not prospective. Data were collected at a single point in time, and the factors examined as possible predictors of fatigue could be considered retrospective in nature—i.e., as potentially existing prior to fatigue.

CHAPTER 9

A. FILL IN THE BLANKS

1. population
2. strata
3. eligibility
4. size
5. Consecutive
6. Quota
7. probability
8. representativeness
9. Convenience
10. random
11. bias
12. systematic
13. power analysis
14. self
15. closed
16. open
17. scale
18. Likert
19. set
20. acquiescence (or yea-sayers)
21. observational
22. checklist
23. Time
24. Measurement
25. Reliability
26. internal consistency
27. test-retest

28. Validity
29. Criterion
30. groups

B. MATCHING EXERCISES

B.1   1. b   2. a   3. d   4. b
          5. d   6. b   7. c   8. d
          9. a   10. b

B.2   1. a, c   2. a, b   3. b, c   4. b
          5. b   6. a, b, c 7. a, b, c 8. a

B.3   1. b   2. a   3. c   4. d
          5. b   6. b

C. STUDY QUESTIONS

C.1   a. Simple random
          b. Convenience
          c. Systematic
          d. Quota
          e. Purposive
          f. Consecutive

C.4   c—Internal consistency reliability
          is only relevant for multi-item
          scales (summated rating scales).

D. APPLICATION EXERCISES

Exercise D.1: Questions of Fact

a. None of the studies in the three appendices used probability samples of participants.
b. The quantitative studies in the Appendices A (Stephens et al.) and D (Eckhardt et al.) used convenience sampling.
c. It appears possible that the evidence-based practice (EBP) project described in Appendix C (Saqe-Rockoff et al.) used consecutive sampling—i.e., all eligible patient charts within a certain time frame.

Exercise D.2: Questions of Fact

a. The studies in Appendices A and D used structured self-reports as a method of data collection. Stephens and colleagues used self-administered questionnaires that incorporated several psychosocial scales (to measure activity levels, 24-hour food consumption, and self-efficacy for healthy eating and exercise). Eckhardt and colleagues administered several psychosocial scales; key variables were measured using multi-item self-report scales (e.g., fatigue, depressive symptoms, and health-related quality of life).
b. None of the studies in these appendices used observational methods of data collection.
c. Stephens and colleagues collected anthropomorphic data on height, weight, body mass index, and waist circumference.
d. In the EBP project by Saqe-Rockoff and colleagues, data from patients' charts were used to evaluate the effects of the evidence-based interventions.

Exercise D.3: Questions of Fact (Appendix D)

a. The target population in Eckhardt et al.'s study could perhaps be described as community-dwelling patients with stable coronary heart disease (CHD) in the United States (or in midwestern United States). The accessible population was patients in cardiology clinics in the state of Illinois.
b. The eligibility criteria for the study included (1) a diagnosis of stable CHD, (2) the ability to speak and read English, and (3) living independently. Exclusion criteria included (1) heart failure with reduced ejection fraction (<40%), (2) terminal illness with prediction of less than 6 months to live, (3) myocardial infarction or a CABG in the previous 2 months, (4) unstable angina, (5) symptoms reflecting worsening or exacerbation of cardiac disease, and (6) hemodialysis. The exclusion criteria were intended to exclude patients with a recent acute event, those with worsening symptoms, and those with comorbid conditions associated with fatigue.
c. The sampling method was nonprobability, specifically, sampling by convenience. However, recruitment of study participants in two sites serving different demographic groups enhanced the representativeness of the sample. One clinic served primarily urban minority patients with CHD, whereas the second clinic served Caucasian

patients from a more rural setting. The authors noted in the Discussion section that a possible limitation of the study was the use of a convenience sample.

d. Specific recruitment strategies were not discussed in the article. For example, there was no information about who did the recruiting, what prospective participants were told, how they were screened for eligibility, or what percentage of those approached actually participated.

e. The researchers increased the likelihood that their sample would be diverse and more representative by recruiting from two sites serving very different demographic and residential groups. In the section of the paper labeled "Strengths and limitations," the authors specifically noted that "sampling an urban and rural population resulted in ethnic and geographic diversity, thus increasing the generalizability of findings."

f. The total sample size was 102 participants.

g. The report made no mention of the researchers having performed a power analysis to estimate sample size needs. No explanation was provided regarding why a sample of 102 patients was selected or is sample size discussed in the Discussion section of the report.

h. Demographic characteristics of the study participants were described in the Results section and summarized in Table 1. Participants ranged in age from 34 to 86 years; the average age was 65 years. The majority of participants were non-Hispanic white (56%), male (64%), married (59%), and retired (52%). About 45% of the sample had at least some college education.

i. The researchers relied on preexisting scales developed by other researchers to measure the key variables of fatigue (the 14-item Fatigue Symptom Inventory), depressive symptoms (the 9-item Patient Health Questionnaire-9), and health-related quality of life (the 36-item SF-36). The researchers also measured several other background variables, such as co-morbid conditions and smoking history. It is possible the researchers developed their own questions, but it is also possible they used or adapted questions from previous studies.

j. The researchers used existing scales, for which evidence about internal consistency reliability and validity was available. For example, for the SF-36 that was used to measure health-related quality of life (HRQoL), the researchers noted, "The SF-36 has been extensively used to measure HRQoL and has established reliability and validity in numerous populations." In addition to *selecting* measures known to have good psychometric properties, the researchers computed internal consistency coefficients using data from their own sample. For example, for the SF-36, they found that internal consistency reliability was good for 7 of the 8 SF-36 subscales. The coefficients ranged from .79 to .88.

CHAPTER 10

A. FILL IN THE BLANKS

1. emergent
2. Ethnonursing
3. participant
4. informants
5. focused
6. lived
7. essence
8. Interpretive; hermeneutics
9. bracketing
10. basic
11. Glaser; Strauss
12. constant
13. case
14. narrative
15. critical
16. action

B. MATCHING EXERCISES

1. b	2. a	3. d	4. c	5. b
6. a	7. b	8. c	9. d	10. c
11. a	12. d			

C. STUDY QUESTIONS

C.1   a. Grounded theory
b. Ethnography
c. Phenomenology
d. Hermeneutics
(phenomenology)

D. APPLICATION EXERCISES

Exercise D.1: Questions of Fact (Appendix B)

a. The study by Ottosen and colleagues was an ethnography. Specifically, it was described as a "medically focused" ethnography that studied the relationship between differing "cultural systems" of clinicians and parents.

b. The central phenomenon of this study was how parents conceptualize patient safety ("safe care") in the neonatal intensive care unit (NICU) environment.

c. No, this study was not longitudinal. Although Ottosen and colleagues conducted the study over an 11-month period (January to November 2014), they were not studying changes in or the evolution of parent's conceptualization of safe care in the NICU.

d. The study took place in "a large academic hospital in Texas that served as a regional neonatal care center for high risk neonates."

e. No, the focus of the study was not on comparisons. However, the authors did recommend that future research on parents' perceptions of safe care in the NICU examine differences in maternal and paternal observations and contributions in promoting patient safety. They also recommended studying whether differences in safety culture across NICUs are related to "differences in the level of partnerships between parents and clinicians."

f. Yes, Ottosen and colleagues used methods consistent with the ethnographic approach. They made detailed observations of parents interacting with clinicians and other parents in the NICU, had informal conversations with parents and health care staff, and conducted in-depth interviews with a sample of parents as well.

g. No, there was no ideological perspective in this study.

Exercise D.2: Questions of Fact (Appendix E)

a. The research by Langegård and colleagues was a grounded theory study.

b. The researchers used the classic Glaser and Strauss approach to grounded theory. The researchers mentioned that they used "classic" grounded theory in their abstract. In the first paragraph of their Methods section, they stated that "the approach described by Glaser and Strauss was used to answer the research questions, 'How do patients manage the symptoms they experience?'"

c. The central phenomenon studied was the management of symptoms by patients with brain tumors.

d. Yes, the study was longitudinal. The researchers collected data from about half of the study participants (12 out of 22) both before and after the proton beam therapy treatment.

e. This study was conducted in three health care facilities—a specialized clinic (the Skandian Clinic) and two university hospitals in Sweden.

f. Yes, in the subsection of the Methods section labeled "Methodology," the researchers stated that they used the constant comparative method "with all units of data." They also elaborated in the "Data Analysis" subsection: "Interviews were transcribed verbatim and consecutively analyzed using the constant comparative method."

g. Yes, the core variable was identified as "The art of living with symptoms."

h. The methods used in this study were congruent with a grounded theory approach. The researchers conducted lengthy conversational interviews with 22 patients who had received proton beam therapy for a brain tumor. Twelve of the 22 sample members were interviewed a second time, after receiving the treatment. As noted previously, constant comparison was used in the analysis of the rich data.

i. No, this study did not have an ideological perspective.

CHAPTER 11

A. FILL IN THE BLANKS

1. Snowball (network)
2. Theoretical
3. purposive
4. maximum variation
5. data saturation

6. topic
7. semi-
8. grand tour
9. Photovoice
10. focus group
11. key informants
12. field; log

B. MATCHING EXERCISES

B.1   1. b   2. c   3. d   4. a
5. b   6. a   7. b   8. a
9. b   10. d

B.2   1. a   2. b   3. c   4. a
5. b   6. c   7. a   8. b
9. a   10. a

D. APPLICATION EXERCISES

Exercise D.1: Questions of Fact (Appendix B)

a. All study participants who were interviewed for this research were parents whose infants were hospitalized in one of two neonatal intensive care units (NICUs) in a large academic hospital in Texas. (Clinicians in those units were observed providing care, but they were not formally interviewed.) Parents were eligible to participate if they spoke English, if their infants were in stable condition, and if their infants had been in the NICU for 3 weeks or more.

b. The article stated that "parents were invited to participate while they were in the NICU by the lead author who described the purpose, procedures, risks and benefits, and voluntary nature of study participation." The report stated that only three parents declined to be interviewed due to time constraints.

c. The article stated that parents were sampled purposively. The researchers made a deliberate effort to "match the age, ethnicity, parity, and infants' gestational age representative of the parents in the NICU." This is an unusual strategy in an ethnographic study, but it ensured that the researchers' conclusions about parents' conceptualization of safe care in the NICU was not skewed by having a markedly atypical

sample. The small number of refusals also enhances confidence in the results.

d. The report did not indicate how many parents and clinicians were observed during the field observations, but 22 "parent informants" participated in in-depth interviews.

e. In the subsection labeled "Sampling Selection," Ottosen and colleagues stated the following: "Participants were enrolled until saturation in the depth and breadth of the interview content was reached, as evidenced by redundancy in the thematic content of responses."

f. The article described background characteristics of the 22 parents in the sample in Table 1. Study participants were predominantly the mothers (82%), and the majority of participants (68%) were married. All but 14% were racial or ethnic minorities. Just over half of the parents were older than 30, and for most parents the infant was their first child. On average, the infants had been in the NICU for more than 3 months at the time of the interview.

g. Yes, the study involved in-depth interviews with the 22 parents. Parents were asked whether they wanted to be interviewed individually, with their partners/spouses, or with other parents. Most wanted to be interviewed with their partner (if there was one). The interviews took place in a conference room adjacent to the NICU.

h. The interviews with 22 parents were described as semi-structured. The questions were developed by the team of research collaborators. NICU clinicians and a NICU parent advisory board reviewed the interview guide. Here is how the authors described the interview: "Interview questions were open-ended and asked parents to describe their overall experience in the NICU, their perceptions of their interactions and communication with the NICU team, their involvement as parents in the NICU, and how they view overall safety in the NICU."

i. Yes, the authors included an appendix to their report that listed the questions in the topic guide. The interviews began with what could be called a "grand tour" question: "Tell me about your experience in the neonatal ICU, how has it been for you?" More focused questions were asked later in the interviews (e.g., "How involved do you feel in the care of your baby?").

j. There was no information in the article about how long the interviews lasted. However, judging from the questions in the topic guide, most interviews likely lasted at least an hour.

k. The interviews were digitally recorded and subsequently transcribed verbatim.

l. Yes, the report indicated that the researchers conducted more than 150 hours of observations and informal conversations with parents and clinical staff. Field observations in the NICU were conducted across all days of the week and all shifts. The observations focused on parents interacting and communicating "with their infants, their families, NICU clinicians, and other parents." The observations were not described as "participant" observations.

m. The article stated that the investigator maintained field notes of the observations. No further information about the notes was provided except a statement that the field observations "provided relevant contextual information and exemplars . . . ."

n. It appears that the lead author of the report, Dr. Madelene Ottosen, collected the study data.

Exercise D.2.: Questions of Fact (Appendix E)

a. The article indicated that participants were adult Swedish patients with primary brain tumors who had been referred for proton beam therapy (PBT).

b. The article stated that patients were informed about the study and invited to participate via a telephone call from the first author, who was a nurse working at the University of Gothenburg.

c. The article described two sampling approaches. The researchers began with purposive (maximum variation) sampling: ". . . participants were strategically selected to provide a broad perspective, with selection based on age, sex, and civil status." Then, purposive sampling was replaced with "theoretical sampling based on the emerging findings."

This was an excellent strategy, appropriate for a grounded theory study.

d. The sample consisted of 22 patients receiving PBT in three Swedish health care centers.

e. The report stated that during theoretical sampling, they selected participants with benign tumors primarily "to gain variation of symptom management during the treatment period and also to confirm saturation."

f. There is no mention of sampling disconfirming cases, but the researchers' comment about "confirming" saturation does suggest the researchers sought confirming cases.

g. Characteristics of the 22 participants were described in Table 1 of the report. There were 10 women and 12 men, who varied in age, education, and marital status. The ages ranged from 5 participants in the 26- to 35-year-old age group to 4 participants who were in the 66- to 75-year-old age group. Half the patients were married with children living at home, and half had a high school education. Fourteen patients had malignant brain tumors, and 8 had a benign tumor.

h. Yes, the primary form of data collection was by means of self-report. The questions focused on the patients' management of their symptoms.

i. In-depth face-to-face interviews were used primarily to collect self-report data. Five interviews were conducted by telephone when face-to-face interviews could not be conducted. Twelve of the 22 sample members were interviewed twice.

j. The report stated that the interviews started with a broad open-ended question as follows: "Can you please tell me about your situation based on your current illness, including how you manage the symptoms you experience?" Follow-up questions included "What does it mean to you in your daily life?"

k. Interviews lasted between 30 and 70 minutes.

l. The report did not specifically state that the interviews were audiorecorded. However, we can infer that they were recorded because there are several references to transcriptions of the interviews.

m. No, the researchers did not observe the study participants. Observational data are sometimes gathered in grounded theory studies, but the more usual procedure is to rely on in-depth interviews.

CHAPTER 12

A. FILL IN THE BLANKS

1. mixed methods
2. sequence; priority
3. qualitative
4. qualitative
5. sequential
6. concurrent
7. pragmatism
8. Quality improvement
9. root cause analysis
10. Plan-Do-Study-Act
11. clinical trial
12. effectiveness
13. randomized
14. intervention theory
15. process
16. economic (or cost)
17. comparative effectiveness
18. Outcomes
19. structure
20. survey
21. secondary
22. methodological

B. MATCHING EXERCISES

1. a, b   2. d   3. c   4. a   5. b
6. d   7. a, b   8. a, b, c, d

D. APPLICATION EXERCISES

Exercise D.1: Questions of Fact

a. Quality improvement (QI) project
   • The Hountz et al. study in Appendix F was a QI project undertaken in a nurse-managed clinic.
b. Clinical trial
   • The Stephens et al. study in Appendix A could be described as a clinical trial—a randomized design was used to test an innovative intervention with clinical applications.

c. Economic analysis
   • None of the studies in the appendices involved an economic analysis (or, if they did, that part of the study was not presented in the reports).
d. Outcomes research
   • None of the studies in the appendices could be described as outcomes research.
e. Survey research
   • The Eckhardt et al. study (Appendix D) is the closest thing to a survey in the appendices, although it is not truly an example of survey research. Surveys typically gather self-report data from a broad population of respondents—like in an opinion poll—rather than from patients with a particular health problem receiving care at particular institutions.
f. Secondary analysis
   • All of the reports in the appendices described studies that collected original data; there are no secondary analyses.
g. Methodological research
   • None of the studies in the appendices could be described as methodological research designed to develop, refine, or test methods of collecting data or designing a study.

Exercise D.2: Questions of Fact (Appendix D)

a. Yes, this was a mixed methods study. As described in the introduction, the study had three purposes: (1) to describe fatigue (intensity, distress, timing, and quality) in patients with stable coronary heart disease (CHD); (2) to determine if specific demographic, physiological, or psychological variables were correlated with fatigue; and (3) to determine if fatigue was associated with health-related quality of life. Quantitative information played a particularly important role in addressing the second and third purposes but was also used to address the first. The qualitative strand was used to enrich the description of fatigue, i.e., the first purpose. No specific mixed methods purpose or question was stated.
b. The quantitative strand had priority in the study design.

c. The design was sequential: Data for the quantitative strand were gathered, followed by the collection of qualitative data.

d. The design used in this study would be described as an explanatory design, using Creswell and Plano-Clark's terminology. Qualitative data were used to explain and elaborate on the results of the quantitative analyses. The authors themselves used a different name for their design: a partially mixed sequential dominant status design. They referenced different authors for their design typology.

e. The authors themselves used notation to depict their design: QUAN → qual.

f. Eckhardt and colleagues used nested sampling. There were 102 CHD patients in the QUAN strand. Using patients' scores on a measure of fatigue (the Fatigue Symptom Inventory [FSI]-Interference Scale), the researchers identified participants with high, moderate, and low levels of interference from fatigue. Thirteen patients in these three groups participated in an in-depth interview in which they were asked to describe their daily lives and the fatigue they experienced.

g. The report did not provide much detail about how the actual integration took place. The report stated that the two strands of data "were compared to determine patterns, enhance description, and address any discrepancies. Qualitative data were used to expand the overall depth of quantitative findings and provide a more thorough description of fatigue." The authors also noted that they paid particular attention to discrepancies and viewed discrepancies as potentially "generative." In their results section, they provided a good example of a discrepancy and how this led to further ideas. One 81-year-old participant in the qualitative strand was in the low fatigue group—a score of zero on scored on the FSI-Interference Scale—and yet in the in-depth interview he stated, "I just get tired. Some days I almost start crawling." The researchers speculated that this incongruence might "represent an accommodation to decreased physical capacity because of CHD.

Exercise D.3: Questions of Fact (Appendix F)

a. The setting for this quality improvement project was a nurse-managed health clinic (NMHC) serving rural areas of the state of Indiana.

b. The authors identified the problem as low colorectal cancer (CRC) screening rates in the NMHC. Figure 1 in the article shows that in 2014, the rate was 33% at the NMHC, substantially lower than the 70% target rate set for the Healthy People 2020 initiative and lower than the U.S. national rate of 62% in 2010.

c. The team identified five goals: (1) reviewing the CRC screening process used at the NMHC, (2) developing interventions to improve the screening rate, (3) implementing the improvement interventions, (4), evaluating whether improvement occurred, and (5) sustaining process changes.

d. Yes, in this project, an Institutional Review Board reviewed and approved the project.

e. The team chose the Plan-Do-Study-Act (PDSA) model for this project. Based on the information in Table 1, which provided a good overview of the methods used, it appears that there were at least two cycles (e.g., there were two Plan cycles from May to June, 2015 and August to September, 2015), but the number of cycles was not explicitly stated. In fact, the word "cycle" was not used in the article.

f. The article did not provide much information about how the team identified underlying causes of the problem. There was no mention of a root cause analysis. However, Table 1 stated that the team developed a process flow map to visualize the current process for encouraging CRC screenings to patients. Table 1 also indicated that the team "analyzed preintervention data with identification of problems" and used the analysis and other sources to shape intervention development.

g. Table 3 of the article described the various components of the QI intervention. This included provider education (not described in Table 3 but noted in the text of the article), provider reminders and decision support tools, patient education, and patient reminders. The text also noted that provider feedback was used in their effort to sustain process changes: "Monthly feedback was given to individual providers and continues to be posted at the NMHC." The importance of performance feedback was discussed at some length in the Discussion section of the report.

h. The authors explicitly stated that they conducted a literature review and identified strategies that had been used to address the problem of CRC screening rates in other QI projects. In Table 1, the authors noted that they incorporated information from the literature review in developing the QI intervention.

i. The basic design for this study was a before–after (pretest–posttest) quasi-experimental design. Data on CRC screening rates were collected for 200 patients prior to the intervention in early 2015 and then for 200 patients after the intervention in January 2016.

j. The team used two outcome measures: the rate for CRC screenings ordered and the rate for CRC screenings completed.

k. Yes, in addition to collecting quantitative data on screening rates during the "Plan" and "Study" phases of the PDSA cycle, the team conducted semi-structured interviews with staff as part of the planning process. These interviews helped the team to identify strengths and weaknesses of the existing process, and staff also had suggestions for process improvements.

l. Yes, the team concluded that the QI interventions were successful in increasing CRC screenings. Over the 1-year period, the number of screenings ordered for eligible patients increased from 38% to 75% of patients and the number of screenings completed increased from 30% to 58% of patients (Figure 2 and Table 5).

CHAPTER 13

A. FILL IN THE BLANKS

1. ordinal
2. ratio
3. nominal
4. interval
5. continuous
6. negative; positive
7. unimodal; bimodal
8. normal
9. mean
10. mode
11. standard
12. crosstabs
13. odds ratio
14. Inferential
15. alpha
16. Type I
17. Type II
18. power
19. level
20. *t*-test
21. confidence
22. analysis of variance (ANOVA)
23. *d* statistic
24. Pearson's *r*
25. positive
26. chi-squared
27. regression
28. predictor
29. square
30. covariate
31. Logistic
32. coefficient alpha (Cronbach's alpha)
33. intraclass correlation
34. Cohen's kappa
35. sensitivity

B. MATCHING EXERCISES

B.1

1. d	2. a	3. d	4. b
5. c	6. a	7. b	8. d
9. c	10. b	11. b	12. a

B.2

1. b	2. a	3. c	4. d
5. b	6. b	7. a	8. a
9. c	10. a		

C. STUDY QUESTIONS

C.1 Unimodal around the mode of 51, fairly symmetric

C.2 Mean: 81.8; median: 83; mode: 84

C.3

Observed Frequencies for Children With Lactose Intolerance						
	Gender					
	Girls		Boys		Total	
Status	n	%	n	%	N	%
Lactose intolerant	16	26.7	12	20.0	28	23.3
Not Lactose intolerant	44	73.3	48	80.0	92	76.7
TOTAL	60	100.0	60	100.0	120	100.0

For the sample as a whole, nearly one out of four children was lactose intolerant. In this sample, boys were less likely than girls to be lactose intolerant (20.0% vs. 26.7%, respectively). To learn if this difference is statistically significant, we would need to perform a chi-squared test.

C.4   a. −.13
       b. Yes, the r of .17 is significant at $p < .01$
       c. Number of doctor visits, physical functioning, and mental health score
       d. Women who had lower physical functioning scores had significantly more doctor visits than women with higher scores.

C.5   a. chi-squared
       b. t-test
       c. Pearson's r
       d. ANOVA

C.6   a. Logistic regression
       b. ANCOVA
       c. Multiple regression

D. APPLICATION EXERCISES

Exercise D.1 (Questions of Fact)

a. All four of the studies reported percentages. Stephens et al. reported some demographic characteristics of their sample as percentages in Table 2 (e.g., percent White, 38.7% in both the intervention and control groups). Saqe-Rockoff et al. reported some demographic and clinical characteristics (e.g., sex, temperature category) in percentages in Table 1 (e.g., 6.4% of patients had hypothermia in 2017). Eckhardt et al. reported many background and clinical characteristics of their sample as percentages. In fact, all of the statistics in Table 1 were percentages (e.g., 86.3% of the sample used aspirin). Hountz et al. compared sample characteristics of pre- and postintervention patients in Table 4 (e.g., 21.5% of the preintervention patients had private insurance).

b. Stephens et al. (Appendix A) did not report means and standard deviations (SDs). The researchers did not state their rationale for using alternative descriptive indexes in the report itself, but Stephens et al. informed us (in a personal communication) that their decision was based on their relatively small sample size. (Their decision was reasonable, but the rationale is too complex to explain here.) Saqe-Rockoff et al. (Appendix C) did not make clear that they reported means, although they likely did. In the text (Results section), they stated that "over the period of 3 months, there was a steady increase in the *average* temperature of the trauma bay"—but they did not indicate what they meant by "average." However, Figure 2 shows average temperatures with standard deviations, which would only be shown with mean values. Eckhardt et al. (Appendix D) reported a few means and SDs. For example, in the "Demographic Characteristics" subsection of the Results section, they reported that the mean age of participants was 65 years (*SD* = 11). They also presented some of their findings with means and *SD*s. For example, for the scores on the fatigue scale, women had a mean of 4.38 (*SD* = 2.16), whereas men had a mean of 3.43 (*SD* = 2.16). This information was presented in the text, not in tables. Hountz et al. (Appendix F) did not report means and *SD*s.

c. The Stephens research team (Appendix A) reported medians rather than means for all outcomes. For example, for the demographic characteristics reported in Table 11, the median age was 20.0 in both the intervention and control group. Tables 3 and 4 presented results of the randomized trial, and again median values (and ranges) were reported. For example, the median pre- and postintervention weight of those in the intervention group were 82.8 and 80.1, respectively. Saqe-Rockoff et al. (Appendix C) reported median age of participants in Table 1: The median age was 52.4 in 2016 and 68.6 in 2017. Neither Eckhardt et al. (Appendix D) nor Hountz et al. (Appendix F) reported medians.

d. None of the articles reported modes.

Exercise D.2 (Questions of Fact)

a. Stephens et al. (Appendix A) did not use *t*-tests in their analyses. Stephens and colleagues did, however, use a repeated measures ANOVA for some analyses. In the section of their report labeled "Evaluation," Saqe-Rockoff et al. (Appendix C) mentioned that the Student *t*-test was used, but actual values of test statistics were not shown in the report. Eckhardt et al. (Appendix D) reported the results of several *t*-tests. For example, men and women were compared with respect to fatigue-related outcomes using *t*-tests. The researchers noted that women reported significantly more interference from fatigue than men (*t* = 2.74, *p* = .007).

b. Stephens and colleagues (Appendix A) used chi-squared tests for some of their analyses, as noted in the subsection labeled "Statistical Analysis." The actual test values were not, however, reported.

For example, in Table 2, it is likely that chi-squared tests were used to compare the proportion male and female in the two study groups. The difference was not statistically significant (*p* = .6322). Saqe-Rockoff et al. (Appendix C) mentioned that chi-squared tests were used, but actual values of test statistics were not shown in the report. Eckhardt and colleagues (Appendix D) reported that they used chi-squared tests in their analysis of demographic data, but the results were not presented in the paper.

c. Stephens et al. (Appendix A) undertook analyses that examined, for the intervention group, the relationship between the number of days logged for exercise activity and the amount of weight lost. However, the researchers did not report the actual values of the correlation coefficients. (In a personal communication, Stephens informed us that they did use Pearson's *r* in this analysis.) Saqe-Rockoff et al. (Appendix C) did not report any correlation coefficients. Eckhardt and colleagues (Appendix D) used correlation procedures extensively. They noted in their subsection labeled "Quantitative Analysis" that Pearson's *r* (and Spearman's rho) were used "to identify factors associated with fatigue." In Table 2, for example, the researchers presented values of *r* for fatigue intensity and fatigue interference with several independent variables. The highest correlations for both outcomes were with scores on a measure of depressive symptoms (*r* = .56 and *r* = .66, respectively, both *p* <. 0001).

Exercise D.3: Questions of Fact (Appendix D)

a. Referring to Table 1:
   - Nominal-level: gender, race/ethnicity, marital status, employment status, presence of comorbid condition, and types of medications taken
   - Ordinal-level: As operationalized in this paper, education was measured on an ordinal scale.
   - Interval-level: none
   - Ratio-level: None. Education *could* have been measured on a ratio scale as the number of years of schooling completed. However, ordinal

categories such as the ones used actually are more informative than presenting mean years of schooling completed.

- The typical study participant was a white (non-Hispanic) male who was married and retired, with at least 12 years of education.
- The 12.7% of the sample had a graduate degree.

b. Referring to Table 2:

- Fatigue intensity scores were significantly correlated with the following variables: gender, PHQ-9 (depressive symptoms) scores, income, and smoking history.
- The correlation between education and fatigue intensity was −.16. This suggests that people who had more education were slightly *less* likely to have high fatigue intensity scores than those with less education. However, this correlation was not statistically significant ($p = .12$) and so it cannot be concluded that education was correlated with fatigue intensity at all.
- Table 2 suffers from a flaw that is very common in research reports— the table does not indicate how the variable gender was coded. If men were coded with a higher value than women (e.g., 1 vs. 0), then the positive and significant correlation of .22 would indicate higher scores for men than for women because the correlation is positive. But if women were coded with a higher value than men (e.g., 2 vs. 1), then the reverse would be true. We know from the text (but not the table) that women had higher fatigue scores. The researchers should have provided coding information for gender, race, and several other variables in Table 2 because without such information the table by itself fails to communicate important information.

c. Eckhardt and colleagues used multiple regression analysis in this study.

d. Yes, in Tables 3 and 4, the researchers presented the results of multiple regression analyses and reported the values of R^2. For example, in Table 4, in the multiple regression equation that involved the prediction of fatigue interference scores on the basis of gender, age, and scores on the measure of depressive symptoms, the value of R^2 was .46.

CHAPTER 14

A. FILL IN THE BLANKS

1. interpretation
2. correlation
3. Effect
4. CONSORT
5. limitations (weaknesses)
6. hypothesis
7. precision
8. discussion
9. significant
10. clinical
11. minimal important change
12. responder

B. MATCHING EXERCISES

1. b   2. a   3. e   4. d
5. c   6. a, d   7. a   8. e

D. APPLICATION EXERCISES

Exercise D.1: Questions of Fact (Appendix A)

a. Yes, Figure 1 was a CONSORT-type flow chart that showed that 87 young adults were screened for the study and 62 were randomized. The chart then showed the number in intervention and control group who were allocated to each group, the number who dropped out, and the number that completed the study and were included in the analysis ($N = 59$).

b. Baseline values on the key demographic and outcome variables were presented in Table 2 for both intervention and control group members, and the last column presents information about the statistical significance of group differences on these variables. None of the group differences was statistically significant at the .05 level. When randomization is used, as in this study, selection bias is seldom a threat to the internal validity of a study—and when differences do occur, it is purely a function of chance.

c. There was little attrition, and the difference in rates of attrition between the two groups was small (6.4% in the intervention group and 3.2% in the control group—only 2 and 1 persons, respectively, dropped out of the study by the time of the 3-month follow-up). The researchers did not do an analysis of potential attrition biases, but such an analysis would not have yielded useful information because the Ns were too small. It should be noted that the researchers did a power analysis to estimate their sample size needs, and in that power analysis, they assumed an attrition rate of 15%. Thus, their attrition rate (overall, 4.8%) was lower than expected. It does not seem likely that their results were biased by attrition.

d. Hypotheses about the effects of the intervention were not formally stated, although they were clearly implied. There were statistically significant differences between the intervention and control groups for the three main outcomes—weight, body mass index (BMI), and waist circumference. For example, the change in median values for weight was +1.5 kg for the control group and −2.7 kg for the intervention group, $p = .026$, as shown in Table 3. Both groups had improvements in self-efficacy and physical activity over the 3-month period; group differences were not statistically significant. In terms of participants' diet (Table 4), only 37 study participants (15 in the intervention group and 22 in the control group) provided information about their diets. The only significant group difference was for the consumption of fiber, which was higher in the intervention group. It is possible that more of the dietary differences would have been significant with a larger sample. For example, those in the intervention group consumed less added sugars ($p = .077$) and more protein ($p = .080$). For these dietary outcomes, the analyses were likely insufficiently powered to detect differences at significant levels.

e. The paper did not provide confidence intervals (CIs) around values for the main outcomes (e.g., differences between group means or medians). In Table 5, 95% CIs are shown around values for the b coefficients for the relationships between the consistency of logging physical activity and weight change. We did not explain b coefficients in the textbook—although they were discussed in the supplement to Chapter 13.

f. Effect size estimates summarizing the magnitude of the intervention effects were not presented in the report.

g. There was no explicit discussion about internal validity in the discussion section, but the authors did note, correctly, that a major strength of this study was the use of a randomized design. Such a design provides a basis for an inference of causality—i.e., that participation in the intervention *caused* improvements in weight, waist circumference, and BMI. There do not appear to be any threats to the internal validity of the study. In experimental designs, attrition can be a major threat, but the rate of attrition in this study was low.

h. Yes, the authors did note in their discussion that generalizability was limited because the study participants were all attending college at an east coast university in the United States. Generalizing the results to, for example, low-income young adults living in poor urban neighborhoods is not warranted without a replication.

i. There was no explicit discussion about statistical conclusion validity in the discussion section. The researchers did, however, note that the sample size was small, and this in turn could have resulted in Type II errors for some of the outcomes—especially those relating to diet.

j. Yes, some of the findings were discussed vis-à-vis findings from earlier research. For example, the researchers stated that "these results are promising when examining other similar research," and then cited two earlier studies.

k. Yes, several limitations of the study were discussed. These included the small sample size, constraints on generalizability, and the inability to identify whether the intervention effects are attributable to the smartphone part of the intervention, or to the health coach. With regard to sample size, we note that in the power analysis, the researchers assumed an effect size of $d = .80$ based on a previous study. However, this is a very large and probably unrealistic effect size estimate. In any event, there was sufficient power for the main outcomes but not for the secondary ones.

l. No, the researchers did not say anything specifically about the clinical significance of their findings. They came to a broad conclusion that the trial provided "valuable information" about the intervention and did say that it had a "meaningful impact" on weight, BMI, and waist circumference. However, they did not define what constituted a "meaningful" effect.

Exercise D.2: Questions of Fact (Appendix D)

a. The researchers mentioned bias twice. First, they stated that they timed the in-depth qualitative interview 3 to 5 weeks after enrollment in the study, specifically to avoid the risk of *recall* biases. Second, participants for the qualitative interviews were purposively selected from patients who were high, moderate, or low on a key research variable level of interference from fatigue. To avoid bias, the researchers analyzed the qualitative data without knowing which of the three fatigue groups the people were in. Thus, they made efforts to avoid something akin to *expectation bias*.

b. Hypotheses were not formally stated in the introduction of this article, and yet hypotheses were implied (by virtue of the researchers' conceptual model) and tested statistically. For example, the framework (Figure 1) implies that fatigue would affect quality of life, and Table 5 shows that both fatigue intensity and fatigue interference were significantly and negatively correlated with all dimensions on the quality of life scale in this sample.

c. In this cross-sectional study, the issue of temporal ambiguity (i.e., whether one variable preceded or followed another) makes it difficult to infer a causal connection. The researchers specifically made a point about this in their discussion section as follows: ". . . it remains to be determined if depression is the cause or consequence of fatigue."

d. Precision information was not reported—i.e., there were no confidence intervals (CIs). CIs around correlation coefficients are almost never presented, and most of the analyses in this study were correlational.

e. The researchers did not specifically use effect size language in discussing their results. However, the value of r and R^2 can be directly interpreted as effect size indexes. For example, the value of $R^2 = .46$ (the prediction of fatigue interference) would be considered high. (The standard convention for a "large" R^2 is .30.) Thus, the three predictors shown in Table 4 (age, gender, and depression scores) had a fairly strong combined relationship with fatigue interference.

f. Yes, the researchers explicitly noted that the generalizability of their findings was likely enhanced by including a diverse mix of participants in terms of ethnicity and urban/rural residence.

g. Yes, some limitations of the study were explicitly noted in the discussion section as well as some strengths. The limitations included the use of a convenience sample and the potential inclusion of patients with undiagnosed heart failure.

h. Yes, the researchers did discuss clinical significance at the individual level. They noted (in the section on "Quantitative measurement—Fatigue") that a previous researcher had established a benchmark—a fatigue intensity score of 3 or higher on the Fatigue Symptom Inventory—as reflective of clinically meaningful fatigue. The researchers then reported that 57% of the men and 78% of the women in their sample had clinically meaningful levels of fatigue. This finding was the first thing they discussed in their discussion because this represents very high levels of fatigue. Indeed, categorizing participants as having or not having clinically significant levels of fatigue is more useful information than simply reporting that the mean fatigue intensity score was 4.4 for women and 3.4 for men. Thus, this study illustrates the value of defining clinical signifi-cance at the individual level and using a benchmark to classify patients.

CHAPTER 15

A. FILL IN THE BLANKS

1. coding
2. content; thematic
3. domain
4. taxonomic
5. descriptive
6. line-by-line
7. metaphor
8. circle
9. exemplars
10. Paradigm
11. open
12. selective
13. memo
14. emergent
15. constructivist

B. MATCHING EXERCISES

1. a, b, c	2. a	3. b	4. a, b, c
5. a	6. c	7. b	8. d

C. STUDY QUESTIONS

C.1

a. A grounded theory analysis would not yield themes; phenomenological stud-ies, for example, involves a thematic analysis.
b. Texts from poetry are used by interpre-tive phenomenologists, not by ethnog-raphers (unless the poetry is a product of the culture under study, which it is not in this case).
c. Phenomenological studies do not focus on domains, ethnographies do.
d. Grounded theory studies do not yield taxonomies, ethnographies do.
e. A paradigm case is a strategy in a her-meneutic analysis, not in an ethno-graphic one.

D. APPLICATION EXERCISES

Exercise D.1: Appendix B and D

a. The findings from Ottosen and col-league's data analysis were organized into several broad themes (e.g., "Parents as partners with clinicians to promote safe care," "Contributing fac-tors to parent-clinician partnership") that were described in major subsec-tions of their Results section. The words *themes* or *thematic* were men-tioned several times—for example, in connection with the description of data saturation and the peer debrief-ing sessions in which "thematic results and exemplars" were presented to four nurse colleagues for review. The quali-tative data in Eckhardt et al.'s mixed methods study also were analyzed for themes. In the section labeled "Qualitative Analysis," the researchers wrote, "Using the theory of unpleas-ant symptoms, themes of situational, psychological, and physiological factors; symptom description . . . , and performance . . . were analyzed. As data were coded, emerging themes were added . . . ."
b. Although the word *taxonomy* was not mentioned in the Ottosen et al.'s report, Table 2 presents what might be described as a taxonomy, or a category system, that identified and described five different roles that parents play in promoting safe care in the neonatal intensive care unit (NICU). Eckhardt et al.'s analysis did not involve the creation of a taxonomy.
c. Neither study involved the develop-ment of a grounded theory. Ottosen et al.'s study was an ethnography, and the Eckhardt et al.'s study involved a mixed methods approach in which the qualitative data were analyzed thematically.
d. Based on their data analysis, Ottosen et al. developed a "Conceptual model of parents as partners in NICU patient safety." The model was presented in Figure 1 of the article. No sche-matic model was developed for the data in the Eckhardt et al.'s study in Appendix D.

Exercise D.2: Questions of Fact (Appendix E)

a. Yes, the report indicates that "interviews were transcribed verbatim." Although Langegård and colleagues did not specifically mention audio-recording the interviews with the 22 participants, transcriptions would not be undertaken if such recordings were not made. In total, there were 34 interviews, which likely resulted in hundreds of pages in the data set that had to be read and reread, coded, and analyzed.

b. Yes, at the beginning of the section labeled "Data Analysis," the authors stated that the interviews were transcribed "and consecutively analyzed using the constant comparative method."

c. The report stated that the widely used software called NVivo was used in this study.

d. No, Langegård and colleagues did not use metaphors; metaphors are more likely to be used in phenomenological studies than in grounded theory studies.

e. Yes, the report indicated that the researchers wrote analytic memos during the process of data analysis. Their Table 2 illustrates memo writing by presenting a direct quote, the coding category, and a memo associated with the quote.

f. The report stated in the "Data Analysis" section that researchers started by using line-by-line coding. The codes were the actual words used by the patients, which is a standard approach to open coding. The report goes on to describe the progression to theoretical coding.

g. The researchers used the classic Glaserian approach to grounded theory analysis.

h. Yes, the researchers created a conceptual map that showed that three main concepts were linked to each other and to the core variable, "The art of living with symptoms."

i. Yes, the researchers provided several quotes in support of their conceptualization. For example, the core category of "The art of living with symptoms"

encompassed three symptom management concepts. Here is a quote for the concept: Adapting to limited ability:

- *What are obvious are the epileptic cramps. And that I get tired in public but otherwise I am not in pain. There are some things I cannot do. I cannot drive a car. I shall not expose myself to some contexts. One shall not be intoxicated. One shall not be a high altitudes. One shall not swim in deep water. So one is a little limited.*

CHAPTER 16

A. FILL IN THE BLANKS

1. Credibility
2. dependability
3. transferability
4. confirmability
5. Authenticity
6. triangulation
7. audit
8. thick description
9. internal
10. observation
11. negative
12. member
13. Investigator
14. peer
15. prolonged

B. MATCHING EXERCISES

1. a   2. b   3. c   4. a   5. b

D. APPLICATION EXERCISES

Exercise D.1: Questions of Fact (Appendix B)

a. No, Ottosen and colleagues did not devote a separate section of their report to their quality-enhancement strategies. They did, however, describe several steps that were taken to enhance trustworthiness in the Methods section.

b. Ottosen et al. used method triangulation in their study. Data were gathered through formal interviews with 22 parents, informal conversation with other parents and clinical staff, and field observations in the neonatal intensive care unit (NICU). The research team also used investigator triangulation. In the subsection on "Data Analysis," the report stated that "the lead author initially coded the data and reviewed the codes with 2 coauthors to reach consensus on interpreted findings."

c. Several strategies were used to enhance rigor in this study.

- We can conclude that both *persistent observation* (the researchers' very thorough and in-depth scrutiny of the safety culture in the NICU) and *prolonged engagement* (continuing to gather data and observe participants over an 11-month period) were used as quality-enhancement strategies in this study.
- The report indicated, in the "Data Analysis" subsection, that "thematic results and exemplars were presented by lead author at a *peer debriefing* of 4 nurse colleagues with NICU and/or qualitative experience to validate the congruency and clarity of the data supporting the findings." Peer review was also mentioned in connection with the development of the interview guide.
- Ottosen et al. did not mention *member checking*. However, the report stated that verification of understandings was sought during the course of data collection: "Throughout data collection, we verified and clarified the interpretations of the participants' comments and behaviors . . . ." The researchers also examined whether their conceptual model "resonated with parents of neonates" by presenting their findings and the model to six members of the NICU's parent advisory council.
- The report did not discuss any efforts to search for disconfirming evidence (although this does not necessarily mean it did not occur).
- Nothing was specifically mentioned about maintaining reflexive notes or journals in the report, but that does not mean that such activity did not occur.

Exercise D.2: Questions of Fact (Appendix E)

a. No, Langegård and colleagues did not have a section of their report specifically devoted to a description of quality-enhancement strategies. They did, however, note some of their strategies in two places as follows: (1) in the "Data Analysis" subsection of their Methods section and (2) a subsection of their discussion labeled "Methodological considerations."

b. Investigator triangulation was the only type of triangulation that the authors noted. In the "Data Analysis" section, they stated that "the analysis process was discussed by 3 of the authors, who read and/or analyzed a sample of the transcripts. Emerging codes and categories were compared and collectively discussed . . . ." Later in the "Methodological considerations" section, the authors noted that "to ensure credibility, two authors started the analysis process and created the concepts together . . . ." (Also, in the "Data Collection" subsection, the report indicated that the two interviewers collaborated on interviewing techniques.) Note that although the researchers interviewed some study participants more than once, their purpose was not time triangulation so much as to understand the unfolding processes of symptom management.

c. The authors commented that the transferability of their findings was enhanced because participants were drawn "from all over Sweden." However, they also noted some limitations to transferability because participants were all required to stay in a special hotel, which could "limit the transferability of the findings to patients treated in ordinary Swedish cancer care facilities." There was no discussion of transferability outside of Sweden.

d. Several strategies were used to enhance rigor in this study.

- Langegård and colleagues did not indicate how much time they spent gathering data, but it seems likely that many months were devoted to data collection. They noted that, consistent with grounded theory, their questioning evolved as their grounded theory emerged. Twelve of the 22 study participants were interviewed twice, suggesting prolonged engagement over the course of treatment for many of the study participants.

- In their subsection labeled "Data Collection," the authors indicated that three participants "were selected to confirm the extracted concepts," indicating that member checking occurred.
- There was no mention of searching for disconfirming evidence.
- Reflexivity was used in this study. In the subsection on "Methodological considerations" near the end of the paper, the authors stated "memos and regular discussions were conducted among the research group. The memos provided a trustworthy data source for the analysis, as they were obtained by regular use of a reflective research diary."
- The report did not state that an audit trail was maintained, although this does not mean that it did not happen.
- The report stated that "all the authors are experienced researchers and one has long experience working with GT (Grounded theory). The authors are either clinically experienced nurses or clinically experienced physicians." There was no mention of a personal connection to brain tumors or to proton beam therapy.

CHAPTER 17

A. FILL IN THE BLANKS

1. meta-analysis
2. scoping
3. grey
4. publication
5. quality
6. effect size
7. heterogeneity
8. difference
9. subgroup
10. forest

11. GRADE
12. aggregative; interpretive
13. qualitative evidence syntheses
14. metasyntheses
15. meta-ethnography
16. meta-summary
17. frequency
18. meta-aggregation

B. MATCHING EXERCISES

1. c	2. d	3. b	4. d
5. b	6. a	7. d	8. b

D. APPLICATION EXERCISES

Exercise D.1: Questions of Fact (Appendix G)

a. The purpose of Chase and colleagues' systematic review was "to determine the overall effectiveness of interventions designed to improve medication adherence (MA) among adults with CAD" (coronary artery disease). The independent variable was receipt versus nonreceipt of a special intervention, and the dependent (outcome) variable was medication adherence. Chase and colleagues articulated two specific research questions: (1) What is the overall effectiveness of medication adherence interventions on MA outcomes among patients with CAD? and (2) Does intervention effectiveness vary as a function of characteristics of the intervention, the sample, or the study design?

b. To be eligible for this systematic review, a primary study had to be a two-group (treatment vs. control group) study that tested the effectiveness of an intervention to increase medication adherence in adult patients aged 18 or older with a diagnosis of CAD. A total of 24 studies (28 comparisons) met these criteria.

c. The reviewers relied primarily on electronic database searches. They searched in about a dozen databases, using a wide array of search terms. They also used "hand searching" of 57 relevant journals, author searches of key researchers in the field, and ancestry searches using the bibliographies of identified studies.

d. No, this study did not present a flow chart summarizing the search and selection process. No information was provided about how many studies were initially identified through their search strategies and how many were eliminated for various reasons. This is not typical in a review with a meta-analyses—recent guidelines for reporting meta-analyses indicate that a flow chart should be provided, much like a CONSORT-type flow chart described in the textbook.

e. It was noted in the abstract and in the Results section that a total of 18,839 people participated in the primary studies.

f. Participants in the primary studies were, on average, 62.9 years old; this was the median of the study mean ages. The majority of study participants were male and, in studies for which ethnicity was reported, white. Many studies reported that their participants had other chronic diseases, such as hypertension and hyperlipidemia.

g. According to the Table 4, 20 of the 28 comparisons involved random assignment to a treatment or a control group. Thus, the review included studies with both experimental ($n = 20$) and quasi-experimental ($n = 8$) designs.

h. Study quality was assessed using a domain approach rather than a scale approach. Each study was coded for the presence or absence of certain features, including randomization, use of a theory, the blinding of data collectors, and the use of the recommended analytic approach called *intention to treat*. All coding was performed by two independent research specialists, who then compared and discussed their ratings until there was 100% agreement.

i. Studies were not excluded on the basis of quality, per se, but they were excluded if they used a weak one-group pretest–posttest design.

j. The effect size used in this study was the standardized mean difference, which we referred to in the textbook as *d*.

k. Yes, the researchers tested for statistical heterogeneity. They opted to use a random effects model, even before learning that the test for heterogeneity was statistically significant, because they expected variation of effects across studies.

l. Yes, Figure 1 presented the main effects on a study-by-study basis in a forest plot.

m. The overall effect size comparing adherence outcomes for those in an intervention group compared to a control group was .229. As shown in Table 2, the 95% confidence interval around this value was .138 to .321, which is significant because the interval does not include zero. We can be 95% confident that the true beneficial effect lies somewhere in the interval between .14 and .32 (rounded values).

n. With regard to Figure 1:
   - The study with the largest effect size (ES) was a small study published in 1985 at the bottom of the forest plot. The ES for this study was 2.521, favoring those in the intervention group.
   - Yes, there were many studies for which intervention effectiveness was nonsignificant—all those where the lines for the 95% CI crosses the vertical line for 0.00. Indeed, this was true for most of the studies in Figure 1.
   - Yes, there were five studies for which the value of *d* was negative, indicating outcomes favoring the control group. However, in none of these cases was the result statistically significant. This can be seen by examining the values of the lower and upper limits of the 95% CI. For these five studies where the value of *d* was negative, the lower limit was negative but the upper limit was positive, thus indicating the possibility that the value of *d* could be 0 (i.e., no intervention effects).

o. Yes, numerous exploratory subgroup analyses were undertaken to assess factors contributing to the heterogeneity of effects across studies. One interesting finding was that MA interventions delivered by nurses were especially effective. Another finding was that interventions in which health care providers were given information about patients' adherence were more effective than interventions without this component. Also, interventions initiated in inpatient settings were especially effective. Many of the subgroup analyses, however, yielded nonsignificant results.

p. No, this systematic review did not include ratings of the team's confidence in the review findings.

Exercise D.2: Questions of Fact (Appendix H)

a. Carr and colleagues conducted a metasynthesis that integrated findings from 16 qualitative studies. The review had both aggregative and interpretive elements, but the focus on women's experiences of breast reconstruction following a mastectomy was primarily interpretive.

b. Carr and colleagues followed procedures developed by Sandelowski and Barroso, although they did not undertake a meta-summary. The metasynthesists used two approaches suggested by Sandelowski and Barroso: taxonomic analysis and constant targeted comparison.

c. The report indicated these objectives: "to explore the qualitative research regarding women's experiences with BR (breast reconstruction) and to synthesize the findings in relation to their information needs." A secondary objective was to learn whether a woman's information needs differ for those who choose immediate versus delayed breast reconstruction.

d. Yes, the multidisciplinary research team articulated four inclusion criteria (e.g., the study used qualitative methods, the women's cancer treatment had to involve breast reconstruction surgery) and three exclusion criteria (e.g., the focus of the study was on aspects of cancer treatment other than breast reconstruction, the report was not written in English).

e. The reviewers relied primarily on electronic database searches. They searched in CINAHL, the Cochrane Library, EMBASE, MEDLINE, PsycINFO, and Scopus. The report stated the search terms that were used.

f. Yes, the reviewers included a PRISMA-type flowchart that indicated that 423 records were retrieved from the six bibliographic databases, only 59 of which were duplicates. Of the remaining 364 studies, 347 were excluded because the study did not meet the eligibility criteria. Thus, 17 studies were included. One of these studies was later excluded (not shown in the flowchart), however, because it was classified as having a low level of elaboration.

g. The primary studies in the review were conducted in the United States, Canada, Australia, Sweden, and Taiwan.

h. The primary studies spanned varied types of qualitative inquiry, including grounded theory, phenomenology, hermeneutics, feminist analysis, and narrative analysis.

i. The report indicated that 201 women from the primary studies underwent breast reconstruction. Data were collected from 193 of these women in one-on-one interviews and 8 women participated in a focus group interview.

j. Two main themes were identified in this metasynthesis as follows: (1) The women's expectations did not match the breast reconstruction experience and (2) the women's information needs. The first theme had several subthemes, such as being overwhelmed by information, getting information that conflicted with the outcome, and getting information that inaccurately reflected the actual process of reconstruction. A subtheme of the second theme was the need for greater patient-centered care.

k. Yes, Carr and colleagues included some powerful verbatim quotes from the primary studies in support of their thematic integration. For example, for the subtheme regarding the conflict between the outcome and the information the women received, here is one quote: "I don't like the way it feels. It still feels like something that's been grafted onto my body. I wasn't prepared for it being quite so fake."

CHAPTER 18

A. FILL IN THE BLANKS

1. Cochrane
2. Knowledge
3. pre-appraised

4. guideline
5. models
6. trigger
7. ask
8. Assess
9. quantity
10. consistency
11. Applicability
12. Patient
13. average
14. heterogeneity
15. Comparative
16. pragmatic
17. PRECIS
18. subgroup
19. Type I
20. interaction

B. MATCHING EXERCISES

1. c   2. b   3. c   4. b
5. a   6. d

D. APPLICATION EXERCISES

Exercise D.1: Questions of Fact (Appendix C)

a. The purpose of this evidence-based project was to develop, implement, and evaluate the effectiveness of a package of strategies for improving thermo-regulation for trauma patients in the emergency department.

b. The setting for the project was the emergency department (ED) of a 450-bed teaching facility (a Level I trauma center) in Brooklyn, New York.

c. The project was guided by the Iowa Model of Evidence-Based Practice to Promote Quality Care. The authors did not provide extensive detail about how the model facilitated the development of the effort, but that does not mean that they did not make extensive use of the model's guidance.

d. The authors specifically described the project as having a problem-focused trigger. In a subsection labeled "Approach," they stated that "it was determined that the trigger is of high priority to the ED and trauma program, which facilitated organizational engagement." As shown in the diagram

of the Iowa Model (Fig. 18.1 of the textbook), an early question for the evidence-based practice (EBP) team is whether the topic is considered a priority.

e. There were four authors of this report, and presumably they were the major team members on this project. Three authors were nurses (Saqe-Rockoff, Ciardiello, and Douglas) and one had a Masters of Public Health degree. One nurse was certified as a critical care nurse, and the other two nurses were certified as emergency room specialists. The lead author has a master's degree in nursing and was an adult-gerontology clinical nurse specialist. The text of the report indicated that the EBP project team was interdisciplinary. In addition to the listed authors, the report also mentioned the involvement of ED management, the ED nurse educator, and the manager of the surgical intensive care unit.

f. The report did not describe the team's evidence-searching efforts in detail. The lead author conducted a search in PubMed. No other bibliographic databases were mentioned. The authors noted that they "found sufficient research with consistent findings to warrant a practice change." This statement suggests that, in appraising the evidence, the team considered the quantity of evidence and its consistency. The report also noted that "evidence-based practice interventions were derived from the best available clinical evidence," suggesting quality of the evidence was an additional criterion.

g. The report indicated that changes that were part of their EBP project were pilot tested for a 3-month period. The authors did not describe any details of the pilot but noted that a focus was to assess feasibility and preliminary signs of improved outcomes.

h. The report described in a fair amount of detail the practice changes that were implemented as part of this EBP effort. The practice changes included the following: (1) encouragement of the use of warm blankets for all trauma patients unless exposure was necessary for medical interventions; (2) elevation of the trauma bay ambient temperature to 80°F; (3) temperature assessment on arrival, with an emphasis on core temperature evaluations; (4) escalation of rewarming measures, using a clear pathway of escalation; and (5) encouragement of the use of a thermoregulation checklist. The team provided staff training and education relating to the changes. In the section labeled "Educational Interventions," the authors stated that "huddles were conducted by the CNS multiple times per day for 1 week before launching the checklist. All ED nurses received a mass email outlining the EBP project and checklist. After go-live, weekly huddles were conducted with staff on all shifts."

i. Yes, the team used a "before–after" design to evaluate whether the practice changes resulted in improved outcomes. A 3-month period in the year prior to the practice changes (2016) was compared to a similar 3-month period after implementation (2017). The goals of the project were "to decrease time to temperature assessment, increase core temperature assessment, and increase implementation of appropriate rewarming methods."

j. Among the key findings were the following: (1) The ambient temperature in the trauma bay was higher after implementing the changes than before—although the report noted that there was some staff resistance to maintaining the higher temperature; (2) there was a significant increase in the assessment of patients' core temperature, from 4% in 2016 to 23% in 2017; and (3) the use of blankets in normothermic patients increased significantly, from 80% in 2016 to 91% in 2017.

Exercise D.2: Questions of Fact (Appendix A)

a. The report did not specifically discuss the involvement of stakeholders in the development of the smartphone and text messaging intervention. However, the article did state that the idea for such an intervention was explored with stakeholders (young adults) in a focus group study conducted by the first author. There may have been other efforts to involve stakeholders that were not mentioned in the article due to page constraints.

b. No, this study would not be considered comparative effectiveness research. The intervention was compared to a "no intervention" control group, not an alternative intervention.

c. The authors of the report did not refer to this RCT as a pragmatic trial, and there is nothing to suggest that "pragmatism" was a feature of the design. This intervention *was* done in community settings with a nonclinical population, but the eligibility criteria were fairly extensive—as is typical in an explanatory trial.

d. No, no subgroup analyses were performed. The sample was too small to undertake subgroup analyses. For example, there were only 8 men in the control group and 10 men in the intervention group.

e. The researchers noted that a limitation of the study was the small sample size and "limited generalizability." Most participants were attending college at one university on the east coast of the United States. In their conclusion, the researchers noted that future trials should include a broader sample—i.e., including young adults who do not attend college, to enhance generalizability.

f. No, the report did not mention the construct of *applicability*. This issue is a fairly recent development in research.